Applied Predictive Modeling

Max Kuhn • Kjell Johnson

Applied Predictive Modeling

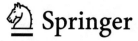 Springer

Max Kuhn
Division of Nonclinical Statistics
Pfizer Global Research and
    Development
Groton, Connecticut, USA

Kjell Johnson
Arbor Analytics
Saline, Michigan, USA

Corrected at 5th printing 2016.

ISBN 978-1-4939-7936-3   ISBN 978-1-4614-6849-3 (eBook)
DOI 10.1007/978-1-4614-6849-3

Printed on acid-free paper

This Springer imprint is published by Springer Nature
The registered company is Springer Science+Business Media LLC New York

To our families:
Miranda and Stefan
Valerie, Truman, and baby Gideon

Preface

This is a book on *data analysis* with a specific focus on the *practice of predictive modeling*. The term predictive modeling may stir associations such as machine learning, pattern recognition, and data mining. Indeed, these associations are appropriate and the methods implied by these terms are an integral piece of the predictive modeling process. But predictive modeling encompasses much more than the tools and techniques for uncovering patterns within data. The practice of predictive modeling defines the process of developing a model in a way that we can understand and quantify the model's prediction accuracy on future, yet-to-be-seen data. The *entire* process is the focus of this book.

We intend this work to be a practitioner's guide to the predictive modeling process and a place where one can come to learn about the approach and to gain intuition about the many commonly used and modern, powerful models. A host of statistical and mathematical techniques are discussed, but our motivation in almost every case is to describe the techniques in a way that helps develop intuition for its strengths and weaknesses instead of its mathematical genesis and underpinnings. For the most part we avoid complex equations, although there are a few necessary exceptions. For more theoretical treatments of predictive modeling, we suggest Hastie et al. (2008) and Bishop (2006). For this text, the reader should have some knowledge of basic statistics, including variance, correlation, simple linear regression, and basic hypothesis testing (e.g. p-values and test statistics).

The predictive modeling process is inherently hands-on. But during our research for this work we found that many articles and texts prevent the reader from reproducing the results either because the data were not freely available or because the software was inaccessible or only available for purchase. Buckheit and Donoho (1995) provide a relevant critique of the traditional scholarly veil:

> An article about computational science in a scientific publication is not the scholarship itself, it is merely advertising of the scholarship. The actual

scholarship is the complete software development environment and the complete set of instructions which generated the figures.

Therefore, it was our goal to be as hands-on as possible, enabling the readers to reproduce the results within reasonable precision as well as being able to naturally extend the predictive modeling approach to their own data. Furthermore, we use the R language (Ihaka and Gentleman 1996; R Development Core Team 2010), a freely accessible software for statistical and mathematical calculations, for all stages of the predictive modeling process. Almost all of the example data sets are available in R packages. The AppliedPredictiveModeling R package contains many of the data sets used here as well as R scripts to reproduce the analyses in each chapter.

We selected R as the computational engine of this text for several reasons. First R is freely available (although commercial versions exist) for multiple operating systems. Second, it is released under the *General Public License* (Free Software Foundation June 2007), which outlines how the program can be redistributed. Under this structure anyone is free to examine and modify the source code. Because of this open-source nature, dozens of predictive models have already been implemented through freely available packages. Moreover R contains extensive, powerful capabilities for the overall predictive modeling process. Readers not familiar with R can find numerous tutorials online. We also provide an introduction and start-up guide for R in the Appendix.

There are a few topics that we didn't have time and/or space to add, most notably: generalized additive models, ensembles of different models, network models, time series models, and a few others.

There is also a web site for the book:

http://appliedpredictivemodeling.com/

that will contain relevant information.

This work would not have been possible without the help and mentoring from many individuals, including: Walter H. Carter, Jim Garrett, Chris Gennings, Paul Harms, Chris Keefer, William Klinger, Daijin Ko, Rich Moore, David Neuhouser, David Potter, David Pyne, William Rayens, Arnold Stromberg, and Thomas Vidmar. We would also like to thank Ross Quinlan for his help with Cubist and C5.0 and vetting our descriptions of the two. At Springer, we would like to thank Marc Strauss and Hannah Bracken as well as the reviewers: Vini Bonato, Thomas Miller, Ross Quinlan, Eric Siegel, Stan Young, and an anonymous reviewer. Lastly, we would like to thank our families for their support: Miranda Kuhn, Stefan Kuhn, Bobby Kuhn, Robert Kuhn, Karen Kuhn, and Mary Ann Kuhn; Warren and Kay Johnson; and Valerie and Truman Johnson.

Groton, CT, USA   Max Kuhn
Saline, MI, USA   Kjell Johnson

Contents

Appendix

Indicies

Chapter 1
Introduction

Every day people are faced with questions such as "What route should I take to work today?" "Should I switch to a different cell phone carrier?" "How should I invest my money?" or "Will I get cancer?" These questions indicate our desire to know future events, and we earnestly want to make the best decisions towards that future.

We usually make decisions based on information. In some cases we have tangible, objective data, such as the morning traffic or weather report. Other times we use intuition and experience like "I should avoid the bridge this morning because it usually gets bogged down when it snows" or "I should have a PSA test because my father got prostate cancer." In either case, we are predicting future events given the information and experience we currently have, and we are making decisions based on those predictions.

As information has become more readily available via the internet and media, our desire to use this information to help us make decisions has intensified. And while the human brain can consciously and subconsciously assemble a vast amount of data, it cannot process the even greater amount of easily obtainable, relevant information for the problem at hand. To aid in our decision-making processes, we now turn to tools like Google to filter billions of web pages to find the most appropriate information for our queries, WebMD to diagnose our illnesses based on our symptoms, and E*TRADE to screen thousands of stocks and identify the best investments for our portfolios.

These sites, as well as many others, use tools that take our current information, sift through data looking for patterns that are relevant to our problem, and return answers. The process of developing these kinds of tools has evolved throughout a number of fields such as chemistry, computer science, physics, and statistics and has been called "machine learning," "artificial intelligence," "pattern recognition," "data mining," "predictive analytics," and "knowledge discovery." While each field approaches the problem using different perspectives and tool sets, the ultimate objective is the same: *to make an accurate prediction*. For this book, we will pool these terms into the commonly used phrase *predictive modeling*.

M. Kuhn and K. Johnson, *Applied Predictive Modeling*,
DOI 10.1007/978-1-4614-6849-3_1,
© Springer Science+Business Media New York 2013

Geisser (1993) defines predictive modeling as "the process by which a model is created or chosen to try to best predict the probability of an outcome." We tweak this definition slightly:

> **Predictive modeling**: the process of developing a mathematical tool or model that generates an accurate prediction

Steve Levy of *Wired* magazine recently wrote of the increasing presence of predictive models (Levy 2010), "Examples [of artificial intelligence] can be found everywhere: The Google global machine uses AI to interpret cryptic human queries. Credit card companies use it to track fraud. Netflix uses it to recommend movies to subscribers. And the financial system uses it to handle billions of trades (with only the occasional meltdown)." Examples of the types of questions one would like to predict are:

- How many copies will this book sell?
- Will this customer move their business to a different company?
- How much will my house sell for in the current market?
- Does a patient have a specific disease?
- Based on past choices, which movies will interest this viewer?
- Should I sell this stock?
- Which people should we match in our online dating service?
- Is an e-mail spam?
- Will this patient respond to this therapy?

Insurance companies, as another example, must predict the risks of potential auto, health, and life policy holders. This information is then used to determine if an individual will receive a policy, and if so, at what premium. Like insurance companies, governments also seek to predict risks, but for the purpose of protecting their citizens. Recent examples of governmental predictive models include biometric models for identifying terror suspects, models of fraud detection (Westphal 2008), and models of unrest and turmoil (Shachtman 2011). Even a trip to the grocery store or gas station [everyday places where our purchase information is collected and analyzed in an attempt to understand who we are and what we want (Duhigg 2012)] brings us into the predictive modeling world, and we're often not even aware that we've entered it. Predictive models now *permeate our existence*.

While predictive models guide us towards more satisfying products, better medical treatments, and more profitable investments, they regularly generate inaccurate predictions and provide the wrong answers. For example, most of us have not received an important e-mail due to a predictive model (a.k.a. e-mail filter) that incorrectly identified the message as spam. Similarly, predictive models (a.k.a. medical diagnostic models) misdiagnose diseases, and predictive models (a.k.a. financial algorithms) erroneously buy and sell stocks predicting profits when, in reality, finding losses. This final example of predictive models gone wrong affected many investors in 2010. Those who follow the stock market are likely familiar with the "flash crash" on May 6, 2010, in which the market rapidly lost more than 600 points, then immediately regained those points. After months of investigation, the Commodity Futures Trading Commission and the Securities and Exchange Commission identified an erroneous algorithmic model as the cause of the crash (U.S. Commodity Futures Trading Commission and U.S. Securities & Exchange Commission 2010).

Stemming in part from the flash crash and other failures of predictive models, Rodriguez (2011) writes, "Predictive modeling, the process by which a model is created or chosen to try to best predict the probability of an outcome has lost credibility as a forecasting tool." He hypothesizes that predictive models regularly fail because they do not account for complex variables such as human behavior. Indeed, our abilities to predict or make decisions are constrained by our present and past knowledge and are affected by factors that we have not considered. These realities are limits of any model, yet these realities should not prevent us from seeking to improve our process and build better models.

There are a number of common reasons why predictive models fail, and we address each of these in subsequent chapters. The common culprits include (1) inadequate pre-processing of the data, (2) inadequate model validation, (3) unjustified extrapolation (e.g., application of the model to data that reside in a space which the model has never seen), or, most importantly, (4) over-fitting the model to the existing data. Furthermore, predictive modelers often only explore relatively few models when searching for predictive relationships. This is usually due to either modelers' preference for, knowledge of, or expertise in, only a few models or the lack of available software that would enable them to explore a wide range of techniques.

This book endeavors to help predictive modelers produce reliable, trustworthy models by providing a step-by-step guide to the model building process and to provide intuitive knowledge of a wide range of common models. The objectives of this book are to provide:

- Foundational principles for building predictive models
- Intuitive explanations of many commonly used predictive modeling methods for both classification and regression problems
- Principles and steps for validating a predictive model
- Computer code to perform the necessary foundational work to build and validate predictive models

To illustrate these principles and methods, we will use a diverse set of real-world examples ranging from finance to pharmaceutical which we describe in detail in Sect. 1.4. But before describing the data, we first explore a reality that confronts predictive modeling techniques: the trade-off between prediction and interpretation.

1.1 Prediction Versus Interpretation

For the examples listed above, historical data likely exist that can be used to create a mathematical tool to predict future, unseen cases. Furthermore, the foremost objective of these examples is not to understand why something will (or will not) occur. Instead, we are primarily interested in accurately projecting the chances that something will (or will not) happen. Notice that the focus of this type of modeling is to optimize prediction accuracy. For example, we don't really care why an e-mail filter thinks a message is spam. Rather, we only care that the filter accurately trashes spam and allows messages we care about to pass through to our mailbox. As another example, if I am selling a house, my primary interest is not how a web site (such as zillow.com) estimated its value. Instead, I am keenly interested that zillow.com has correctly priced the home. An undervaluation will yield lower bids and a lower sale price; alternatively, an overvaluation may drive away potential buyers.

The tension between prediction and interpretation is also present in the medical field. For example, consider the process that a cancer patient and physician encounter when contemplating changing treatment therapies. There are many factors for the physician and patient to consider such as dosing schedule, potential side effects, and survival rates. However, if enough patients have taken the alternative therapy, then data could be collected on these patients related to their disease, treatment history, and demographics. Also, laboratory tests could be collected related to patients' genetic background or other biological data (e.g., protein measurements). Given their outcome, a predictive model could be created to predict the response to the alternative therapy based on these data. The critical question for the doctor and patient is a prediction of *how* the patient will react to a change in therapy. Above all, this prediction needs to be accurate. If a model is created to make this prediction, it should not be constrained by the requirement of interpretability. A strong argument could be made that this would be unethical. As long as the model can be appropriately validated, it should not matter whether it is a black box or a simple, interpretable model.

While the primary interest of predictive modeling is to generate accurate predictions, a secondary interest may be to interpret the model and understand why it works. The unfortunate reality is that as we push towards higher accuracy, models become more complex and their interpretability becomes more difficult. This is almost always the trade-off we make when prediction accuracy is the primary goal.

1.2 Key Ingredients of Predictive Models

The colloquial examples thus far have illustrated that data, in fact very large data sets, can now be easily generated in an attempt to answer almost any type of research question. Furthermore, free or relatively inexpensive model building software such as JMP, WEKA, and many packages in R, as well as powerful personal computers, make it relatively easy for anyone with some computing knowledge to begin to develop predictive models. But as Rodriguez (2011) accurately points out, the credibility of model building has weakened especially as the window to data access and analysis tools has widened.

As we will see throughout this text, if a predictive signal exists in a set of data, many models will find some degree of that signal regardless of the technique or care placed in developing the model. Naïve model application can therefore be effective to an extent; as the saying goes, "even a blind squirrel finds a nut." But the best, most predictive models are fundamentally influenced by a modeler with expert knowledge and context of the problem. This expert knowledge should first be applied in obtaining *relevant* data for the desired research objectives. While vast databases of information can be used as substrate for constructing predictions, irrelevant information can drive down predictive performance of many models. Subject-specific knowledge can help separate potentially meaningful information from irrelevant information, eliminating detrimental noise and strengthening the underlying signal. Undesirable, confounding signal may also exist in the data and may not be able to be identified without expert knowledge. As an extreme example of misleading signal and the need for an expert understanding of the problem, consider the U.S. Food and Drug Administration's Adverse Event Reporting System database which provides information on millions of reported occurrences of drugs and their reported side effects. Obvious biases abound in this collection of data; for example, a search on a drug for treating nausea may reflect that a large proportion of the patients using the treatment had leukemia. An uninformed analysis may identify leukemia as a potential side effect of the drug. The more likely explanation is that the subjects were taking the nausea medication to mitigate the side effects of the cancer therapy. This may be intuitively obvious, but clearly the availability of large quantities of records is not a protection against an uninformed use of the data.

Ayres (2007) extensively studies the interplay between expert opinion and empirical, data-driven models makes two important observations bolstering the need for problem-specific knowledge. Firstly,

> "In the end, [predictive modeling] is not a substitute for intuition, but rather a complement"

Simply put, neither data-driven models nor the expert relying solely on intuition will do better than a combination of the two. Secondly,

> "Traditional experts make better decisions when they are provided with the results of statistical prediction. Those who cling to the authority of traditional

experts tend to embrace the idea of combining the two forms of 'knowledge' by
giving the experts 'statistical support' ... Humans usually make better predictions when they are provided with the results of statistical prediction."

In some cases, such as spam detection, it may be acceptable to let computers
do most of the thinking. When the consequences are more serious, such as
predicting patient response, a combined approach often leads to better results.

To summarize, the foundation of an effective predictive model is laid with
intuition and *deep knowledge of the problem context*, which are entirely vi-
tal for driving decisions about model development. That process begins with
relevant data, another key ingredient. The third ingredient is a *versatile* computational toolbox which includes techniques for data pre-processing and visualization as well as a suite of modeling tools for handling a range of possible
scenarios such as those that are described in Table 1.1.

1.3 Terminology

As previously noted, "predictive modeling" is one of the many names that
refers to the process of uncovering relationships within data for predicting
some desired outcome. Since many scientific domains have contributed to
this field, there are synonyms for different entities:

- The terms *sample, data point, observation*, or *instance* refer to a single,
  independent unit of data, such as a customer, patient, or compound.
  The term *sample* can also refer to a subset of data points, such as the
  training set sample. The text will clarify the appropriate context when
  this term is used.
- The *training set* consists of the data used to develop models while the *test*
  or *validation* sets are used solely for evaluating the performance of a final
  set of candidate models.
- The *predictors, independent variables, attributes*, or *descriptors* are the
  data used as input for the prediction equation.
- *Outcome, dependent variable, target, class*, or *response* refer to the outcome
  event or quantity that is being predicted.
- *Continuous* data have natural, numeric scales. Blood pressure, the cost of
  an item, or the number of bathrooms are all continuous. In the last case,
  the counts cannot be a fractional number, but is still treated as continuous
  data.
- *Categorical* data, otherwise known as *nominal, attribute*, or *discrete* data,
  take on specific values that have no scale. Credit status ("good" or "bad")
  or color ("red," "blue," etc.) are examples of these data.
- *Model building, model training*, and *parameter estimation* all refer to the
  process of using data to determine values of model equations.

1.4 Example Data Sets and Typical Data Scenarios

In later chapters, case studies are used to illustrate techniques. Before proceeding, it may be instructive to briefly explore a few examples of predictive modeling problems and the types of data used to solve them. The focus here is on the diversity of the problems as well as the characteristics of the collected data. Several example data sets originate from machine learning competitions, which provide real-world problems with an (often monetary) incentive for providing the best solution. Such competitions have a long history in predictive modeling and have greatly stimulated the field.

Music Genre

This data set was published as a contest data set on the TunedIT web site (http://tunedit.org/challenge/music-retrieval/genres). In this competition, the objective was to develop a predictive model for classifying music into six categories. In total, there were 12,495 music samples for which 191 characteristics were determined. The response categories were not balanced (Fig. 1.1), with the smallest segment coming from the heavy metal category (7 %) and the largest coming from the classical category (28 %). All predictors were continuous; many were highly correlated and the predictors spanned different scales of measurement. This data collection was created using 60 performers from which 15–20 pieces of music were selected for each performer. Then 20 segments of each piece were parameterized in order to create the final data set. Hence, the samples are inherently not independent of each other.

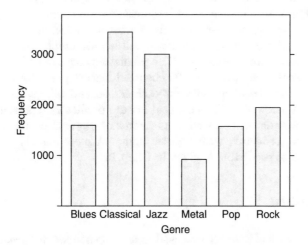

Fig. 1.1: The frequency distribution of genres in the music data

Grant Applications

This data set was also published for a competition on the **Kaggle** web site (http://www.kaggle.com). For this competition, the objective was to develop a predictive model for the probability of success of a grant application. The historical database consisted of 8,707 University of Melbourne grant applications from 2009 and 2010 with 249 predictors. Grant status (either "unsuccessful" or "successful") was the response and was fairly balanced (46 % successful). The web site notes that current Australian grant success rates are less than 25 %. Hence the historical database rates are not representative of Australian rates. Predictors include measurements and categories such as Sponsor ID, Grant Category, Grant Value Range, Research Field, and Department and were continuous, count, and categorical. Another notable characteristic of this data set is that many predictor values were missing (83 %). Furthermore, the samples were not independent since the same grant writers occurred multiple times throughout the data. These data are used throughout the text to demonstrate different classification modeling techniques.

We will use these data extensively throughout Chaps. 12 through 15, and a more detailed explanation and summary of the data can be found in Sect. 12.1.

Hepatic Injury

A data set from the pharmaceutical industry was used to develop a model for predicting compounds' probability of causing hepatic injury (i.e., liver damage). This data set consisted of 281 unique compounds; 376 predictors were measured or computed for each. The response was categorical (either "does not cause injury," "mild injury," or "severe injury") and was highly unbalanced (Fig. 1.2). This variety of response often occurs in pharmaceutical data because companies steer away from creating molecules that have undesirable safety characteristics. Therefore, well-behaved molecules often greatly outnumber undesirable molecules. The predictors consisted of measurements from 184 biological screens and 192 chemical feature predictors. The biological predictors represent activity for each screen and take values between 0 and 10 with a mode of 4. The chemical feature predictors represent counts of important substructures as well as measures of physical properties that are thought to be associated with hepatic injury. A more extensive description of these types of predictors is given in Chap. 5.

Permeability

This pharmaceutical data set was used to develop a model for predicting compounds' permeability. In short, permeability is the measure of a molecule's ability to cross a membrane. The body, for example, has notable membranes between the body and brain, known as the blood–brain barrier, and between

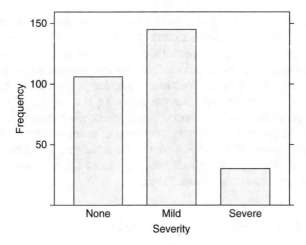

Fig. 1.2: Distribution of hepatic injury type

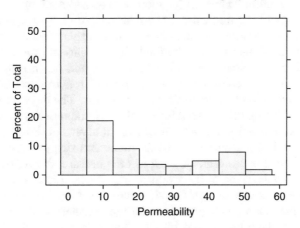

Fig. 1.3: Distribution of permeability values

the gut and body in the intestines. These membranes help the body guard critical regions from receiving undesirable or detrimental substances. For an orally taken drug to be effective in the brain, it first must pass through the intestinal wall and then must pass through the blood–brain barrier in order to be present for the desired neurological target. Therefore, a compound's ability to permeate relevant biological membranes is critically important to understand early in the drug discovery process. Compounds that appear to be effective for a particular disease in research screening experiments but appear to be poorly permeable may need to be altered in order to improve permeability and thus the compound's ability to reach the desired target. Identifying permeability problems can help guide chemists towards better molecules.

Permeability assays such as PAMPA and Caco-2 have been developed to help measure compounds' permeability (Kansy et al. 1998). These screens are effective at quantifying a compound's permeability, but the assay is expensive labor intensive. Given a sufficient number of compounds that have been screened, we could develop a predictive model for permeability in an attempt to potentially reduce the need for the assay. In this project there were 165 unique compounds; 1,107 molecular fingerprints were determined for each. A molecular fingerprint is a binary sequence of numbers that represents the presence or absence of a specific molecular substructure. The response is highly skewed (Fig. 1.3), the predictors are sparse (15.5 % are present), and many predictors are strongly associated.

Chemical Manufacturing Process

This data set contains information about a chemical manufacturing process, in which the goal is to understand the relationship between the process and the resulting final product yield. Raw material in this process is put through a sequence of 27 steps to make the final pharmaceutical product. The starting material is generated from a biological unit and has a range of quality and characteristics. The objective in this project was to develop a model to predict percent yield of the manufacturing process. The data set consisted of 177 samples of biological material for which 57 characteristics were measured. Of the 57 characteristics, there were 12 measurements of the biological starting material and 45 measurements of the manufacturing process. The process variables included measurements such as temperature, drying time, washing time, and concentrations of by-products at various steps. Some of the process measurements can be controlled, while others are observed. Predictors are continuous, count, categorical; some are correlated, and some contain missing values. Samples are not independent because sets of samples come from the same batch of biological starting material.

Fraudulent Financial Statements

Fanning and Cogger (1998) describe a data set used to predict management fraud for publicly traded companies. Using public data sources, such as U.S. Securities and Exchange Commission documents, the authors were able to identify 102 fraudulent financial statements. Given that a small percentage of statements are fraudulent, they chose to sample an equivalent number[1] of non-fraudulent companies, which were sampled to control for important factors (e.g., company size and industry type). Of these data, 150 data points were used to train models and the remaining 54 were used to evaluate them.

---

[1] This type of sampling is very similar to *case-control studies* in the medical field.

The authors started the analysis with an unidentified number of predictors derived from key areas, such as executive turnover rates, litigation, and debt structure. In the end, they used 20 predictors in their models. Examples include the ratio of accounts receivable to sales, the ratio of inventory to sales, and changes in the gross margins between years. Many of the predictor variables of ratios share common denominators (e.g., the ratio of accounts receivable to sales and the ratio of inventory to sales). Although the actual data points were not published, there is likely to be strong correlations between predictors.

From a modeling perspective, this example is interesting for several reasons. First, because of the large class imbalance, the frequencies of the two classes in the data sets were very different from the population that will be predicted with severe imbalances. This is a common strategy to minimize the consequences of such an imbalance and is sometimes referred to as "down-sampling" the data. Second, the number of possible predictors was large compared to the number of samples. In this situation, the selection of predictors for the models is delicate as there are only a small number of samples for selecting predictors, building models, and evaluating their performance. Later chapters discuss the problem of over-fitting, where trends in the training data are not found in other samples of the population. With a large number of predictors and a small number of data points, there is a risk that a relevant predictor found in this data set will not be reproducible.

Comparisons Between Data Sets

These examples illustrate characteristics that are common to most data sets. First, the response may be continuous or categorical, and for categorical responses there may be more than two categories. For continuous response data, the distribution of the response may be symmetric (e.g., chemical manufacturing) or skewed (e.g., permeability); for categorical response data, the distribution may be balanced (e.g., grant applications) or unbalanced (e.g., music genre, hepatic injury). As we will show in Chap. 4, understanding the distribution of the response is critically necessary for one of the first steps in the predictive modeling process: splitting the data into training and testing sets. Understanding the response distribution will guide the modeler towards better ways of partitioning the data; not understanding response characteristics can lead to computational difficulties for certain kinds of models and to models that have less-than-optimal predictive ability.

The data sets summarized in Table 1.1 also highlight characteristics of predictors that are universal to most data sets. Specifically, the values of predictors may be continuous, count, and/or categorical; they may have missing values and could be on different scales of measurement. Additionally, predictors within a data set may have high correlation or association, thus indicating that the predictor set contains numerically redundant information.

Furthermore, predictors may be sparse, meaning that a majority of samples contain the same information while only a few contain unique information. Like the response, predictors can follow a symmetric or skewed distribution (for continuous predictors) or be balanced or unbalanced (for categorical predictors). Lastly, predictors within a data set may or may not have an underlying relationship with the response.

Different kinds of models handle these types of predictor characteristics in different ways. For example, partial least squares naturally manages correlated predictors but is numerically more stable if the predictors are on similar scales. Recursive partitioning, on the other hand, is unaffected by predictors of different scales but has a less stable partitioning structure when predictors are correlated. As another example of predictor characteristics' impact on models, multiple linear regression cannot handle missing predictor information, but recursive partitioning can be used when predictors contain moderate amounts of missing information. In either of these example scenarios, failure to appropriately adjust the predictors prior to modeling (known as pre-processing) will produce models that have less-than-optimal predictive performance. Assessing predictor characteristics and addressing them through pre-processing is covered in Chap. 3.

Finally, each of these data sets illustrates another fundamental characteristic that must be considered when building a predictive model: the relationship between the number of samples (n) and number of predictors (P). In the case of the music genre data set, the number of samples ($n = 12{,}496$) is much greater than the number of predictors ($P = 191$). All predictive models handle this scenario, but computational time will vary among models and will likely increase as the number of samples and predictors increase. Alternatively, the permeability data set has significantly fewer samples ($n = 165$) than predictors ($P = 1{,}107$). When this occurs, predictive models such as multiple linear regression or linear discriminant analysis cannot be directly used. Yet, some models [e.g., recursive partitioning and K-nearest neighbors (KNNs)] can be used directly under this condition. As we discuss each method in later chapters, we will identify the method's ability to handle data sets where $n < P$. For those that cannot operate under this condition, we will suggest alternative modeling methods or pre-processing steps that will effectively reduce the dimension of the predictor space.

In summary, we must have a detailed understanding of the predictors and the response for any data set prior to attempting to build a model. Lack of understanding can lead to computational difficulties and less than optimal model performance. Furthermore, most data sets will require some degree of pre-processing in order to expand the universe of possible predictive models and to optimize each model's predictive performance.

Table 1.1: A comparison of several characteristics of the example data sets

Data characteristic	Data set					
	Music genre	Grant applications	Hepatic injury	Fraud detection	Permeability	Chemical manufacturing
Dimensions						
# Samples	12,495	8,707	281	204	165	177
# Predictors	191	249	376	20	1,107	57
Response characteristics						
Categorical or continuous	Categorical	Categorical	Categorical	Categorical	Continuous	Continuous
Balanced/symmetric	×	×				×
Unbalanced/skewed			×	×	×	
Independent			×			
Predictor Characteristics						
Continuous	×	×	×	×		×
Count	×	×	×			×
Categorical		×	×	×	×	×
Correlated/associated	×	×	×	×	×	×
Different scales	×	×	×	×	×	×
Missing values		×	×			×
Sparse					×	×

1.5 Overview

This book consists of four parts that walk the reader through the process of building and critically evaluating predictive models. Because most readers will likely desire to implement these concepts, we provide a computing section at the end of each chapter that contains code for implementing the topics covered in that chapter. Throughout the text, we focus on the R programming language (R Development Core Team 2010). For those readers who are not familiar with R, we provide an introduction to this software in Appendix B. The goal of Appendix B is to supply an overview and quick reference for the primary R programming constructs. However, this text may not contain enough information for those who are new to R. In this case, many other tutorials exist in print and on the web; for additional instruction, we recommend Verzani (2002); Venables et al. (2003); Maindonald and Braun (2007); Muenchen (2009), and Spector (2008).

In Part I, we explain approaches for laying strong foundations onto which models can be built. The cornerstone concepts of data pre-processing (Chap. 3) and resampling (Chap. 4) should be well understood before attempting to model any data. Chapter 3 explains common methods of preprocessing such as data transformations, the addition and/or removal of variables, and binning continuous variables. This chapter also details why most models require data to be preprocessed prior to modeling. Chapter 4 will introduce the idea of data spending and methods for spending data in order to appropriately tune a model and assess its performance. Furthermore, this chapter illustrates that the practitioner should always try a diverse set of models for any given problem.

Upon laying the foundation for predictive modeling, we survey traditional and modern regression techniques in Part II. This portion of the book begins with ways to measure performance when modeling a continuous outcome (Chap. 5). Chapter 6 provides a working understanding and intuition for regression models that seek the underlying structure of the data using linear combinations of the predictors. These models include linear regression, partial least squares, and L_1 regularization. Subsequently (Chap. 7), we present an explanation of regression models that are not based on simple linear combinations of the predictors, which include neural networks, multivariate adaptive regression splines (MARS), support vector machines (SVMs), and KNNs. Tree-based models also do not rely on linear combinations of the predictors. Because of their popularity and because of their use in ensemble methods, we have devoted a separate chapter to these techniques (Chap. 8). In this chapter we give an overview of regression trees, bagged trees, random forests, boosting, and Cubist. We end Part II with a case study (Chap. 10) which compares and contrasts all of the above techniques on a specific problem: modeling the compressive strength of concrete to obtain formulations with better properties.

Predictive classification models naturally follow an explanation of regression models and are covered in Part III. Measures of performance for classification problems are different than regression; we define these metrics in Chap. 11. Following the same structure as in Part II, we then supply a working understanding and intuition for classification models (Chap. 12) that are based on linear combinations of the predictors such as linear, quadratic, regularized, and partial least squares discriminant analysis. We additionally review penalized methods for classification. In Chap. 13, we explore classification methods that are highly nonlinear functions of the predictors. These include flexible discriminant analysis, neural networks, SVMs, KNNs, Naïve Bayes, and nearest shrunken centroids. Parallel to Part II, tree-based methods for classification are addressed in Chap. 14, and a classification case study and method comparison are presented in Chap. 17.

We conclude this work in Part IV by addressing other important considerations when building a model or evaluating its performance. In an attempt to find only the most relevant predictors in a given problem, many different types of feature selection methods have been proposed. While these methods have the potential to uncover practically meaningful information, they often help the user to understand the data's noise rather than its structure. Chapter 18 illustrates various methods for quantifying predictor importance while Chap. 19 provides an introduction and guide to properly utilizing feature selection techniques. Also, an array of elements can affect model performance and mislead the practitioner into believing that either the model has poor predictive performance (when it truly has good performance) or the model has good predictive performance (when the opposite is true). Some common factors affecting model performance are excess noise in the predictor set and/or response and predictive extrapolation. These topics are covered in Chap. 20.

1.6 Notation

One goal of this text is to provide intuitive descriptions of many techniques. Whenever possible, words are used in place of equations. Many models can be described in algorithmic terms, but others require more mathematical explanations. Generally, the characters x and y in their various fonts and case types represent the predictors and the response, respectively. Here are the specific forms they take in this text:

$n =$ the number of data points

$P =$ the number of predictors

$y_i =$ the ith observed value of the outcome, $i = 1 \ldots n$

$\widehat{y}_i =$ the predicted outcome of the ith data point, $i = 1 \ldots n$

$\bar{y} =$ the average or sample mean of the n observed values of the outcome

$\mathbf{y} =$ a vector of all n outcome values

$x_{ij} =$ the value of the jth predictor for the ith data point, $i = 1 \ldots n$ and
$\quad\quad j = 1 \ldots P$

$\bar{x}_j =$ the average or sample mean of n data points for the jth predictor,
$\quad\quad j = 1 \ldots P$

$\mathbf{x}_i =$ a collection (i.e., vector) of the P predictors for the ith data point,
$\quad\quad i = 1 \ldots n$

$\mathbf{X} =$ a matrix of P predictors for all data points; this matrix has n rows
and P columns

$\mathbf{X}' =$ the transpose of $\mathbf{X}$; this matrix has P rows and n columns

Other notational guidelines used in equations throughout the text are:

$C =$ the number of classes in a categorical outcome

$C_\ell =$ the value of the ℓth class level

$p =$ the probability of an event

$p_\ell =$ the probability of the ℓth event

$Pr[.] =$ the probability of event

$\sum_{i=1}^{n} =$ the summation operator over the index i

$\mathbf{\Sigma} =$ the theoretical covariance matrix

$E[\cdot] =$ the expected value of $\cdot$

$f(\cdot) =$ a function of $.$; $g(\cdot)$ and $h(\cdot)$ also represent functions throughout
the text

$\beta =$ an unknown or theoretical model coefficient

$b =$ an estimated model coefficient based on a sample of data points

The reader should note that we use other symbols throughout the text that may be unique to a specific topic or model. In these cases we define that notation locally.

Part I
General Strategies

Chapter 2
A Short Tour of the Predictive Modeling Process

Before diving in to the formal components of model building, we present a simple example that illustrates the broad concepts of model building. Specifically, the following example demonstrates the concepts of data "spending," building candidate models, and selecting the optimal model.

2.1 Case Study: Predicting Fuel Economy

The fueleconomy.gov web site, run by the U.S. Department of Energy's Office of Energy Efficiency and Renewable Energy and the U.S. Environmental Protection Agency, lists different estimates of fuel economy for passenger cars and trucks. For each vehicle, various characteristics are recorded such as the engine displacement or number of cylinders. Along with these values, laboratory measurements are made for the city and highway miles per gallon (MPG) of the car.

In practice, we would build a model on as many vehicle characteristics as possible in order to find the most predictive model. However, this introductory illustration will focus high-level concepts of model building by using a single predictor, engine displacement (the volume inside the engine cylinders), and a single response, unadjusted highway MPG for 2010–2011 model year cars.

The first step in any model building process is to understand the data, which can most easily be done through a graph. Since we have just one predictor and one response, these data can be visualized with a scatter plot (Fig. 2.1). This figure shows the relationship between engine displacement and fuel economy. The "2010 model year" panel contains all the 2010 data while the other panel shows the data only for new 2011 vehicles. Clearly, as engine displacement increases, the fuel efficiency drops regardless of year. The relationship is somewhat linear but does exhibit some curvature towards the extreme ends of the displacement axis.

M. Kuhn and K. Johnson, *Applied Predictive Modeling*,
DOI 10.1007/978-1-4614-6849-3_2,
© Springer Science+Business Media New York 2013

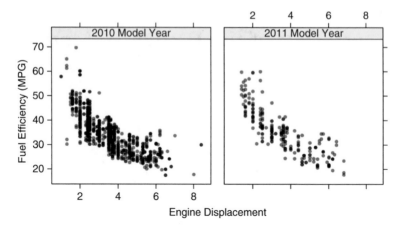

Fig. 2.1: The relationship between engine displacement and fuel efficiency of all 2010 model year vehicles and new 2011 car lines

If we had more than one predictor, we would need to further understand characteristics of the predictors and the relationships among the predictors. These characteristics may suggest important and necessary pre-processing steps that must be taken prior to building a model (Chap. 3).

After first understanding the data, the next step is to build and evaluate a model on the data. A standard approach is to take a random sample of the data for model building and use the rest to understand model performance. However, suppose we want to predict the MPG for a *new* car line. In this situation, models can be created using the 2010 data (containing 1,107 vehicles) and tested on the 245 new 2011 cars. The common terminology would be that the 2010 data are used as the model "training set" and the 2011 values are the "test" or "validation" set.

Now that we have defined the data used for model building and evaluation, we should decide how to measure performance of the model. For regression problems where we try to predict a numeric value, the residuals are important sources of information. Residuals are computed as the observed value minus the predicted value (i.e., $y_i - \widehat{y}_i$). When predicting numeric values, the root mean squared error (RMSE) is commonly used to evaluate models. Described in more detail in Chap. 7, RMSE is interpreted as how far, on average, the residuals are from zero.

At this point, the modeler will try various techniques to mathematically define the relationship between the predictor and outcome. To do this, the training set is used to estimate the various values needed by the model equations. The test set will be used only when a few strong candidate models have been finalized (repeatedly using the test set in the model build process negates its utility as a final arbitrator of the models).

Suppose a linear regression model was created where the predicted MPG is a basic slope and intercept model. Using the training data, we estimate the

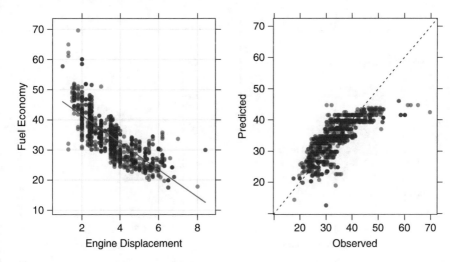

Fig. 2.2: Quality of fit diagnostics for the linear regression model. The training set data and its associated predictions are used to understand how well the model works

intercept to be 50.6 and the slope to be -4.5 MPG/liters using the method of least squares (Sect. 6.2). The model fit is shown in Fig. 2.2 for the training set data.[1] The left-hand panel shows the training set data with a linear model fit defined by the estimated slope and intercept. The right-hand panel plots the observed and predicted MPG. These plots demonstrate that this model misses some of the patterns in the data, such as under-predicting fuel efficiency when the displacement is less than 2 L or above 6 L.

When working with the training set, one must be careful not to simply evaluate model performance using the same data used to build the model. If we simply re-predict the training set data, there is the potential to produce overly optimistic estimates of how well the model works, especially if the model is highly adaptable. An alternative approach for quantifying how well the model operates is to use *resampling*, where different subversions of the training data set are used to fit the model. Resampling techniques are discussed in Chap. 4. For these data, we used a form of resampling called 10-fold cross-validation to estimate the model RMSE to be 4.6 MPG.

Looking at Fig. 2.2, it is conceivable that the problem might be solved by introducing some nonlinearity in the model. There are many ways to do this. The most basic approach is to supplement the previous linear regression model with additional complexity. Adding a squared term for engine displacement would mean estimating an additional slope parameter associated with the square of the predictor. In doing this, the model equation changes to

---

[1] One of our graduate professors once said "the only way to be comfortable with your data is to never look at it."

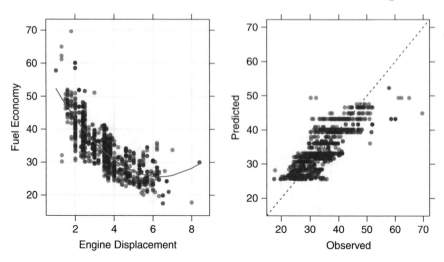

Fig. 2.3: Quality of fit diagnostics for the quadratic regression model (using the training set)

$$\text{efficiency} = 63.2 - 11.9 \times \text{displacement} + 0.94 \times \text{displacement}^2$$

This is referred to as a *quadratic model* since it includes a squared term; the model fit is shown in Fig. 2.3. Unquestionably, the addition of the quadratic term improves the model fit. The RMSE is now estimated to be 4.2 MPG using cross-validation. One issue with quadratic models is that they can perform poorly on the extremes of the predictor. In Fig. 2.3, there may be a hint of this for the vehicles with very high displacement values. The model appears to be bending upwards unrealistically. Predicting new vehicles with large displacement values may produce significantly inaccurate results.

Chapters 6–8 discuss many other techniques for creating sophisticated relationships between the predictors and outcome. One such approach is the multivariate adaptive regression spline (MARS) model (Friedman 1991). When used with a single predictor, MARS can fit separate linear regression lines for different ranges of engine displacement. The slopes and intercepts are estimated for this model, as well as the number and size of the separate regions for the linear models. Unlike the linear regression models, this technique has a *tuning parameter* which cannot be directly estimated from the data. There is no analytical equation that can be used to determine how many segments should be used to model the data. While the MARS model has internal algorithms for making this determination, the user can try different values and use resampling to determine the appropriate value. Once the value is found, a final MARS model would be fit using all the training set data and used for prediction.

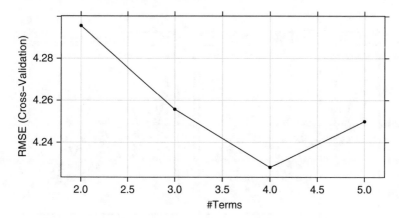

Fig. 2.4: The cross-validation profile for the MARS tuning parameter

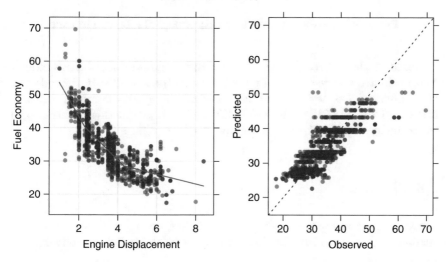

Fig. 2.5: Quality of fit diagnostics for the MARS model (using the training set). The MARS model creates several linear regression fits with change points at 2.3, 3.5, and 4.3 L

For a single predictor, MARS can allow for up to five model terms (similar to the previous slopes and intercepts). Using cross-validation, we evaluated four candidate values for this tuning parameter to create the resampling profile which is shown in Fig. 2.4. The lowest RMSE value is associated with four terms, although the scale of change in the RMSE values indicates that there is some insensitivity to this tuning parameter. The RMSE associated with the optimal model was 4.2 MPG. After fitting the final MARS model with four terms, the training set fit is shown in Fig. 2.5 where several linear segments were predicted.

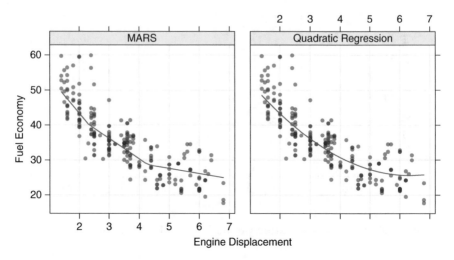

Fig. 2.6: The test set data and with model fits for two models

Based on these three models, the quadratic regression and MARS models were evaluated on the test set. Figure 2.6 shows these results. Both models fit very similarly. The test set RMSE values for the quadratic model was 4.72 MPG and the MARS model was 4.69 MPG. Based on this, either model would be appropriate for the prediction of new car lines.

2.2 Themes

There are several aspects of the model building process that are worth discussing further, especially for those who are new to predictive modeling.

Data Splitting

Although discussed in the next chapter, how we allocate data to certain tasks (e.g., model building, evaluating performance) is an important aspect of modeling. For this example, the primary interest is to predict the fuel economy of *new* vehicles, which is not the same population as the data used to build the model. This means that, to some degree, we are testing how well the model *extrapolates* to a different population. If we were interested in predicting from the same population of vehicles (i.e., *interpolation*), taking a simple random sample of the data would be more appropriate. How the training and test sets are determined should reflect how the model will be applied.

How much data should be allocated to the training and test sets? It generally depends on the situation. If the pool of data is small, the data splitting decisions can be critical. A small test would have limited utility as a judge of performance. In this case, a sole reliance on resampling techniques (i.e., no test set) might be more effective. Large data sets reduce the criticality of these decisions.

Predictor Data

This example has revolved around one of many predictors: the engine displacement. The original data contain many other factors, such as the number of cylinders, the type of transmission, and the manufacturer. An earnest attempt to predict the fuel economy would examine as many predictors as possible to improve performance. Using more predictors, it is likely that the RMSE for the new model cars can be driven down further. Some investigation into the data can also help. For example, none of the models were effective at predicting fuel economy when the engine displacement was small. Inclusion of predictors that target these types of vehicles would help improve performance.

An aspect of modeling that was not discussed here was feature selection: the process of determining the minimum set of relevant predictors needed by the model. This common task is discussed in Chap. 19.

Estimating Performance

Before using the test set, two techniques were employed to determine the effectiveness of the model. First, quantitative assessments of statistics (i.e., the RMSE) using resampling help the user understand how each technique would perform on new data. The other tool was to create simple visualizations of a model, such as plotting the observed and predicted values, to discover areas of the data where the model does particularly good or bad. This type of qualitative information is critical for improving models and is lost when the model is gauged only on summary statistics.

Evaluating Several Models

For these data, three different models were evaluated. It is our experience that some modeling practitioners have a favorite model that is relied on indiscriminately. The "No Free Lunch" Theorem (Wolpert 1996) argues that, without having substantive information about the modeling problem, there is no single model that will always do better than any other model. Because of this, a strong case can be made to try a wide variety of techniques, then determine which model to focus on. In our example, a simple plot of the data shows that there is a nonlinear relationship between the outcome and the predictor. Given this knowledge, we might exclude linear models from consideration, but there is still a wide variety of techniques to evaluate. One might say that "model X is always the best performing model" but, for these data, a simple quadratic model is extremely competitive.

Model Selection

At some point in the process, a specific model must be chosen. This example demonstrated two types of model selection. First, we chose some models over others: the linear regression model did not fit well and was dropped. In this case, we chose *between models*. There was also a second type of model selection shown. For MARS, the tuning parameter was chosen using cross-validation. This was also model selection where we decided on the *type of MARS model* to use. In this case, we did the selection *within* different MARS models.

In either case, we relied on cross-validation and the test set to produce quantitative assessments of the models to help us make the choice. Because we focused on a single predictor, which will not often be the case, we also made visualizations of the model fit to help inform us. At the end of the process, the MARS and quadratic models appear to give equivalent performance. However, knowing that the quadratic model might not do well for vehicles with very large displacements, our intuition might tell us to favor the MARS model. One goal of this book is to help the user gain intuition regarding the strengths and weakness of different models to make informed decisions.

2.3 Summary

At face value, model building appears straightforward: pick a modeling technique, plug in data, and generate a prediction. While this approach will generate a predictive model, it will most likely *not* generate a reliable, trustworthy model for predicting new samples. To get this type of model, we must first understand the data *and* the objective of the modeling. Upon understanding the data and objectives, we then pre-process and split the data. Only after these steps do we finally proceed to building, evaluating, and selecting models.

Chapter 3
Data Pre-processing

Data pre-processing techniques generally refer to the addition, deletion, or transformation of training set data. Although this text is primarily concerned with modeling techniques, data preparation can make or break a model's predictive ability. Different models have different sensitivities to the type of predictors in the model; *how* the predictors enter the model is also important. Transformations of the data to reduce the impact of data skewness or outliers can lead to significant improvements in performance. Feature extraction, discussed in Sect. 3.3, is one empirical technique for creating surrogate variables that are combinations of multiple predictors. Additionally, simpler strategies such as removing predictors based on their lack of information content can also be effective.

The need for data pre-processing is determined by the type of model being used. Some procedures, such as tree-based models, are notably insensitive to the characteristics of the predictor data. Others, like linear regression, are not. In this chapter, a wide array of *possible* methodologies are discussed. For modeling techniques described in subsequent chapters, we will also discuss which, if any, pre-processing techniques can be useful.

This chapter outlines approaches to *unsupervised* data processing: the outcome variable is not considered by the pre-processing techniques. In other chapters, *supervised* methods, where the outcome is utilized to pre-process the data, are also discussed. For example, partial least squares (PLS) models are essentially supervised versions of principal component analysis (PCA). We also describe strategies for removing predictors without considering how those variables might be related to the outcome. Chapter 19 discusses techniques for finding subsets of predictors that optimize the ability of the model to predict the response.

How the predictors are encoded, called *feature engineering*, can have a significant impact on model performance. For example, using combinations of predictors can sometimes be more effective than using the individual values: the ratio of two predictors may be more effective than using two independent

M. Kuhn and K. Johnson, *Applied Predictive Modeling*,
DOI 10.1007/978-1-4614-6849-3_3,
© Springer Science+Business Media New York 2013

predictors. Often the most effective encoding of the data is informed by the modeler's understanding of the problem and thus is not derived from any mathematical technique.

There are usually several different methods for encoding predictor data. For example, in Chaps. 12 through 15, an illustrative data set is described for predicting the success of academic grants. One piece of information in the data is the submission date of the grant. This date can be represented in myriad ways:

- The number of days since a reference date
- Isolating the month, year, and day of the week as separate predictors
- The numeric day of the year (ignoring the calendar year)
- Whether the date was within the school year (as opposed to holiday or summer sessions)

The "correct" feature engineering depends on several factors. First, some encodings may be optimal for some models and poor for others. For example, tree-based models will partition the data into two or more bins. Theoretically, if the month were important, the tree would split the numeric day of the year accordingly. Also, in some models, multiple encodings of the same data may cause problems. As will be illustrated several times in later chapters, some models contain built-in *feature selection*, meaning that the model will only include predictors that help maximize accuracy. In these cases, the model can pick and choose which representation of the data is best.

The relationship between the predictor and the outcome is a second factor. For example, if there were a seasonal component to these data, and it appears that there is, then the numeric day of the year would be best. Also, if some months showed higher success rates than others, then the encoding based on the month is preferable.

As with many questions of statistics, the answer to "which feature engineering methods are the best?" is that *it depends*. Specifically, it depends on the model being used and the true relationship with the outcome. A broad discussion regarding how the data were encoded for our analyses is given in Sect. 12.1.

Prior to delving into specific techniques, an illustrative data set that is used throughout the chapter is introduced.

3.1 Case Study: Cell Segmentation in High-Content Screening

Medical researchers often seek to understand the effects of medicines or diseases on the size, shape, development status, and number of cells in a living organism or plant. To do this, experts can examine the target serum or tissue under a microscope and manually assess the desired cell characteristics.

This work is tedious and requires expert knowledge of the cell type and characteristics.

Another way to measure the cell characteristics from these kinds of samples is by using high-content screening (Giuliano et al. 1997). Briefly, a sample is first dyed with a substance that will bind to the desired characteristic of the cells. For example, if a researcher wants to quantify the size or shape of cell nuclei, then a stain can be applied to the sample that attaches to the cells' DNA. The cells can be fixed in a substance that preserves the nature state of the cell. The sample is then interrogated by an instrument (such as a confocal microscope) where the dye deflects light and the detectors quantify the degree of scattering for that specific wavelength. If multiple characteristics of the cells are desired, then multiple dyes and multiple light frequencies can be used simultaneously. The light scattering measurements are then processed through imaging software to quantify the desired cell characteristics.

Using an automated, high-throughput approach to assess samples' cell characteristics can sometimes produce misleading results. Hill et al. (2007) describe a research project that used high-content screening to measure several aspects of cells. They observed that the imaging software used to determine the location and shape of the cell had difficulty segmenting cells (i.e., defining cells' boundaries). Consider Fig. 3.1, which depicts several example cells from this study. In these images, the bright green boundaries identify the cell nucleus, while the blue boundaries define the cell perimeter. Clearly some cells are *well segmented*, while others are not. Cells that are poorly segmented appear to be damaged, when in reality they are not. If cell size, shape, and/or quantity are the endpoints of interest in a study, then it is important that the instrument and imaging software can correctly segment cells.

For this research, Hill et al. (2007) assembled a data set consisting of 2,019 cells. Of these cells, 1,300 were judged to be poorly segmented (PS) and 719 were well segmented (WS); 1,009 cells were reserved for the training set.[1]

For a particular type of cell, the researchers used different stains that would be visible to different optical channels. Channel one was associated with the cell body and can be used to determine the cell perimeter, area, and other qualities. Channel two interrogated the cell nucleus by staining the nuclear DNA (shown in blue shading in Fig. 3.1). Channels three and four were stained to detect actin and tubulin, respectively. These are two types of filaments that transverse the cells in scaffolds and are part of the cell's cytoskeleton. For all cells, 116 features (e.g., cell area, spot fiber count) were measured and were used to predict the segmentation quality of cells.[2]

---

[1] The individual data points can be found on the journal web site or in the R Applied-PredictiveModeling package. See the Computing section at the end of this chapter.

[2] The original authors included several "status" features that are binary representations of other features in the data set. We excluded these from the analysis in this chapter.

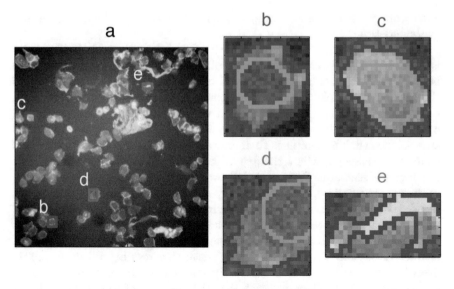

Fig. 3.1: An image showing cell segmentation from Hill et al. (2007). The *red boxes* [panels (**d**) and (**e**)] show poorly segmented cells while the cells in the *blue boxes* are examples of proper segmentation

This chapter will use the training set samples identified by the original authors to demonstrate data pre-processing techniques.

3.2 Data Transformations for Individual Predictors

Transformations of predictor variables may be needed for several reasons. Some modeling techniques may have strict requirements, such as the predictors having a common scale. In other cases, creating a good model may be difficult due to specific characteristics of the data (e.g., outliers). Here we discuss centering, scaling, and skewness transformations.

Centering and Scaling

The most straightforward and common data transformation is to center scale the predictor variables. To center a predictor variable, the average predictor value is subtracted from all the values. As a result of centering, the predictor has a zero mean. Similarly, to scale the data, each value of the predictor variable is divided by its standard deviation. Scaling the data coerce the values to have a common standard deviation of one. These manipulations are generally used to improve the numerical stability of some calculations. Some models, such as PLS (Sects. 6.3 and 12.4), benefit from the predictors being on a common scale. The only real downside to these transformations is a loss of interpretability of the individual values since the data are no longer in the original units.

Transformations to Resolve Skewness

Another common reason for transformations is to remove distributional skewness. An un-skewed distribution is one that is roughly symmetric. This means that the probability of falling on either side of the distribution's mean is roughly equal. A right-skewed distribution has a large number of points on the left side of the distribution (smaller values) than on the right side (larger values). For example, the cell segmentation data contain a predictor that measures the standard deviation of the intensity of the pixels in the actin filaments. In the natural units, the data exhibit a strong right skewness; there is a greater concentration of data points at relatively small values and small number of large values. Figure 3.2 shows a histogram of the data in the natural units (left panel).

A general rule of thumb to consider is that skewed data whose ratio of the highest value to the lowest value is greater than 20 have significant skewness. Also, the skewness statistic can be used as a diagnostic. If the predictor distribution is roughly symmetric, the skewness values will be close to zero. As the distribution becomes more right skewed, the skewness statistic becomes larger. Similarly, as the distribution becomes more left skewed, the value becomes negative. The formula for the sample skewness statistic is

$$\text{skewness} = \frac{\sum (x_i - \bar{x})^3}{(n-1)v^{3/2}}$$

$$\text{where} \quad v = \frac{\sum (x_i - \bar{x})^2}{(n-1)},$$

where x is the predictor variable, n is the number of values, and $\bar{x}$ is the sample mean of the predictor. For the actin filament data shown in Fig. 3.2, the skewness statistic was calculated to be 2.39 while the ratio to the largest and smallest value was 870.

Replacing the data with the log, square root, or inverse may help to remove the skew. For the data in Fig. 3.2, the right panel shows the distribution of the data once a log transformation has been applied. After the transformation, the distribution is not entirely symmetric but these data are better behaved than when they were in the natural units.

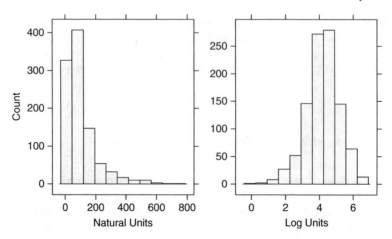

Fig. 3.2: *Left*: a histogram of the standard deviation of the intensity of the pixels in actin filaments. This predictor has a strong right skewness with a concentration of points with low values. For this variable, the ratio of the smallest to largest value is 870 and a skewness value of 2.39. *Right*: the same data after a log transformation. The skewness value for the logged data was -0.4

Alternatively, statistical methods can be used to empirically identify an appropriate transformation. Box and Cox (1964) propose a *family* of transformations[3] that are indexed by a parameter, denoted as λ:

$$x^* = \begin{cases} \frac{x^\lambda - 1}{\lambda} & \text{if } \lambda \neq 0 \\ \log(x) & \text{if } \lambda = 0 \end{cases}$$

In addition to the log transformation, this family can identify square transformation ($\lambda = 2$), square root ($\lambda = 0.5$), inverse ($\lambda = -1$), and others in-between. Using the training data, λ can be estimated. Box and Cox (1964) show how to use maximum likelihood estimation to determine the transformation parameter. This procedure would be applied independently to each predictor data that contain values greater than zero.

For the segmentation data, 69 predictors were not transformed due to zero or negative values and 3 predictors had λ estimates within 1 ± 0.02, so no transformation was applied. The remaining 44 predictors had values estimated between -2 and 2. For example, the predictor data shown in Fig. 3.2 have an estimated transformation value of 0.1, indicating the log

---

[3] Some readers familiar with Box and Cox (1964) will know that this transformation was developed for *outcome* data while Box and Tidwell (1962) describe similar methods for transforming a set of predictors in a linear model. Our experience is that the Box–Cox transformation is more straightforward, less prone to numerical issues, and just as effective for transforming individual predictor variables.

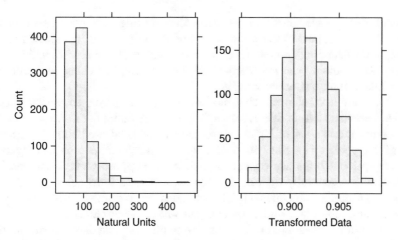

Fig. 3.3: *Left*: a histogram of the cell perimeter predictor. *Right*: the same data after a Box–Cox transformation with λ estimated to be -1.1

transformation is reasonable. Another predictor, the estimated cell perimeter, had a λ estimate of -1.1. For these data, the original and transformed values are shown in Fig. 3.3.

3.3 Data Transformations for Multiple Predictors

These transformations act on groups of predictors, typically the entire set under consideration. Of primary importance are methods to resolve outliers and reduce the dimension of the data.

Transformations to Resolve Outliers

We will generally define outliers as samples that are exceptionally far from the mainstream of the data. Under certain assumptions, there are formal statistical definitions of an outlier. Even with a thorough understanding of the data, outliers can be hard to define. However, we can often identify an unusual value by looking at a figure. When one or more samples are suspected to be outliers, the first step is to make sure that the values are scientifically valid (e.g., positive blood pressure) and that no data recording errors have occurred. Great care should be taken not to hastily remove or change values, especially if the sample size is small. With small sample sizes, apparent outliers might be a result of a skewed distribution where there are not yet

enough data to see the skewness. Also, the outlying data may be an indication of a special part of the population under study that is just starting to be
sampled. Depending on how the data were collected, a "cluster" of valid points
that reside outside the mainstream of the data might belong to a different
population than the other samples.[4]

There are several predictive models that are resistant to outliers. Tree-
based classification models create splits of the training data and the prediction equation is a set of logical statements such as "if predictor A is greater
than X, predict the class to be Y," so the outlier does not usually have
an exceptional influence on the model. Also, support vector machines for
classification generally disregard a portion of the training set samples when
creating a prediction equation. The excluded samples may be far away from
the decision boundary and outside of the data mainstream.

If a model is considered to be sensitive to outliers, one data transformation
that can minimize the problem is the *spatial sign* (Serneels et al. 2006). This
procedure projects the predictor values onto a multidimensional sphere. This
has the effect of making all the samples the same distance from the center of
the sphere. Mathematically, each sample is divided by its squared norm:

$$x_{ij}^* = \frac{x_{ij}}{\sqrt{\sum_{j=1}^{P} x_{ij}^2}}.$$

Since the denominator is intended to measure the squared distance to the
center of the predictor's distribution, it is important to center and scale the
predictor data prior to using this transformation. Note that, unlike centering
or scaling, this manipulation of the predictors transforms them as a group.
Removing predictor variables after applying the spatial sign transformation
may be problematic.

Figure 3.4 shows another data set with two correlated predictors. In these
data, at least eight samples cluster away from the majority of other data.
These data points are likely a valid, but poorly sampled subpopulation of the
data. The modeler would investigate why these points are different; perhaps
they represent a group of interest, such as highly profitable customers. The
spatial sign transformation is shown on the right-hand panel where all the
data points are projected to be a common distance away from the origin.
The outliers still reside in the Northwest section of the distribution but are
contracted inwards. This mitigates the effect of the samples on model training.

---

[4] Section 20.5 discusses model *extrapolation*—where the model predicts samples outside of the mainstream of the training data. Another concept is the *applicability
domain* of the model, which is the population of samples that can be effectively predicted by the model.

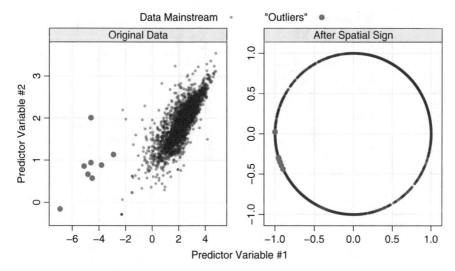

Fig. 3.4: *Left*: An illustrative example with a group of outlying data points. *Right*: When the original data are transformed, the results bring the outliers towards the majority of the data

Data Reduction and Feature Extraction

Data reduction techniques are another class of predictor transformations. These methods reduce the data by generating a smaller set of predictors that seek to capture a majority of the information in the original variables. In this way, fewer variables can be used that provide reasonable fidelity to the original data. For most data reduction techniques, the new predictors are functions of the original predictors; therefore, all the original predictors are still needed to create the surrogate variables. This class of methods is often called *signal extraction* or *feature extraction* techniques.

PCA is a commonly used data reduction technique (Abdi and Williams 2010). This method seeks to find linear combinations of the predictors, known as principal components (PCs), which capture the most possible variance. The first PC is defined as the linear combination of the predictors that captures the most variability of all possible linear combinations. Then, subsequent PCs are derived such that these linear combinations capture the most remaining variability while also being uncorrelated with all previous PCs. Mathematically, the jth PC can be written as:

$$\text{PC}_j = (a_{j1} \times \text{Predictor 1}) + (a_{j2} \times \text{Predictor 2}) + \cdots + (a_{jP} \times \text{Predictor } P).$$

P is the number of predictors. The coefficients $a_{j1}, a_{j2}, \ldots, a_{jP}$ are called component weights and help us understand which predictors are most important to each PC.

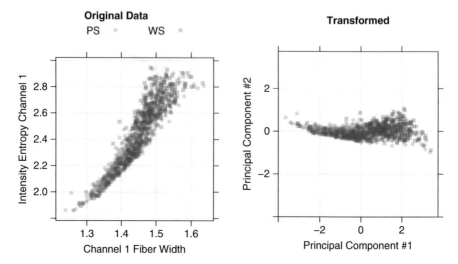

Fig. 3.5: An example of the principal component transformation for the cell segmentation data. The *shapes* and *colors* indicate which cells were poorly segmented or well segmented

To illustrate PCA, consider the data in Fig. 3.5. This set contains a subset of two correlated predictors, average pixel intensity of channel 1 and entropy of intensity values in the cell (a measure of cell shape), and a categorical response. Given the high correlation between the predictors (0.93), we could infer that average pixel intensity and entropy of intensity values measure redundant information about the cells and that either predictor or a linear combination of these predictors could be used in place of the original predictors. In this example, two PCs can be derived (right plot in Fig. 3.5); this transformation represents a rotation of the data about the axis of greatest variation. The first PC summarizes 97 % of the original variability, while the second summarizes 3 %. Hence, it is reasonable to use only the first PC for modeling since it accounts for the majority of information in the data.

The primary advantage of PCA, and the reason that it has retained its popularity as a data reduction method, is that it creates components that are uncorrelated. As mentioned earlier in this chapter, some predictive models prefer predictors to be uncorrelated (or at least low correlation) in order to find solutions and to improve the model's numerical stability. PCA preprocessing creates new predictors with desirable characteristics for these kinds of models.

While PCA delivers new predictors with desirable characteristics, it must be used with understanding and care. Notably, practitioners must understand that PCA seeks predictor-set variation without regard to any further understanding of the predictors (i.e., measurement scales or distributions)

or to knowledge of the modeling objectives (i.e., response variable). Hence, without proper guidance, PCA can generate components that summarize characteristics of the data that are irrelevant to the underlying structure of the data and also to the ultimate modeling objective.

Because PCA seeks linear combinations of predictors that maximize variability, it will naturally first be drawn to summarizing predictors that have more variation. If the original predictors are on measurement scales that differ in orders of magnitude [consider demographic predictors such as income level (in dollars) and height (in feet)], then the first few components will focus on summarizing the higher magnitude predictors (e.g., income), while latter components will summarize lower variance predictors (e.g., height). This means that the PC weights will be larger for the higher variability predictors on the first few components. In addition, it means that PCA will be focusing its efforts on identifying the data structure based on measurement scales rather than based on the important relationships within the data for the current problem.

For most data sets, predictors are on different scales. In addition, predictors may have skewed distributions. Hence, to help PCA avoid summarizing distributional differences and predictor scale information, it is best to first transform skewed predictors (Sect. 3.2) and then center and scale the predictors prior to performing PCA. Centering and scaling enables PCA to find the underlying relationships in the data without being influenced by the original measurement scales.

The second caveat of PCA is that it does not consider the modeling objective or response variable when summarizing variability. Because PCA is blind to the response, it is an *unsupervised technique*. If the predictive relationship between the predictors and response is not connected to the predictors' variability, then the derived PCs will not provide a suitable relationship with the response. In this case, a *supervised technique*, like PLS (Sects. 6.3 and 12.4), will derive components while simultaneously considering the corresponding response.

Once we have decided on the appropriate transformations of the predictor variables, we can then apply PCA. For data sets with many predictor variables, we must decide how many components to retain. A heuristic approach for determining the number of components to retain is to create a scree plot, which contains the ordered component number (x-axis) and the amount of summarized variability (y-axis) (Fig. 3.6). For most data sets, the first few PCs will summarize a majority of the variability, and the plot will show a steep descent; variation will then taper off for the remaining components. Generally, the component number prior to the tapering off of variation is the maximal component that is retained. In Fig. 3.6, the variation tapers off at component 5. Using this rule of thumb, four PCs would be retained. In an automated model building process, the optimal number of components can be determined by cross-validation (see Sect. 4.4).

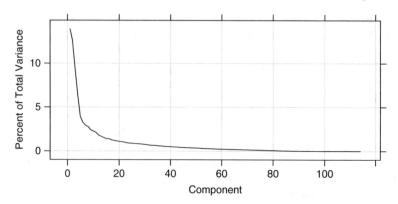

Fig. 3.6: A "scree plot" where the percentage of the total variance explained by each component is shown

Visually examining the principal components is a critical step for assessing data quality and gaining intuition for the problem. To do this, the first few principal components can be plotted against each other and the plot symbols can be colored by relevant characteristics, such as the class labels. If PCA has captured a sufficient amount of information in the data, this type of plot can demonstrate clusters of samples or outliers that may prompt a closer examination of the individual data points. For classification problems, the PCA plot can show potential separation of classes (if there is a separation). This can set the initial expectations of the modeler; if there is little clustering of the classes, the plot of the principal component values will show a significant overlap of the points for each class. Care should be taken when plotting the components; the scale of the components tend to become smaller as they account for less and less variation in the data. For example, in Fig. 3.5, the values of component one range from -3.7 to 3.4 while the component two ranges from -1 to 1.1. If the axes are displayed on separate scales, there is the potential to over-interpret any patterns that might be seen for components that account for small amounts of variation. See Geladi, Manley, and Lestander (2003) for other examples of this issue.

PCA was applied to the entire set of segmentation data predictors. As previously demonstrated, there are some predictors with significant skewness. Since skewed predictors can have an impact on PCA, there were 44 variables that were transformed using the Box–Cox procedure previously described. After the transformations, the predictors were centered and scaled prior to conducting PCA.

Figure 3.6 shows the percentage of the total variation in the data which was accounted for by each component. Notice that the percentages decrease as more components are added. The first three components accounted for 14 %, 12.6 %, and 9.4 % of the total variance, respectively. After four components,

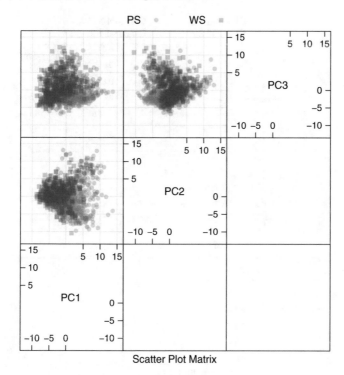

Fig. 3.7: A plot of the first three principal components for the cell segmentation data, colored by cell type

there is a sharp decline in the percentage of variation being explained, although these four components describe only 42.4 % of the information in the data set.

Figure 3.7 shows a scatter plot matrix for the first three principal components. The points are colored by class (segmentation quality). Since the percentages of variation explained are not large for the first three components, it is important not to over-interpret the resulting image. From this plot, there appears to be some separation between the classes when plotting the first and second components. However, the distribution of the well-segmented cells is roughly contained within the distribution of the poorly identified cells. One conclusion to infer from this image is that the cell types are not *easily* separated. However, this does not mean that other models, especially those which can accommodate highly nonlinear relationships, will reach the same conclusion. Also, while there are some cells in the data that are not completely within the data mainstream, there are no blatant outliers.

Another exploratory use of PCA is characterizing which predictors are associated with each component. Recall that each component is a linear combination of the predictors and the coefficient for each predictor is called the

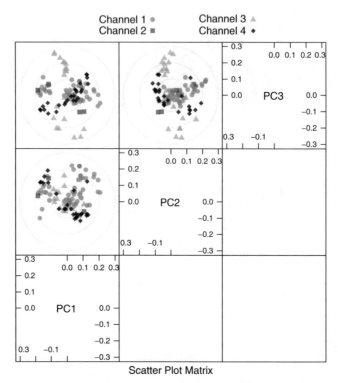

Fig. 3.8: A plot of the loadings of the first three principal components for the
cell segmentation data, colored by optical channel. Recall that channel one
was associated with the cell body, channel two with the cell nucleus, channel
three with actin, and channel four with tubulin

loading. Loadings close to zero indicate that the predictor variable did not
contribute much to that component. Figure 3.8 shows the loadings for the
first three components in the cell segmentation data. Each point corresponds
to a predictor variable and is colored by the optical channel used in the experiment. For the first principal component, the loadings for the first channel
(associated with the cell body) are on the extremes. This indicates that cell
body characteristics have the largest effect on the first principal component
and by extension the predictor values. Also note that the majority of the loadings for the third channel (measuring actin and tubulin) are closer to zero
for the first component. Conversely, the third principal component is mostly
associated with the third channel while the cell body channel plays a minor
role here. Even though the cell body measurements account for more variation in the data, this does not imply that these variables will be associated
with predicting the segmentation quality.

3.4 Dealing with Missing Values

In many cases, some predictors have no values for a given sample. These missing data could be *structurally missing*, such as the number of children a man has given birth to. In other cases, the value cannot or was not determined at the time of model building.

It is important to understand *why* the values are missing. First and foremost, it is important to know if the pattern of missing data is related to the outcome. This is called "informative missingness" since the missing data pattern is instructional on its own. Informative missingness can induce significant bias in the model. In the introductory chapter, a short example was given regarding predicting a patient's response to a drug. Suppose the drug was extremely ineffective or had significant side effects. The patient may be likely to miss doctor visits or to drop out of the study. In this case, there clearly is a relationship between the probability of missing values and the treatment. Customer ratings can often have informative missingness; people are more compelled to rate products when they have strong opinions (good or bad). In this case, the data are more likely to be polarized by having few values in the middle of the rating scale. In the Netflix Prize machine learning competition to predict which movies people will like based on their previous ratings, the "Napoleon Dynamite Effect" confounded many of the contestants because people who did rate the movie *Napoleon Dynamite* either loved or hated it.

Missing data should not be confused with *censored* data where the exact value is missing but something is known about its value. For example, a company that rents movie disks by mail may use the duration that a customer has kept a movie in their models. If a customer has not yet returned a movie, we do not know the actual time span, only that it is as least as long as the current duration. Censored data can also be common when using laboratory measurements. Some assays cannot measure below their limit of detection. In such cases, we know that the value is smaller than the limit but was not precisely measured.

Are censored data treated differently than missing data? When building traditional statistical models focused on interpretation or inference, the censoring is usually taken into account in a formal manner by making assumptions about the censoring mechanism. For predictive models, it is more common to treat these data as simple missing data or use the censored value as the observed value. For example, when a sample has a value below the limit of detection, the actual limit can be used in place of the real value. For this situation, it is also common to use a random number between zero and the limit of detection.

In our experience, missing values are more often related to predictor variables than the sample. Because of this, amount of missing data may be concentrated in a subset of predictors rather than occurring randomly across all the predictors. In some cases, the percentage of missing data is substantial enough to remove this predictor from subsequent modeling activities.

There are cases where the missing values might be concentrated in specific samples. For large data sets, removal of samples based on missing values is not a problem, assuming that the missingness is not informative. In smaller data sets, there is a steep price in removing samples; some of the alternative approaches described below may be more appropriate.

If we do not remove the missing data, there are two general approaches. First, a few predictive models, especially tree-based techniques, can specifically account for missing data. These are discussed further in Chap. 8.

Alternatively, missing data can be imputed. In this case, we can use information in the training set predictors to, in essence, estimate the values of other predictors. This amounts to a predictive model within a predictive model.

Imputation has been extensively studied in the statistical literature, but in the context of generating correct hypothesis testing procedures in the presence of missing data. This is a separate problem; for predictive models we are concerned about accuracy of the predictions rather than making valid inferences. There is a small literature on imputation for predictive models. Saar-Tsechansky and Provost (2007b) examine the issue of missing values and delve into how specific models deal with the issue. Jerez et al. (2010) also look at a wide variety of imputation methods for a specific data set.

As previously mentioned, imputation is just another layer of modeling where we try to estimate values of the predictor variables based on other predictor variables. The most relevant scheme for accomplishing this is to use the training set to built an imputation model for each predictor in the data set. Prior to model training or the prediction of new samples, missing values are filled in using imputation. Note that this extra layer of models adds uncertainty. If we are using resampling to select tuning parameter values or to estimate performance, the imputation should be incorporated within the resampling. This will increase the computational time for building models, but it will also provide honest estimates of model performance.

If the number of predictors affected by missing values is small, an exploratory analysis of the relationships between the predictors is a good idea. For example, visualizations or methods like PCA can be used to determine if there are strong relationships between the predictors. If a variable with missing values is highly correlated with another predictor that has few missing values, a focused model can often be effective for imputation (see the example below).

One popular technique for imputation is a K-nearest neighbor model. A new sample is imputed by finding the samples in the training set "closest" to it and averages these nearby points to fill in the value. Troyanskaya et al. (2001) examine this approach for high-dimensional data with small sample sizes. One advantage of this approach is that the imputed data are confined to be within the range of the training set values. One disadvantage is that the entire training set is required every time a missing value needs to be imputed. Also, the number of neighbors is a tuning parameter, as is the method for de-

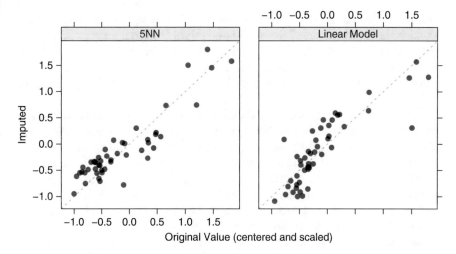

Fig. 3.9: After simulating 50 missing test set values at random for the cell perimeter data, two different imputation models were built with the training set and applied to the missing test set values. This plot shows the centered and scaled values before and after imputation

termining "closeness" of two points. However, Troyanskaya et al. (2001) found the nearest neighbor approach to be fairly robust to the tuning parameters, as well as the amount of missing data.

In Sect. 3.2, a predictor that measures the cell perimeter was used to illustrate skewness (see Fig. 3.3). As an illustration, a 5-nearest neighbor model was created using the training set values. In the test set, missing values were randomly induced in 50 test set cell perimeter values and then imputed using the model. Figure 3.9 shows a scatter plot of the samples set to missing. The left-hand panel shows the results of the 5-nearest neighbor approach. This imputation model does a good job predicting the absent samples; the correlation between the real and imputed values is 0.91.

Alternatively, a simpler approach can be used to impute the cell perimeter. The cell fiber length, another predictor associated with cell size, has a very high correlation (0.99) with the cell perimeter data. We can create a simple linear regression model using these data to predict the missing values. These results are in the right-hand panel of Fig. 3.9. For this approach, the correlation between the real and imputed values is 0.85.

3.5 Removing Predictors

There are potential advantages to removing predictors prior to modeling. First, fewer predictors means decreased computational time and complexity. Second, if two predictors are highly correlated, this implies that they are measuring the same underlying information. Removing one should not compromise the performance of the model and might lead to a more parsimonious and interpretable model. Third, some models can be crippled by predictors with degenerate distributions. In these cases, there can be a significant improvement in model performance and/or stability without the problematic variables.

Consider a predictor variable that has a single unique value; we refer to this type of data as a zero variance predictor. For some models, such an uninformative variable may have little effect on the calculations. A tree-based model (Sects. 8.1 and 14.1) is impervious to this type of predictor since it would never be used in a split. However, a model such as linear regression would find these data problematic and is likely to cause an error in the computations. In either case, these data have no information and can easily be discarded. Similarly, some predictors might have only a handful of unique values that occur with very low frequencies. These "near-zero variance predictors" may have a single value for the vast majority of the samples.

Consider a text mining application where keyword counts are collected for a large set of documents. After filtering out commonly used "stop words," such as *the* and *of*, predictor variables can be created for interesting keywords. Suppose a keyword occurs in a small group of documents but is otherwise unused. A hypothetical distribution of such a word count distribution is given in Table 3.1. Of the 531 documents that were searched, there were only four unique counts. The majority of the documents (523) do not have the keyword; while six documents have two occurrences, one document has three and another has six occurrences. Since 98 % of the data have values of zero, a minority of documents might have an undue influence on the model. Also, if any resampling is used (Sect. 4.4), there is a strong possibility that one of the resampled data sets (Sect. 4.4) will only contain documents without the keyword, so this predictor would only have one unique value.

How can the user diagnose this mode of problematic data? First, the number of unique points in the data must be small relative to the number of samples. In the document example, there were 531 documents in the data set, but only four unique values, so the percentage of unique values is 0.8 %. A small percentage of unique values is, in itself, not a cause for concern as many "dummy variables" (Sect. 3.6 below) generated from categorical predictors would fit this description. The problem occurs when the frequency of these unique values is severely disproportionate. The ratio of the most common frequency to the second most common reflects the imbalance in the frequencies. Most of the documents in the data set ($n = 523$) do not have the keyword. After this, the most frequent case is documents with two occurrences ($n = 6$). The ratio of these frequencies, $523/6 = 87$, is rather high and is indicative of a strong imbalance.

Given this, a rule of thumb for detecting near-zero variance predictors is:

Table 3.1: A predictor describing the number of documents where a keyword occurred

	#Documents
Occurrences: 0	523
Occurrences: 2	6
Occurrences: 3	1
Occurrences: 6	1

- The fraction of unique values over the sample size is low (say 10 %).
- The ratio of the frequency of the most prevalent value to the frequency of the second most prevalent value is large (say around 20).

If both of these criteria are true and the model in question is susceptible to this type of predictor, it may be advantageous to remove the variable from the model.

Between-Predictor Correlations

Collinearity is the technical term for the situation where a pair of predictor variables have a substantial correlation with each other. It is also possible to have relationships between multiple predictors at once (called *multicollinearity*).

For example, the cell segmentation data have a number of predictors that reflect the size of the cell. There are measurements of the cell perimeter, width, and length as well as other, more complex calculations. There are also features that measure cell morphology (i.e., shape), such as the roughness of the cell.

Figure 3.10 shows a correlation matrix of the training set. Each pairwise correlation is computed from the training data and colored according to its magnitude. This visualization is symmetric: the top and bottom diagonals show identical information. Dark blue colors indicate strong positive correlations, dark red is used for strong negative correlations, and white implies no empirical relationship between the predictors. In this figure, the predictor variables have been grouped using a clustering technique (Everitt et al. 2011) so that collinear groups of predictors are adjacent to one another. Looking along the diagonal, there are blocks of strong positive correlations that indicate "clusters" of collinearity. Near the center of the diagonal is a large block of predictors from the first channel. These predictors are related to cell size, such as the width and length of the cell.

When the data set consists of too many predictors to examine visually, techniques such as PCA can be used to characterize the magnitude of the problem. For example, if the first principal component accounts for a large

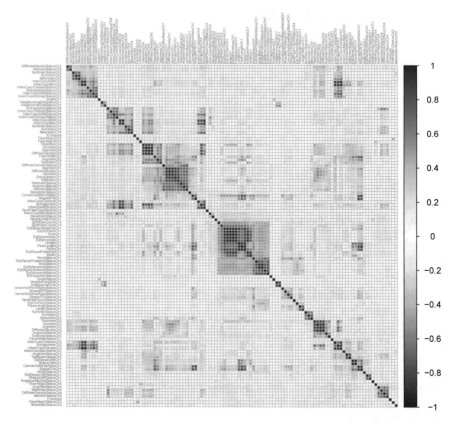

Fig. 3.10: A visualization of the cell segmentation correlation matrix. The order of the variables is based on a clustering algorithm

percentage of the variance, this implies that there is at least one group of predictors that represent the same information. For example, Fig. 3.6 indicates that the first 3–4 components have relative contributions to the total variance. This would indicate that there are at least 3–4 significant relationships between the predictors. The PCA loadings can be used to understand which predictors are associated with each component to tease out this relationships.

In general, there are good reasons to avoid data with highly correlated predictors. First, redundant predictors frequently add more complexity to the model than information they provide to the model. In situations where obtaining the predictor data is costly (either in time or money), fewer variables is obviously better. While this argument is mostly philosophical, there are mathematical disadvantages to having correlated predictor data. Using highly correlated predictors in techniques like linear regression can result in highly unstable models, numerical errors, and degraded predictive performance.

Classical regression analysis has several tools to diagnose multicollinearity for linear regression. Since collinear predictors can impact the variance of parameter estimates in this model, a statistic called the variance inflation factor (VIF) can be used to identify predictors that are impacted (Myers 1994). Beyond linear regression, this method may be inadequate for several reasons: it was developed for linear models, it requires more samples than predictor variables, and, while it does identify collinear predictors, it does not determine which should be removed to resolve the problem.

A less theoretical, more heuristic approach to dealing with this issue is to remove the minimum number of predictors to ensure that all pairwise correlations are below a certain threshold. While this method only identify collinearities in two dimensions, it can have a significantly positive effect on the performance of some models.

The algorithm is as follows:

1. Calculate the correlation matrix of the predictors.
2. Determine the two predictors associated with the largest absolute pairwise correlation (call them predictors A and B).
3. Determine the average correlation between A and the other variables. Do the same for predictor B.
4. If A has a larger average correlation, remove it; otherwise, remove predictor B.
5. Repeat Steps 2–4 until no absolute correlations are above the threshold.

The idea is to first remove the predictors that have the most correlated relationships.

Suppose we wanted to use a model that is particularly sensitive to between-predictor correlations, we might apply a threshold of 0.75. This means that we want to eliminate the minimum number of predictors to achieve all pairwise correlations less than 0.75. For the segmentation data, this algorithm would suggest removing 43 predictors.

As previously mentioned, feature extraction methods (e.g., principal components) are another technique for mitigating the effect of strong correlations between predictors. However, these techniques make the connection between the predictors and the outcome more complex. Additionally, since signal extraction methods are usually unsupervised, there is no guarantee that the resulting surrogate predictors have any relationship with the outcome.

3.6 Adding Predictors

When a predictor is categorical, such as gender or race, it is common to decompose the predictor into a set of more specific variables. For example, the credit scoring data discussed in Sect. 4.5 contains a predictor based on how much money was in the applicant's savings account. These data were

Table 3.2: A categorical predictor with five distinct groups from the credit scoring case study. The values are the amount in the savings account (in Deutsche Marks)

		Dummy variables				
Value	n	<100	100–500	500–1,000	>1,000	Unknown
<100 DM	103	1	0	0	0	0
100–500 DM	603	0	1	0	0	0
500–1,000 DM	48	0	0	1	0	0
>1,000 DM	63	0	0	0	1	0
Unknown	183	0	0	0	0	1

encoded into several groups, including a group for "unknown." Table 3.2 shows the values of this predictor and the number of applicants falling into each bin.

To use these data in models, the categories are re-encoded into smaller bits of information called "dummy variables." Usually, each category get its own dummy variable that is a zero/one indicator for that group. Table 3.2 shows the possible dummy variables for these data. Only four dummy variables are needed here; once you know the value of four of the dummy variables, the fifth can be inferred. However, the decision to include all of the dummy variables can depend on the choice of the model. Models that include an intercept term, such as simple linear regression (Sect. 6.2), would have numerical issues if each dummy variable was included in the model. The reason is that, for each sample, these variables all add up to one and this would provide the same information as the intercept. If the model is insensitive to this type of issue, using the complete set of dummy variables would help improve interpretation of the model.

Many of the models described in this text automatically generate highly complex, nonlinear relationships between the predictors and the outcome. More simplistic models do not unless the user manually specifies which predictors should be nonlinear and in what way. For example, logistic regression is a well-known classification model that, by default, generates linear classification boundaries. Figure 3.11 shows another illustrative example with two predictors and two classes. The left-hand panel shows the basic logistic regression classification boundaries when the predictors are added in the usual (linear) manner. The right-hand panel shows a logistic model with the basic linear terms and an additional term with the square of predictor B. Since logistic regression is a well-characterized and stable model, using this model with some additional nonlinear terms may be preferable to highly complex techniques (which may overfit).

Additionally, Forina et al. (2009) demonstrate one technique for augmenting the prediction data with addition of complex combinations of the data.

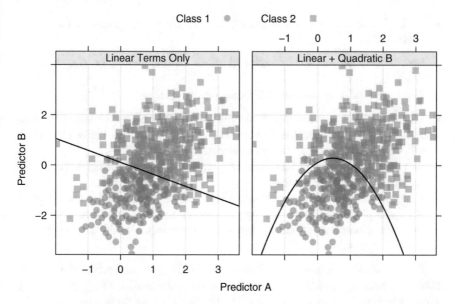

Fig. 3.11: Classification boundaries from two logistic regression models. The *left panel* has linear terms for the two predictors while the *right panel* has an additional quadratic term for predictor B. This model is discussed in more detail in Chap. 12

For classification models, they calculate the "class centroids," which are the centers of the predictor data for each class. Then for each predictor, the distance to each class centroid can be calculated and these distances can be added to the model.

3.7 Binning Predictors

While there are recommended techniques for pre-processing data, there are also methods to *avoid*. One common approach to simplifying a data set is to take a numeric predictor and pre-categorize or "bin" it into two or more groups prior to data analysis. For example, Bone et al. (1992) define a set of clinical symptoms to diagnose Systemic Inflammatory Response Syndrome (SIRS). SIRS can occur after a person is subjected to some sort of physical trauma (e.g., car crash). A simplified version of the clinical criteria for SIRS are:

- Temperature less than 36 °C or greater than 38 °C.
- Heart rate greater than 90 beats per minute.
- Respiratory rate greater than 20 breaths per minute.

- White blood cell count less than 4,000 cells/mm^3 or greater than 12,000 cells/mm^3.

A person who shows two or more of these criteria would be diagnosed as having SIRS.

The perceived advantages to this approach are:

- The ability to make seemingly simple statements, either for sake of having a simple decision rule (as in the SIRS example) or the belief that there will be a simple interpretation of the model.
- The modeler does not have to know the exact relationship between the predictors and the outcome.
- A higher response rate for survey questions where the choices are binned. For example, asking the date of a person's last tetanus shot is likely to have fewer responses than asking for a range (e.g., in the last 2 years, in the last 4 years).

There are many issues with the manual binning of continuous data. First, there can be a significant loss of performance in the model. Many of the modeling techniques discussed in this text are very good at determining complex relationships between the predictors and outcomes. Manually binning the predictors limits this potential. Second, there is a loss of precision in the predictions when the predictors are categorized. For example, if there are two binned predictors, only four combinations exist in the data set, so only simple predictions can be made. Third, research has shown (Austin and Brunner 2004) that categorizing predictors can lead to a high rate of false positives (i.e., noise predictors determined to be informative).

Unfortunately, the predictive models that are most powerful are usually the least interpretable. The bottom line is that the perceived improvement in interpretability gained by manual categorization is usually offset by a significant loss in performance. Since this book is concerned with predictive models (where interpretation is not the primary goal), loss of performance should be avoided. In fact, in some cases it may be unethical to arbitrarily categorize predictors. For example, there is a great deal of research on predicting aspects of disease (e.g., response to treatment, screening patients). If a medical diagnostic is used for such important determinations, patients desire the most accurate prediction possible. As long as complex models are properly validated, it may be improper to use a model that is built for interpretation rather than predictive performance.

Note that the argument here is related to the *manual* categorization of predictors prior to model building. There are several models, such as classification/regression trees and multivariate adaptive regression splines, that estimate cut points in the process of model building. The difference between these methodologies and manual binning is that the models use all the predictors to derive bins based on a single objective (such as maximizing accuracy). They evaluate many variables simultaneously and are usually based on statistically sound methodologies.

3.8 Computing

This section uses data from the AppliedPredictiveModeling package and functions from the caret, corrplot, e1071, and lattice packages.

There are two locations where relevant R code can be found:

- The **chapters** directory of the AppliedPredictiveModeling package contains specific code to reproduce the specific models used in the chapter. This is intended to allow the reader to see exactly how the models used here were created.
- Many chapters in this book contain sections at the end of the chapter that detail how of the computations can be performed in R more generally. For example, there are individual functions that correspond to the data pre-processing methods shown in this chapter. While the computing section provides these details, the individual functions might not be used directly in practice. For example, when using the train function, the pre-processing steps are specified in a single argument and the individual functions are not utilized. These sections do relate to the models created in each chapter, but as discussion points for the functions.

As such, the Computing sections in each chapter explains how to generally do the computations while the code in the **chapters** directory of the AppliedPredictiveModeling package is the best source for the calculations for the specific models in each chapter.

As discussed in Appendix B, there are a few useful R functions that can be used to find existing functions or classes of interest. The function apropos will search any loaded R packages for a given term. For example, to find functions for creating a confusion matrix within the currently loaded packages:

```
> apropos("confusion")
  [1] "confusionMatrix"        "confusionMatrix.train"
```

To find such a function in any package, the RSiteSearch function can help. Running the command:

```
> RSiteSearch("confusion", restrict = "functions")
```

will search online to find matches and will open a web browser to display the results.

The raw segmentation data set is contained in the AppliedPredictiveModeling package.[5] To load the data set into R:

```
> library(AppliedPredictiveModeling)
> data(segmentationOriginal)
```

There were fields that identified each cell (called Cell) and a factor vector that indicated which cells were well segmented (Class). The variable Case

---

[5] A preprocessed version of these data can also be found in the caret package and is used in later chapters.

indicated which cells were originally used for the training and test sets. The analysis in this chapter focused on the training set samples, so the data are filtered for these cells:

```
> segData <- subset(segmentationOriginal, Case == "Train")
```

The Class and Cell fields will be saved into separate vectors, then removed from the main object:

```
> cellID <- segData$Cell
> class <- segData$Class
> case <- segData$Case
> # Now remove the columns
> segData <- segData[, -(1:3)]
```

The original data contained several "status" columns which were binary versions of the predictors. To remove these, we find the column names containing "Status" and remove them:

```
> statusColNum <- grep("Status", names(segData))
> statusColNum
 [1]   2   4   9  10  11  12  14  16  20  21  22  26  27  28  30  32  34
[18]  36  38  40  43  44  46  48  51  52  55  56  59  60  63  64  68  69
[35]  70  72  73  74  76  78  80  82  84  86  88  92  93  94  97  98 103
[52] 104 105 106 110 111 112 114
> segData <- segData[, -statusColNum]
```

Transformations

As previously discussed, some features exhibited significantly skewness. The skewness function in the e1071 package calculates the sample skewness statistic for each predictor:

```
> library(e1071)
> # For one predictor:
> skewness(segData$AngleCh1)
 [1] -0.0243
> # Since all the predictors are numeric columns, the apply function can
> # be used to compute the skewness across columns.
> skewValues <- apply(segData, 2, skewness)
> head(skewValues)
  AngleCh1   AreaCh1 AvgIntenCh1 AvgIntenCh2 AvgIntenCh3 AvgIntenCh4
   -0.0243    3.5251      2.9592      0.8482      2.2023      1.9005
```

Using these values as a guide, the variables can be prioritized for visualizing the distribution. The basic R function hist or the histogram function in the lattice can be used to assess the shape of the distribution.

To determine which type of transformation should be used, the MASS package contains the boxcox function. Although this function estimates λ, it does not create the transformed variable(s). A **caret** function, `BoxCoxTrans`, can find the appropriate transformation and apply them to the new data:

```
> library(caret)
> Ch1AreaTrans <- BoxCoxTrans(segData$AreaCh1)
> Ch1AreaTrans

  Box-Cox Transformation

  1009 data points used to estimate Lambda

  Input data summary:
     Min. 1st Qu.  Median   Mean 3rd Qu.    Max.
      150     194     256    325     376    2190

  Largest/Smallest: 14.6
  Sample Skewness: 3.53

  Estimated Lambda: -0.9
> # The original data
> head(segData$AreaCh1)

  [1] 819 431 298 256 258 358
> # After transformation
> predict(Ch1AreaTrans, head(segData$AreaCh1))

  [1] 1.1085 1.1064 1.1045 1.1036 1.1036 1.1055
> (819^(-.9) - 1)/(-.9)

  [1] 1.1085
```

Another **caret** function, `preProcess`, applies this transformation to a set of predictors. This function is discussed below. The base R function `prcomp` can be used for PCA. In the code below, the data are centered and scaled prior to PCA.

```
> pcaObject <- prcomp(segData,
+                     center = TRUE, scale. = TRUE)
> # Calculate the cumulative percentage of variance which each component
> # accounts for.
> percentVariance <- pcaObject$sd^2/sum(pcaObject$sd^2)*100
> percentVariance[1:3]
  [1] 20.9 17.0 11.9
```

The transformed values are stored in `pcaObject` as a sub-object called x:

```
> head(pcaObject$x[, 1:5])
        PC1     PC2     PC3    PC4    PC5
2     5.099   4.551 -0.0335 -2.64  1.278
3    -0.255   1.198 -1.0206 -3.73  0.999
4     1.293  -1.864 -1.2511 -2.41 -1.491
12   -1.465  -1.566  0.4696 -3.39 -0.330
15   -0.876  -1.279 -1.3379 -3.52  0.394
16   -0.862  -0.329 -0.1555 -2.21  1.473
```

The another sub-object called `rotation` stores the variable loadings, where rows correspond to predictor variables and columns are associated with the components:

```
> head(pcaObject$rotation[, 1:3])
                  PC1      PC2      PC3
AngleCh1      0.00121 -0.0128  0.00682
AreaCh1       0.22917  0.1606  0.08981
AvgIntenCh1  -0.10271  0.1797  0.06770
AvgIntenCh2  -0.15483  0.1638  0.07353
AvgIntenCh3  -0.05804  0.1120 -0.18547
AvgIntenCh4  -0.11734  0.2104 -0.10506
```

The caret package class `spatialSign` contains functionality for the spatial sign transformation. Although we will not apply this technique to these data, the basic syntax would be `spatialSign(segData)`.

Also, these data do not have missing values for imputation. To impute missing values, the impute package has a function, `impute.knn`, that uses K-nearest neighbors to estimate the missing data. The previously mentioned `preProcess` function applies imputation methods based on K-nearest neighbors or bagged trees.

To administer a series of transformations to multiple data sets, the caret class `preProcess` has the ability to transform, center, scale, or impute values, as well as apply the spatial sign transformation and feature extraction. The function calculates the required quantities for the transformation. After calling the `preProcess` function, the `predict` method applies the results to a set of data. For example, to Box–Cox transform, center, and scale the data, then execute PCA for signal extraction, the syntax would be:

```
> trans <- preProcess(segData,
+                     method = c("BoxCox", "center", "scale", "pca"))
> trans
  Call:
  preProcess.default(x = segData, method = c("BoxCox", "center",
    "scale", "pca"))

  Created from 1009 samples and 58 variables
  Pre-processing: Box-Cox transformation, centered, scaled,
   principal component signal extraction

  Lambda estimates for Box-Cox transformation:
    Min. 1st Qu.  Median    Mean 3rd Qu.    Max.    NA's
   -2.00   -0.50   -0.10    0.05    0.30    2.00      11

  PCA needed 19 components to capture 95 percent of the variance
> # Apply the transformations:
> transformed <- predict(trans, segData)
> # These values are different than the previous PCA components since
> # they were transformed prior to PCA
> head(transformed[, 1:5])
```

```
          PC1     PC2     PC3    PC4     PC5
 2      1.568   6.291  -0.333  -3.06  -1.342
 3     -0.666   2.046  -1.442  -4.70  -1.742
 4      3.750  -0.392  -0.669  -4.02   1.793
12      0.377  -2.190   1.438  -5.33  -0.407
15      1.064  -1.465  -0.990  -5.63  -0.865
16     -0.380   0.217   0.439  -2.07  -1.936
```

The order in which the possible transformation are applied is transformation, centering, scaling, imputation, feature extraction, and then spatial sign.

Many of the modeling functions have options to center and scale prior to modeling. For example, when using the train function (discussed in later chapters), there is an option to use preProcess prior to modeling within the resampling iterations.

Filtering

To filter for near-zero variance predictors, the caret package function nearZero Var will return the column numbers of any predictors that fulfill the conditions outlined in Sect. 3.5. For the cell segmentation data, there are no problematic predictors:

```
> nearZeroVar(segData)
  integer(0)
> # When predictors should be removed, a vector of integers is
> # returned that indicates which columns should be removed.
```

Similarly, to filter on between-predictor correlations, the cor function can calculate the correlations between predictor variables:

```
> correlations <- cor(segData)
> dim(correlations)
  [1] 58 58
> correlations[1:4, 1:4]
             AngleCh1  AreaCh1 AvgIntenCh1 AvgIntenCh2
AngleCh1      1.00000 -0.00263     -0.0430     -0.0194
AreaCh1      -0.00263  1.00000     -0.0253     -0.1533
AvgIntenCh1  -0.04301 -0.02530      1.0000      0.5252
AvgIntenCh2  -0.01945 -0.15330      0.5252      1.0000
```

To visually examine the correlation structure of the data, the corrplot package contains an excellent function of the same name. The function has many options including one that will reorder the variables in a way that reveals clusters of highly correlated predictors. The following command was used to produce Fig. 3.10:

```
> library(corrplot)
> corrplot(correlations, order = "hclust")
```

The size and color of the points are associated with the strength of correlation between two predictor variables.

To filter based on correlations, the `findCorrelation` function will apply the algorithm in Sect. 3.5. For a given threshold of pairwise correlations, the function returns column numbers denoting the predictors that are recommended for deletion:

```
> highCorr <- findCorrelation(correlations, cutoff = .75)
> length(highCorr)
  [1] 33
> head(highCorr)

  [1] 23 40 43 36  7 15
> filteredSegData <- segData[, -highCorr]
```

There are also several functions in the subselect package that can accomplish the same goal.

Creating Dummy Variables

Several methods exist for creating dummy variables based on a particular model. Section 4.9 discusses different methods for specifying how the predictors enter into the model. One approach, the formula method, allows great flexibility to create the model function. Using formulas in model functions parameterizes the predictors such that not all categories have dummy variables. This approach will be shown in greater detail for linear regression.

As previously mentioned, there are occasions when a complete set of dummy variables is useful. For example, the splits in a tree-based model are more interpretable when the dummy variables encode all the information for that predictor. We recommend using the full set if dummy variables when working with tree-based models.

To illustrate the code, we will take a subset of the `cars` data set in the caret package. For 2005, Kelly Blue Book resale data for 804 GM cars were collected (Kuiper 2008). The object of the model was to predict the price of the car based on known characteristics. This demonstration will focus on the price, mileage, and car type (e.g., sedan) for a subset of vehicles:

```
> head(carSubset)
      Price Mileage   Type
  214 19981   24323 sedan
  299 21757    1853 sedan
  460 15047   12305 sedan
  728 15327    4318 sedan
  162 20628   20770 sedan
  718 16714   26328 sedan
> levels(carSubset$Type)

  [1] "convertible" "coupe"      "hatchback"   "sedan"      "wagon"
```

To model the price as a function of mileage and type of car, we can use the function dummyVars to determine encodings for the predictors. Suppose our first model assumes that the price can be modeled as a simple additive function of the mileage and type:

```
> simpleMod <- dummyVars(~Mileage + Type,
+                        data = carSubset,
+                        ## Remove the variable name from the
+                        ## column name
+                        levelsOnly = TRUE)
> simpleMod
  Dummy Variable Object

  Formula: ~Mileage + Type
  2 variables, 1 factors
  Factor variable names will be removed
```

To generate the dummy variables for the training set or any new samples, the predict method is used in conjunction with the dummyVars object:

```
> predict(simpleMod, head(carSubset))
    Mileage convertible coupe hatchback sedan wagon
214   24323           0     0         0     1     0
299    1853           0     0         0     1     0
460   12305           0     0         0     1     0
728    4318           0     0         0     1     0
162   20770           0     0         0     1     0
718   26328           0     0         0     1     0
```

The type field was expanded into five variables for five factor levels. The model is simple because it assumes that effect of the mileage is the same for every type of car. To fit a more advance model, we could assume that there is a *joint* effect of mileage and car type. This type of effect is referred to as an interaction. In the model formula, a colon between factors indicates that an interaction should be generated. For these data, this adds another five predictors to the data frame:

```
> withInteraction <- dummyVars(~Mileage + Type + Mileage:Type,
+                              data = carSubset,
+                              levelsOnly = TRUE)
> withInteraction
  Dummy Variable Object

  Formula: ~Mileage + Type + Mileage:Type
  2 variables, 1 factors
  Factor variable names will be removed
> predict(withInteraction, head(carSubset))
    Mileage convertible coupe hatchback sedan wagon Mileage:convertible
214   24323           0     0         0     1     0                   0
299    1853           0     0         0     1     0                   0
460   12305           0     0         0     1     0                   0
728    4318           0     0         0     1     0                   0
```

162	20770	0	0	0	1	0		0
718	26328	0	0	0	1	0		0

	Mileage:coupe	Mileage:hatchback	Mileage:sedan	Mileage:wagon
214	0	0	24323	0
299	0	0	1853	0
460	0	0	12305	0
728	0	0	4318	0
162	0	0	20770	0
718	0	0	26328	0

Exercises

3.1. The UC Irvine Machine Learning Repository[6] contains a data set related to glass identification. The data consist of 214 glass samples labeled as one of seven class categories. There are nine predictors, including the refractive index and percentages of eight elements: Na, Mg, Al, Si, K, Ca, Ba, and Fe.

The data can be accessed via:

```
> library(mlbench)
> data(Glass)
> str(Glass)
  'data.frame':        214 obs. of  10 variables:
   $ RI  : num  1.52 1.52 1.52 1.52 1.52 ...
   $ Na  : num  13.6 13.9 13.5 13.2 13.3 ...
   $ Mg  : num  4.49 3.6 3.55 3.69 3.62 3.61 3.6 3.61 3.58 3.6 ...
   $ Al  : num  1.1 1.36 1.54 1.29 1.24 1.62 1.14 1.05 1.37 1.36 ...
   $ Si  : num  71.8 72.7 73 72.6 73.1 ...
   $ K   : num  0.06 0.48 0.39 0.57 0.55 0.64 0.58 0.57 0.56 0.57 ...
   $ Ca  : num  8.75 7.83 7.78 8.22 8.07 8.07 8.17 8.24 8.3 8.4 ...
   $ Ba  : num  0 0 0 0 0 0 0 0 0 0 ...
   $ Fe  : num  0 0 0 0 0 0.26 0 0 0 0.11 ...
   $ Type: Factor w/ 6 levels "1","2","3","5",..: 1 1 1 1 1 1 1 1 1 1 ...
```

(a) Using visualizations, explore the predictor variables to understand their distributions as well as the relationships between predictors.
(b) Do there appear to be any outliers in the data? Are any predictors skewed?
(c) Are there any relevant transformations of one or more predictors that might improve the classification model?

3.2. The soybean data can also be found at the UC Irvine Machine Learning Repository. Data were collected to predict disease in 683 soybeans. The 35 predictors are mostly categorical and include information on the environmental conditions (e.g., temperature, precipitation) and plant conditions (e.g., left spots, mold growth). The outcome labels consist of 19 distinct classes.

---

[6] http://archive.ics.uci.edu/ml/index.html.

The data can be loaded via:

```
> library(mlbench)
> data(Soybean)
> ## See ?Soybean for details
```

(a) Investigate the frequency distributions for the categorical predictors. Are any of the distributions degenerate in the ways discussed earlier in this chapter?

(b) Roughly 18 % of the data are missing. Are there particular predictors that are more likely to be missing? Is the pattern of missing data related to the classes?

(c) Develop a strategy for handling missing data, either by eliminating predictors or imputation.

3.3. Chapter 5 introduces Quantitative Structure-Activity Relationship (QSAR) modeling where the characteristics of a chemical compound are used to predict other chemical properties. The caret package contains a QSAR data set from Mente and Lombardo (2005). Here, the ability of a chemical to permeate the blood-brain barrier was experimentally determined for 208 compounds. 134 descriptors were measured for each compound.

(a) Start R and use these commands to load the data:

```
> library(caret)
> data(BloodBrain)
> # use ?BloodBrain to see more details
```

The numeric outcome is contained in the vector logBBB while the predictors are in the data frame bbbDescr.

(b) Do any of the individual predictors have degenerate distributions?

(c) Generally speaking, are there strong relationships between the predictor data? If so, how could correlations in the predictor set be reduced? Does this have a dramatic effect on the number of predictors available for modeling?

Chapter 4
Over-Fitting and Model Tuning

Many modern classification and regression models are highly adaptable; they are capable of modeling complex relationships. However, they can very easily overemphasize patterns that are not reproducible. Without a methodological approach to evaluating models, the modeler will not know about the problem until the next set of samples are predicted.

Over-fitting has been discussed in the fields of forecasting (Clark 2004), medical research (Simon et al. 2003; Steyerberg 2010), chemometrics (Gowen et al. 2010; Hawkins 2004; Defernez and Kemsley 1997), meteorology (Hsieh and Tang 1998), finance (Dwyer 2005), and marital research (Heyman and Slep 2001) to name a few. These references illustrate that over-fitting is a concern for any predictive model regardless of field of research. The aim of this chapter is to explain and illustrate key principles of laying a foundation onto which trustworthy models can be built and subsequently used for prediction. More specifically, we will describe strategies that enable us to have confidence that the model we build will predict new samples with a similar degree of accuracy on the set of data for which the model was evaluated. Without this confidence, the model's predictions are *useless*.

On a practical note, all model building efforts are constrained by the existing data. For many problems, the data may have a limited number of samples, may be of less-than-desirable quality, and/or may be unrepresentative of future samples. While there are ways to build predictive models on small data sets, which we will describe in this chapter, we will assume that data quality is sufficient and that it is representative of the entire sample population.

Working under these assumptions, we must use the data at hand to find the best predictive model. Almost all predictive modeling techniques have tuning parameters that enable the model to flex to find the structure in the data. Hence, we must use the existing data to identify settings for the model's parameters that yield the best and most realistic predictive performance (known as model tuning). Traditionally, this has been achieved by splitting the existing data into training and test sets. The training set is used to build and tune the model and the test set is used to estimate the model's

M. Kuhn and K. Johnson, *Applied Predictive Modeling*,
DOI 10.1007/978-1-4614-6849-3_4,
© Springer Science+Business Media New York 2013

predictive performance. Modern approaches to model building split the data into multiple training and testing sets, which have been shown to often find more optimal tuning parameters and give a more accurate representation of the model's predictive performance.

To begin this chapter we will illustrate the concept of over-fitting through an easily visualized example. To avoid over-fitting, we propose a general model building approach that encompasses model tuning and model evaluation with the ultimate goal of finding the reproducible structure in the data. This approach entails splitting existing data into distinct sets for the purposes of tuning model parameters and evaluating model performance. The choice of data splitting method depends on characteristics of the existing data such as its size and structure. In Sect. 4.4, we define and explain the most versatile data splitting techniques and explore the advantages and disadvantages of each. Finally, we end the chapter with a computing section that provides code for implementing the general model building strategy.

4.1 The Problem of Over-Fitting

There now exist many techniques that can learn the structure of a set of data so well that when the model is applied to the data on which the model was built, it correctly predicts every sample. In addition to learning the general patterns in the data, the model has also learned the characteristics of each sample's unique noise. This type of model is said to be over-fit and will usually have poor accuracy when predicting a new sample. To illustrate over-fitting and other concepts in this chapter, consider the simple classification example in Fig. 4.1 that has two predictor variables (i.e., independent variables). These data contain 208 samples that are designated either as "Class 1" or "Class 2." The classes are fairly balanced; there are 111 samples in the first class and 97 in the second. Furthermore, there is a significant overlap between the classes which is often the case for most applied modeling problems.

One objective for a data set such as this would be to develop a model to classify new samples. In this two-dimensional example, the classification models or rules can be represented by boundary lines. Figure 4.2 shows example class boundaries from two distinct classification models. The lines envelop the area where each model predicts the data to be the second class (blue squares). The left-hand panel ("Model #1") shows a boundary that is complex and attempts to encircle every possible data point. The pattern in this panel is not likely to generalize to new data. The right-hand panel shows an alternative model fit where the boundary is fairly smooth and does not overextend itself to correctly classify every data point in the training set.

To gauge how well the model is classifying samples, one might use the training set. In doing so, the estimated error rate for the model in the left-hand panel would be overly optimistic. Estimating the utility of a model

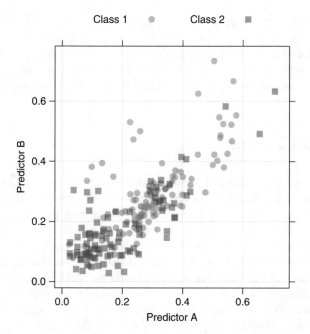

Fig. 4.1: An example of classification data that is used throughout the chapter

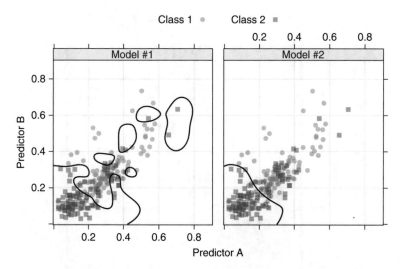

Fig. 4.2: An example of a training set with two classes and two predictors. The panels show two different classification models and their associated class boundaries

by re-predicting the training set is referred to *apparent performance* of the
model (e.g., the apparent error rate). In two dimensions, it is not difficult to
visualize that one model is over-fitting, but most modeling problems are in
much higher dimensions. In these situations, it is very important to have a
tool for characterizing how much a model is over-fitting the training data.

4.2 Model Tuning

Many models have important parameters which cannot be directly estimated
from the data. For example, in the K-nearest neighbor classification model,
a new sample is predicted based on the K-closest data points in the training
set. An illustration of a 5-nearest neighbor model is shown in Fig. 4.3. Here,
two new samples (denoted by the solid dot and filled triangle) are being
predicted. One sample (•) is near a mixture of the two classes; three of the
five neighbors indicate that the sample should be predicted as the first class.
The other sample (▲) has all five points indicating the second class should
be predicted. The question remains as to how many neighbors should be
used. A choice of too few neighbors may over-fit the individual points of the
training set while too many neighbors may not be sensitive enough to yield

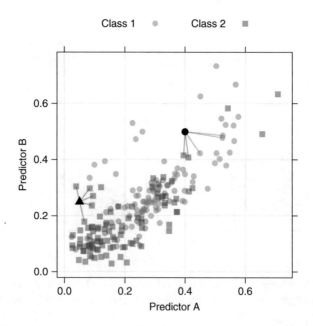

Fig. 4.3: The K-nearest neighbor classification model. Two new points, sym-
bolized by *filled triangle* and *solid dot*, are predicted using the training set

reasonable performance. This type of model parameter is referred to as a *tuning parameter* because there is no analytical formula available to calculate an appropriate value.

Several models discussed in this text have at least one tuning parameter. Since many of these parameters control the complexity of the model, poor choices for the values can result in over-fitting. Figure 4.2 illustrates this point. A support vector machine (Sect. 13.4) was used to generate the class boundaries in each panel. One of the tuning parameters for this model sets the price for misclassified samples in the training set and is generally referred to as the "cost" parameter. When the cost is large, the model will go to great lengths to correctly label every point (as in the left panel) while smaller values produce models that are not as aggressive. The class boundary in the left panel was created by manually setting the cost parameter to a very high number. In the right panel, the cost value was determined using cross-validation (Sect. 4.4).

There are different approaches to searching for the best parameters. A general approach that can be applied to almost any model is to define a set of candidate values, generate reliable estimates of model utility across the candidates values, then choose the optimal settings. A flowchart of this process is shown in Fig. 4.4.

Once a candidate set of parameter values has been selected, then we must obtain trustworthy estimates of model performance. The performance on the hold-out samples is then aggregated into a performance profile which is then used to determine the final tuning parameters. We then build a final model with all of the training data using the selected tuning parameters. Using the K-nearest neighbor example to illustrate the procedure of Fig. 4.4, the candidate set might include all odd values of K between 1 and 9 (odd values are used in the two-class situation to avoid ties). The training data would then be resampled and evaluated many times for each tuning parameter value. These results would then be aggregated to find the optimal value of K.

The procedure defined in Fig. 4.4 uses a set of candidate models that are defined by the tuning parameters. Other approaches such as genetic algorithms (Mitchell 1998) or simplex search methods (Olsson and Nelson 1975) can also find optimal tuning parameters. These procedures algorithmically determine appropriate values for tuning parameters and iterate until they arrive at parameter settings with optimal performance. These techniques tend to evaluate a large number of candidate models and can be superior to a defined set of tuning parameters when model performance can be efficiently calculated. Cohen et al. (2005) provides a comparison of search routines for tuning a support vector machine model.

A more difficult problem is obtaining trustworthy estimates of model performance for these candidate models. As previously discussed, the apparent error rate can produce extremely optimistic performance estimates. A better approach is to test the model on samples that were not used for training.

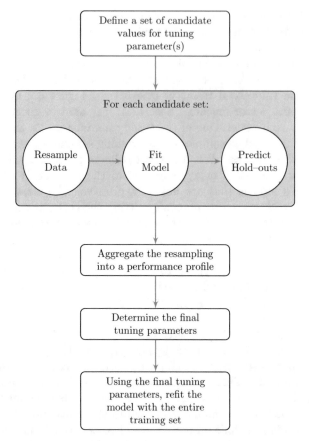

Fig. 4.4: A schematic of the parameter tuning process. An example of a candidate set of tuning parameter values for K-nearest neighbors might be odd numbers between 1 and 9. For each of these values, the data would be resampled multiple times to assess model performance for each value

Evaluating the model on a test set is the obvious choice, but, to get reasonable precision of the performance values, the size of the test set may need to be large.

An alternate approach to evaluating a model on a single test set is to *resample* the training set. This process uses several modified versions of the training set to build multiple models and then uses statistical methods to provide honest estimates of model performance (i.e., not overly optimistic). Section 4.4 illustrates several resampling techniques, and Sect. 4.6 discusses approaches to choose the final parameters using the resampling results.

4.3 Data Splitting

Now that we have outlined the general procedure for finding optimal tuning parameters, we turn to discussing the heart of the process: data splitting. A few of the common steps in model building are:

- Pre-processing the predictor data
- Estimating model parameters
- Selecting predictors for the model
- Evaluating model performance
- Fine tuning class prediction rules (via ROC curves, etc.)

Given a fixed amount of data, the modeler must decide how to "spend" their data points to accommodate these activities.

One of the first decisions to make when modeling is to decide which samples will be used to evaluate performance. Ideally, the model should be evaluated on samples that were not used to build or fine-tune the model, so that they provide an unbiased sense of model effectiveness. When a large amount of data is at hand, a set of samples can be set aside to evaluate the final model. The "training" data set is the general term for the samples used to create the model, while the "test" or "validation" data set is used to qualify performance.

However, when the number of samples is not large, a strong case can be made that a test set should be avoided because every sample may be needed for model building. Additionally, the size of the test set may not have sufficient power or precision to make reasonable judgements. Several researchers (Molinaro 2005; Martin and Hirschberg 1996; Hawkins et al. 2003) show that validation using a single test set can be a poor choice. Hawkins et al. (2003) concisely summarize this point: "holdout samples of tolerable size [...] do not match the cross-validation itself for reliability in assessing model fit and are hard to motivate." Resampling methods, such as cross-validation, can be used to produce appropriate estimates of model performance using the training set. These are discussed in length in Sect. 4.4. Although resampling techniques can be misapplied, such as the example shown in Ambroise and McLachlan (2002), they often produce performance estimates superior to a single test set because they evaluate many alternate versions of the data.

If a test set is deemed necessary, there are several methods for splitting the samples. Nonrandom approaches to splitting the data are sometimes appropriate. For example,

- If a model was being used to predict patient outcomes, the model may be created using certain patient sets (e.g., from the same clinical site or disease stage), and then tested on a different sample population to understand how well the model generalizes.
- In chemical modeling for drug discovery, new "chemical space" is constantly being explored. We are most interested in accurate predictions in the chemical space that is currently being investigated rather than the space that

was evaluated years prior. The same could be said for spam filtering; it is more important for the model to catch the new spamming techniques rather than prior spamming schemes.

However, in most cases, there is the desire to make the training and test sets as homogeneous as possible. Random sampling methods can be used to create similar data sets.

The simplest way to split the data into a training and test set is to take a simple random sample. This does not control for any of the data attributes, such as the percentage of data in the classes. When one class has a disproportionately small frequency compared to the others, there is a chance that the distribution of the outcomes may be substantially different between the training and test sets.

To account for the outcome when splitting the data, stratified random sampling applies random sampling within subgroups (such as the classes). In this way, there is a higher likelihood that the outcome distributions will match. When the outcome is a number, a similar strategy can be used; the numeric values are broken into similar groups (e.g., low, medium, and high) and the randomization is executed within these groups.

Alternatively, the data can be split on the basis of the predictor values. Willett (1999) and Clark (1997) propose data splitting based on *maximum dissimilarity sampling*. Dissimilarity between two samples can be measured in a number of ways. The simplest method is to use the distance between the predictor values for two samples. If the distance is small, the points are in close proximity. Larger distances between points are indicative of dissimilarity. To use dissimilarity as a tool for data splitting, suppose the test set is initialized with a single sample. The dissimilarity between this initial sample and the unallocated samples can be calculated. The unallocated sample that is most dissimilar would then be added to the test set. To allocate more samples to the test set, a method is needed to determine the dissimilarities between *groups* of points (i.e., the two in the test set and the unallocated points). One approach is to use the average or minimum of the dissimilarities. For example, to measure the dissimilarities between the two samples in the test set and a single unallocated point, we can determine the two dissimilarities and average them. The third point added to the test set would be chosen as having the maximum average dissimilarity to the existing set. This process would continue until the targeted test set size is achieved.

Figure 4.5 illustrates this process for the example classification data. Dissimilarity sampling was conducted separately within each class. First, a sample within each class was chosen to start the process (designated as ■ and ● in the figure). The dissimilarity of the initial sample to the unallocated samples within the class was computed and the most dissimilar point was added to the test set. For the first class, the most dissimilar point was in the extreme Southwest of the initial sample. On the second round, the dissimilarities were aggregated using the minimum (as opposed to the average). Again,

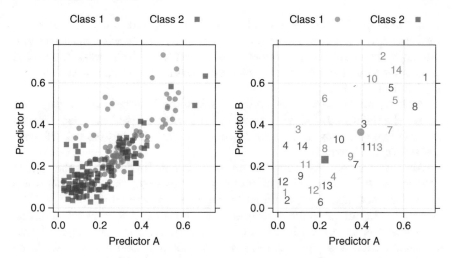

Fig. 4.5: An example of maximum dissimilarity sampling to create a test set. After choosing an initial sample within a class, 14 more samples were added

for the first class, the chosen point was far in the Northeast of the predictor space. As the sampling proceeds, samples were selected on the periphery of the data then work inward.

Martin et al. (2012) compares different methods of splitting data, including random sampling, dissimilarity sampling, and other methods.

4.4 Resampling Techniques

Generally, resampling techniques for estimating model performance operate similarly: a subset of samples are used to fit a model and the remaining samples are used to estimate the efficacy of the model. This process is repeated multiple times and the results are aggregated and summarized. The differences in techniques usually center around the method in which subsamples are chosen. We will consider the main flavors of resampling in the next few subsections.

k-Fold Cross-Validation

The samples are randomly partitioned into k sets of roughly equal size. A model is fit using the all samples except the first subset (called the first *fold*). The held-out samples are predicted by this model and used to estimate performance measures. The first subset is returned to the training set and procedure repeats with the second subset held out, and so on. The k resampled estimates of performance are summarized (usually with the mean and standard error) and used to understand the relationship between the tuning parameter(s) and model utility. The cross-validation process with $k = 3$ is depicted in Fig. 4.6.

A slight variant of this method is to select the k partitions in a way that makes the folds balanced with respect to the outcome (Kohavi 1995). Stratified random sampling, previously discussed in Sect. 4.3, creates balance with respect to the outcome.

Another version, leave-one-out cross-validation (LOOCV), is the special case where k is the number of samples. In this case, since only one sample is held-out at a time, the final performance is calculated from the k individual held-out predictions. Additionally, repeated k-fold cross-validation replicates the procedure in Fig. 4.6 multiple times. For example, if 10-fold cross-validation was repeated five times, 50 different held-out sets would be used to estimate model efficacy.

The choice of k is usually 5 or 10, but there is no formal rule. As k gets larger, the difference in size between the training set and the resampling subsets gets smaller. As this difference decreases, the *bias* of the technique becomes smaller (i.e., the bias is smaller for $k = 10$ than $k = 5$). In this context, the bias is the difference between the estimated and true values of performance.

Another important aspect of a resampling technique is the uncertainty (i.e., variance or noise). An unbiased method may be estimating the correct value (e.g., the true theoretical performance) but may pay a high price in uncertainty. This means that repeating the resampling procedure may produce a very different value (but done enough times, it will estimate the true value). k-fold cross-validation generally has high variance compared to other methods and, for this reason, might not be attractive. It should be said that for large training sets, the potential issues with variance and bias become negligible.

From a practical viewpoint, larger values of k are more computationally burdensome. In the extreme, LOOCV is most computationally taxing because it requires as many model fits as data points and each model fit uses a subset that is nearly the same size of the training set. Molinaro (2005) found that leave-one-out and k =10-fold cross-validation yielded similar results, indicating that $k = 10$ is more attractive from the perspective of computational efficiency. Also, small values of k, say 2 or 3, have high bias but are very computationally efficient. However, the bias that comes with small values of k is about the same as the bias produced by the bootstrap (see below), but with much larger variance.

Research (Molinaro 2005; Kim 2009) indicates that repeating k-fold cross-validation can be used to effectively increase the precision of the estimates while still maintaining a small bias.

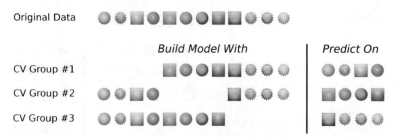

Fig. 4.6: A schematic of threefold cross-validation. Twelve training set samples are represented as symbols and are allocated to three groups. These groups are left out in turn as models are fit. Performance estimates, such as the error rate or R^2 are calculated from each set of held-out samples. The average of the three performance estimates would be the cross-validation estimate of model performance. In practice, the number of samples in the held-out subsets can vary but are roughly equal size

Generalized Cross-Validation

For linear regression models, there is a formula for approximating the leave-one-out error rate. The generalized cross-validation (GCV) statistic (Golub et al. 1979) does not require iterative refitting of the model to different data subsets. The formula for this statistic is the i_{th} training set outcome

$$\text{GCV} = \frac{1}{n} \sum_{i=1}^{n} \left(\frac{y_i - \hat{y}_i}{1 - df/n} \right)^2,$$

where y_i is the ith in the training set set outcome, $\hat{y}_i$ is the model prediction of that outcome, and df is the degrees of freedom of the model. The degrees of freedom are an accounting of how many parameters are estimated by the model and, by extension, a measure of complexity for linear regression models. Based on this equation, two models with the same sums of square errors (the numerator) would have different GCV values if the complexities of the models were different.

Repeated Training/Test Splits

Repeated training/test splits is also known as "leave-group-out cross-validation" or "Monte Carlo cross-validation." This technique simply creates multiple splits of the data into modeling and prediction sets (see Fig. 4.7). The proportion of the data going into each subset is controlled by the practitioner as is the number of repetitions. As previously discussed, the bias

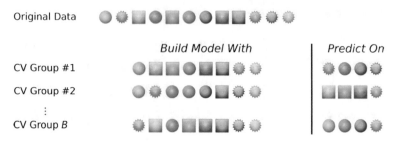

Fig. 4.7: A schematic of B repeated training and test set partitions. Twelve training set samples are represented as symbols and are allocated to B subsets that are 2/3 of the original training set. One difference between this procedure and k-fold cross-validation are that samples can be represented in multiple held-out subsets. Also, the number of repetitions is usually larger than in k-fold cross-validation

of the resampling technique decreases as the amount of data in the subset approaches the amount in the modeling set. A good rule of thumb is about 75–80 %. Higher proportions are a good idea if the number of repetitions is large.

The number of repetitions is important. Increasing the number of subsets has the effect of decreasing the uncertainty of the performance estimates. For example, to get a gross estimate of model performance, 25 repetitions will be adequate if the user is willing to accept some instability in the resulting values. However, to get stable estimates of performance, it is suggested to choose a larger number of repetitions (say 50–200). This is also a function of the proportion of samples being randomly allocated to the prediction set; the larger the percentage, the more repetitions are needed to reduce the uncertainty in the performance estimates.

The Bootstrap

A bootstrap sample is a random sample of the data taken *with replacement* (Efron and Tibshirani 1986). This means that, after a data point is selected for the subset, it is still available for further selection. The bootstrap sample is the same size as the original data set. As a result, some samples will be represented multiple times in the bootstrap sample while others will not be selected at all. The samples not selected are usually referred to as the "out-of-bag" samples. For a given iteration of bootstrap resampling, a model is built on the selected samples and is used to predict the out-of-bag samples (Fig. 4.8).

In general, bootstrap error rates tend to have less uncertainty than k-fold cross-validation (Efron 1983). However, on average, 63.2 % of the data points the bootstrap sample are represented at least once, so this technique has bias

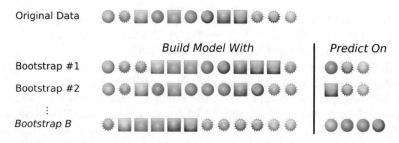

Fig. 4.8: A schematic of bootstrap resampling. Twelve training set samples are represented as symbols and are allocated to B subsets. Each subset is the same size as the original and can contain multiple instances of the same data point. Samples not selected by the bootstrap are predicted and used to estimate model performance

similar to k-fold cross-validation when $k \approx 2$. If the training set size is small, this bias may be problematic, but will decrease as the training set sample size becomes larger.

A few modifications of the simple bootstrap procedure have been devised to eliminate this bias. The "632 method" (Efron 1983) addresses this issue by creating a performance estimate that is a combination of the simple bootstrap estimate and the estimate from re-predicting the training set (e.g., the apparent error rate). For example, if a classification model was characterized by its error rate, the 632 method would use

$$(0.632 \times \text{simple bootstrap estimate}) + (0.368 \times \text{apparent error rate}).$$

The modified bootstrap estimate reduces the bias, but can be unstable with small samples sizes. This estimate can also result in unduly optimistic results when the model severely over-fits the data, since the apparent error rate will be close to zero. Efron and Tibshirani (1997) discuss another technique, called the "632+ method," for adjusting the bootstrap estimates.

4.5 Case Study: Credit Scoring

A straightforward application of predictive models is credit scoring. Existing data can be used to create a model to predict the probability that applicants have good credit. This information can be used to quantify the risk to the lender.

The German credit data set is a popular tool for benchmarking machine learning algorithms. It contains 1,000 samples that have been given labels of good and bad credit. In the data set, 70 % were rated as having good credit. As discussed in Sect. 11.2, when evaluating the accuracy of a model, the baseline accuracy rate to beat would be 70 % (which we could achieve by simply predicting all samples to have good credit).

Along with these outcomes, data were collected related to credit history, employment, account status, and so on. Some predictors are numeric, such as the loan amount. However, most of the predictors are categorical in nature, such as the purpose of the loan, gender, or marital status. The categorical predictors were converted to "dummy variables" that related to a single category. For example, the applicant's residence information was categorized as either "rent," "own," or "free housing." This predictor would be converted to three yes/no bits of information for each category. For example, one predictor would have a value of one if the applicant rented and is zero otherwise. Creation of dummy variables is discussed at length in Sect. 3.6. In all, there were 41 predictors used to model the credit status of an individual.

We will use these data to demonstrate the process of tuning models using resampling, as defined in Fig. 4.4. For illustration, we took a stratified random sample of 800 customers to use for training models. The remaining samples will be used as a test set to verify performance when a final model is determined. Section 11.2 will discuss the results of the test set in more detail.

4.6 Choosing Final Tuning Parameters

Once model performance has been quantified across sets of tuning parameters, there are several philosophies on how to choose the final settings. The simplest approach is to pick the settings associated with the numerically best performance estimates.

For the credit scoring example, a nonlinear support vector machine model[1] was evaluated over cost values ranging from 2^{-2} to 2^7. Each model was evaluated using five repeats of 10-fold cross-validation. Figure 4.9 and Table 4.1 show the accuracy profile across the candidate values of the cost parameter. For each model, cross-validation generated 50 different estimates of the accuracy; the solid points in Fig. 4.9 are the average of these estimates. The bars reflect the average plus/minus two-standard errors of the mean. The profile shows an increase in accuracy until the cost value is one. Models with cost values between 1 and 16 are relatively constant; after which, the accuracy decreases (likely due to over-fitting). The numerically optimal value of the cost parameter is 8, with a corresponding accuracy rate of 75 %. Notice that the apparent accuracy rate, determined by re-predicting the training set samples, indicates that the model improves as the cost is increased, although more complex models over-fit the training set.

---

[1] This model uses a radial basis function kernel, defined in Sect. 13.4. Although not explored here, we used the analytical approach discussed later for determining the kernel parameter and fixed this value for all resampling techniques.

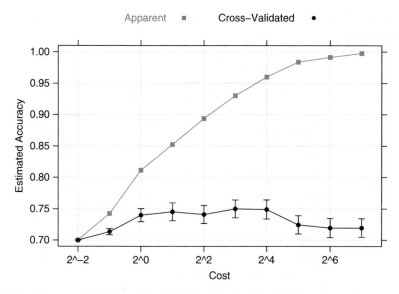

Fig. 4.9: The performance profile of a radial basis function support vector machine for the credit scoring example over different values of the cost parameter. The *vertical lines* indicate ± two-standard errors of the accuracy

In general, it may be a good idea to favor simpler models over more complex ones and choosing the tuning parameters based on the numerically optimal value may lead to models that are overly complicated. Other schemes for choosing less complex models should be investigated as they might lead to simpler models that provide acceptable performance (relative to the numerically optimal settings).

The "one-standard error" method for choosing simpler models finds the numerically optimal value and its corresponding standard error and then seeks the simplest model whose performance is within a single standard error of the numerically best value. This procedure originated with classification and regression trees (Breiman et al. (1984) and Sects. 8.1 and 14.1). In Fig. 4.10, the standard error of the accuracy values when the cost is 8 is about 0.7 %. This technique would find the simplest tuning parameter settings associated with accuracy no less than 74.3 % (75 %–0.7 %). This procedure would choose a value of 2 for the cost parameter.

Another approach is to choose a simpler model that is within a certain tolerance of the numerically best value. The percent decrease in performance could be quantified by $(X - O)/O$ where X is the performance value and O is the numerically optimal value. For example, in Fig. 4.9, the best accuracy value across the profile was 75 %. If a 4 % loss in accuracy was acceptable as a trade-off for a simpler model, accuracy values greater than 71.2 % would

Table 4.1: Repeated cross-validation accuracy results for the support vector machine model

	Resampled accuracy (%)		
Cost	Mean	Std. error	% Tolerance
0.25	70.0	0.0	−6.67
0.50	71.3	0.2	−4.90
1.00	74.0	0.5	−1.33
2.00	74.5	0.7	−0.63
4.00	74.1	0.7	−1.20
8.00	75.0	0.7	0.00
16.00	74.9	0.8	−0.13
32.00	72.5	0.7	−3.40
64.00	72.0	0.8	−4.07
128.00	72.0	0.8	−4.07

The one-standard error rule would select the simplest model with accuracy no less than 74.3 % (75 %–0.7 %). This corresponds to a cost value of 2. The "pick-the-best" solution is shown in bold

be acceptable. For the profile in Fig. 4.9, a cost value of 1 would be chosen using this approach.

As an illustration, additional resampling methods were applied to the same data: repeated 10-fold cross-validation, LOOCV, the bootstrap (with and without the 632 adjustment), and repeated training/test splits (with 20 % held-out). The latter two methods used 50 resamples to estimate performance.

The results are shown in Fig. 4.10. A common pattern within the cross-validation methods is seen where accuracy peaks at cost values between 4 and 16 and stays roughly constant within this window.

In each case, performance rapidly increases with the cost value and then, after the peak, decreases at a slower rate as over-fitting begins to occur. The cross-validation techniques estimate the accuracy to be between 74.5 % and 76.6 %. Compared to the other methods, the simple bootstrap is slightly pessimistic, estimating the accuracy to be 74.2 % while the 632 rule appears to overcompensate for the bias and estimates the accuracy to be 82.3 %. Note that the standard error bands of the simple 10-fold cross-validation technique are larger than the other methods, mostly because the standard error is a function of the number of resamples used (10 versus the 50 used by the bootstrap or repeated splitting).

The computational times varied considerably. The fastest was 10-fold cross-validation, which clocked in at 0.82 min. Repeated cross-validation, the bootstrap, and repeated training-test splits fit the same number of models and, on average, took about 5-fold more time to finish. LOOCV, which fits as many models as there are samples in the training set, took 86-fold longer and should only be considered when the number of samples is very small.

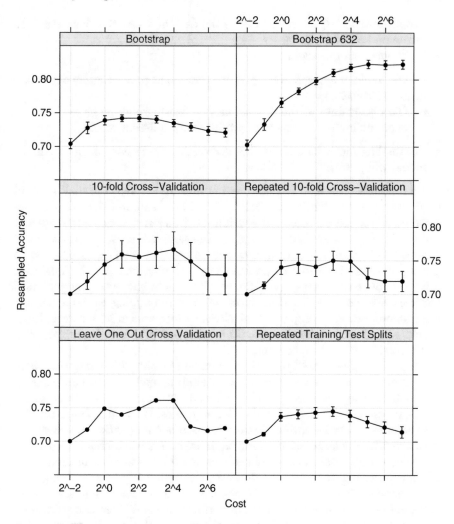

Fig. 4.10: The performance profile of nonlinear support vector machine over different values of the cost parameter for the credit scoring example using several different resampling procedures. The *vertical lines* indicate ± two-standard errors of the accuracy

4.7 Data Splitting Recommendations

As previously discussed, there is a strong technical case to be made against a single, independent test set:

- A test set is a single evaluation of the model and has limited ability to characterize the uncertainty in the results.

- Proportionally large test sets divide the data in a way that increases bias in the performance estimates.
- With small sample sizes:
  - The model may need every possible data point to adequately determine model values.
  - The uncertainty of the test set can be considerably large to the point where different test sets may produce very different results.

- Resampling methods can produce reasonable predictions of how well the model will perform on future samples.

No resampling method is uniformly better than another; the choice should be made while considering several factors. If the samples size is small, we recommend repeated 10-fold cross-validation for several reasons: the bias and variance properties are good and, given the sample size, the computational costs are not large. If the goal is to choose between models, as opposed to getting the best indicator of performance, a strong case can be made for using one of the bootstrap procedures since these have very low variance. For large sample sizes, the differences between resampling methods become less pronounced, and computational efficiency increases in importance. Here, simple 10-fold cross-validation should provide acceptable variance, low bias, and is relatively quick to compute.

Varma and Simon (2006) and Boulesteix and Strobl (2009) note that there is a potential bias that can occur when estimating model performance during parameter tuning. Suppose that the final model is chosen to correspond to the tuning parameter value associated with the smallest error rate. This error rate has the potential to be optimistic since it is a random quantity that is chosen from a potentially large set of tuning parameters. Their research is focused on scenarios with a small number of samples and a large number of predictors, which exacerbates the problem. However, for moderately large training sets, our experience is that this bias is small. In later sections, comparisons are made between resampled estimates of performance and those derived from a test set. For these particular data sets, the *optimization bias* is insubstantial.

4.8 Choosing Between Models

Once the settings for the tuning parameters have been determined for each model, the question remains: how do we choose between multiple models? Again, this largely depends on the characteristics of the data and the type of questions being answered. However, predicting which model is most fit for purpose can be difficult. Given this, we suggest the following scheme for finalizing the type of model:

1. Start with several models that are the least interpretable and most flexible, such as boosted trees or support vector machines. Across many problem domains, these models have a high likelihood of producing the empirically optimum results (i.e., most accurate).
2. Investigate simpler models that are less opaque (e.g., not complete black boxes), such as multivariate adaptive regression splines (MARS), partial least squares, generalized additive models, or naïve Bayes models.
3. Consider using the simplest model that reasonably approximates the performance of the more complex methods.

Using this methodology, the modeler can discover the "performance ceiling" for the data set before settling on a model. In many cases, a range of models will be equivalent in terms of performance so the practitioner can weight the benefits of different methodologies (e.g., computational complexity, easy of prediction, interpretability). For example, a nonlinear support vector machine or random forest model might have superior accuracy, but the complexity and scope of the prediction equation may prohibit exporting the prediction equation to a production system. However, if a more interpretable model, such as a MARS model, yielded similar accuracy, the implementation of the prediction equation would be trivial and would also have superior execution time.

Consider the credit scoring support vector machine classification model that was characterized using resampling in Sect. 4.6. Using repeated 10-fold cross-validation, the accuracy for this model was estimated to be 75 % with most of the resampling results between 66 % and 82 %.

Logistic regression (Sect. 12.2) is a more simplistic technique than the nonlinear support vector machine model for estimating a classification boundary. It has no tuning parameters and its prediction equation is simple and easy to implement using most software. Using the same cross-validation scheme, the estimated accuracy for this model was 74.9 % with most of the resampling results between 66 % and 82 %.

The same 50 resamples were used to evaluate each model. Figure 4.11 uses box plots to illustrate the distribution of the resampled accuracy estimates. Clearly, there is no performance loss by using a more straightforward model for these data.

Hothorn et al. (2005) and Eugster et al. (2008) describe statistical methods for comparing methodologies based on resampling results. Since the accuracies were measured using identically resampled data sets, statistical methods for *paired comparisons* can be used to determine if the differences between models are statistically significant. A paired t-test can be used to evaluate the hypothesis that the models have equivalent accuracies (on average) or, analogously, that the mean difference in accuracy for the resampled data sets is zero. For these two models, the average difference in model accuracy was 0.1 %, with the logistic regression supplying the better results. The 95 % confidence interval for this difference was $(-1.2 \%, 1 \%)$, indicating that there

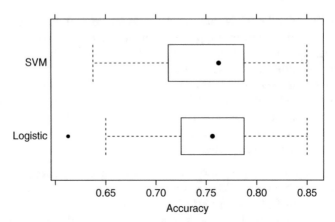

Fig. 4.11: A comparison of the cross-validated accuracy estimates from a support vector machine model and a logistic regression model for the credit scoring data described in Sect. 4.5

is no evidence to support the idea that the accuracy for either model is significantly better. This makes intuitive sense; the resampled accuracies in Fig. 4.11 range from 61.3 % to 85 %; given this amount of variation in the results, a 0.1 % improvement of accuracy is not meaningful.

When a model is characterized in multiple ways, there is a possibility that comparisons between models can lead to different conclusions. For example, if a model is created to predict two classes, sensitivity and specificity may be used to characterize the efficacy of models (see Chap. 11). If the data set includes more events than nonevents, the sensitivity can be estimated with greater precision than the specificity. With increased precision, there is a higher likelihood that models can be differentiated in terms of sensitivity than for specificity.

4.9 Computing

The R language is used to demonstrate modeling techniques. A concise review of R and its basic usage are found in Appendix B. Those new to R should review these materials prior to proceeding. The following sections will reference functions from the AppliedPredictiveModeling, caret, Design, e1071, ipred and MASS packages. Syntax will be demonstrated using the simple two-class example shown in Figs. 4.2 and 4.3 and the data from the credit scoring case study.

Data Splitting

The two-class data shown in Fig. 4.1 are contained in the AppliedPredictive-
Modeling package and can be obtained using

```
> library(AppliedPredictiveModeling)
> data(twoClassData)
```

The predictors for the example data are stored in a data frame called
predictors. There are two columns for the predictors and 208 samples in
rows. The outcome classes are contained in a factor vector called classes.

```
> str(predictors)
   'data.frame':          208 obs. of  2 variables:
    $ PredictorA: num  0.158 0.655 0.706 0.199 0.395 ...
    $ PredictorB: num  0.1609 0.4918 0.6333 0.0881 0.4152 ...
> str(classes)
   Factor w/ 2 levels "Class1","Class2": 2 2 2 2 2 2 2 2 2 2 ...
```

The base R function sample can create simple random splits of the data.
To create stratified random splits of the data (based on the classes), the
createDataPartition function in the **caret** package can be used. The percent
of data that will be allocated to the training set should be specified.

```
> # Set the random number seed so we can reproduce the results
> set.seed(1)
> # By default, the numbers are returned as a list. Using
> # list = FALSE, a matrix of row numbers is generated.
> # These samples are allocated to the training set.
> trainingRows <- createDataPartition(classes,
+                                      p = .80,
+                                      list= FALSE)
> head(trainingRows)
        Resample1
  [1,]         99
  [2,]        100
  [3,]        101
  [4,]        102
  [5,]        103
  [6,]        104


> # Subset the data into objects for training using
> # integer sub-setting.
> trainPredictors <- predictors[trainingRows, ]
> trainClasses <- classes[trainingRows]
> # Do the same for the test set using negative integers.
> testPredictors <- predictors[-trainingRows, ]
> testClasses <- classes[-trainingRows]


> str(trainPredictors)
```

```
  'data.frame':          167 obs. of  2 variables:
   $ PredictorA: num  0.226 0.262 0.52 0.577 0.426 ...
   $ PredictorB: num  0.291 0.225 0.547 0.553 0.321 ...
> str(testPredictors)
  'data.frame':          41 obs. of  2 variables:
   $ PredictorA: num  0.0658 0.1056 0.2909 0.4129 0.0472 ...
   $ PredictorB: num  0.1786 0.0801 0.3021 0.2869 0.0414 ...
```

To generate a test set using maximum dissimilarity sampling, the caret function tion maxdissim can be used to sequentially sample the data.

Resampling

The caret package has various functions for data splitting. For example, to use repeated training/test splits, the function createDataPartition could be used again with an additional argument named times to generate multiple splits.

```
> set.seed(1)
> # For illustration, generate the information needed for three
> # resampled versions of the training set.
> repeatedSplits <- createDataPartition(trainClasses, p = .80,
+                                        times = 3)
> str(repeatedSplits)
  List of 3
   $ Resample1: int [1:135] 1 2 3 4 5 6 7 9 11 12 ...
   $ Resample2: int [1:135] 4 6 7 8 9 10 11 12 13 14 ...
   $ Resample3: int [1:135] 2 3 4 6 7 8 9 10 11 12 ...
```

Similarly, the caret package has functions createResamples (for bootstrapping), createFolds (for k-old cross-validation) and createMultiFolds (for repeated cross-validation). To create indicators for 10-fold cross-validation,

```
> set.seed(1)
> cvSplits <- createFolds(trainClasses, k = 10,
+                         returnTrain = TRUE)
> str(cvSplits)
  List of 10
   $ Fold01: int [1:151] 1 2 3 4 5 6 7 8 9 11 ...
   $ Fold02: int [1:150] 1 2 3 4 5 6 8 9 10 12 ...
   $ Fold03: int [1:150] 1 2 3 4 6 7 8 10 11 13 ...
   $ Fold04: int [1:151] 1 2 3 4 5 6 7 8 9 10 ...
   $ Fold05: int [1:150] 1 2 3 4 5 7 8 9 10 11 ...
   $ Fold06: int [1:150] 2 4 5 6 7 8 9 10 11 12 ...
   $ Fold07: int [1:150] 1 2 3 4 5 6 7 8 9 10 ...
   $ Fold08: int [1:151] 1 2 3 4 5 6 7 8 9 10 ...
   $ Fold09: int [1:150] 1 3 4 5 6 7 9 10 11 12 ...
   $ Fold10: int [1:150] 1 2 3 5 6 7 8 9 10 11 ...
> # Get the first set of row numbers from the list.
> fold1 <- cvSplits[[1]]
```

To get the first 90 % of the data (the first fold):

```
> cvPredictors1 <- trainPredictors[fold1,]
> cvClasses1 <- trainClasses[fold1]
> nrow(trainPredictors)
  [1] 167
> nrow(cvPredictors1)
  [1] 151
```

In practice, functions discussed in the next section can be used to automatically create the resampled data sets, fit the models, and evaluate performance.

Basic Model Building in R

Now that we have training and test sets, we could fit a 5-nearest neighbor classification model (Fig. 4.3) to the training data and use it to predict the test set. There are multiple R functions for building this model: the knn function in the MASS package, the ipredknn function in the ipred package, and the knn3 function in caret. The knn3 function can produce class predictions as well as the proportion of neighbors for each class.

There are two main conventions for specifying models in R: the formula interface and the non-formula (or "matrix") interface. For the former, the predictors are explicitly listed. A basic R formula has two sides: the left-hand side denotes the outcome and the right-hand side describes how the predictors are used. These are separated with a tilde ($\sim$). For example, the formula

```
> modelFunction(price ~ numBedrooms + numBaths + acres,
+               data = housingData)
```

would predict the closing price of a house using three quantitative characteristics. The formula $y \sim .$ can be used to indicate that all of the columns in the data set (except y) should be used as a predictor. The formula interface has many conveniences. For example, transformations such as log(acres) can be specified in-line. Unfortunately, R does not efficiently store the information about the formula. Using this interface with data sets that contain a large number of predictors may unnecessarily slow the computations.

The non-formula interface specifies the predictors for the model using a matrix or data frame (all the predictors in the object are used in the model). The outcome data are usually passed into the model as a vector object. For example,

```
> modelFunction(x = housePredictors, y = price)
```

Note that not all R functions have both interfaces.

For `knn3`, we can estimate the 5-nearest neighbor model with

```
> trainPredictors <- as.matrix(trainPredictors)
> knnFit <- knn3(x = trainPredictors, y = trainClasses, k = 5)
> knnFit
  5-nearest neighbor classification model

  Call:
  knn3.matrix(x = trainPredictors, y = trainClasses, k = 5)

  Training set class distribution:

  Class1 Class2
      89     78
```

At this point, the `knn3` object is ready to predict new samples. To assign new samples to classes, the `predict` method is used with the model object. The standard convention is

```
> testPredictions <- predict(knnFit, newdata = testPredictors,
+                            type = "class")
> head(testPredictions)
  [1] Class2 Class2 Class1 Class1 Class2 Class2
  Levels: Class1 Class2
> str(testPredictions)
   Factor w/ 2 levels "Class1","Class2": 2 2 1 1 2 2 2 2 2 2 ...
```

The value of the `type` argument varies across different modeling functions.

Determination of Tuning Parameters

To choose tuning parameters using resampling, sets of candidate values are evaluated using different resamples of the data. A profile can be created to understand the relationship between performance and the parameter values. R has several functions and packages for this task. The e1071 package contains the `tune` function, which can evaluate four types of models across a range of parameters. Similarly, the `errorest` function in the ipred package can resample single models. The `train` function in the caret package has built-in modules for 144 models and includes capabilities for different resampling methods, performances measures, and algorithms for choosing the best model from the profile. This function also has capabilities for parallel processing so that the resampled model fits can be executed across multiple computers or processors. Our focus will be on the `train` function.

Section 4.6 illustrated parameter tuning for a support vector machine using the credit scoring data. Using resampling, a value of the cost parameter was estimated. As discussed in later chapters, the SVM model is characterized by what type of *kernel function* the model uses. For example, the linear kernel function specifies a linear relationship between the predictors and the outcome. For the credit scoring data, a radial basis function (RBF) kernel function was used. This kernel function has an additional tuning parameter associated with it denoted as σ, which impacts the smoothness of the decision boundary. Normally, several combinations of both tuning parameters would be evaluated using resampling. However, Caputo et al. (2002) describe an analytical formula that can be used to get reasonable estimates of σ. The caret function train uses this approach to estimate the kernel parameter, leaving only the cost parameter for tuning.

To tune an SVM model using the credit scoring training set samples, the train function can be used. Both the training set predictors and outcome are contained in an R data frame called GermanCreditTrain.

```
> library(caret)
> data(GermanCredit)
```

The **chapters** directory of the AppliedPredictiveModeling package contains the code for creating the training and test sets. These data sets are contained in the data frames GermanCreditTrain and GermanCreditTest, respectively.

We will use all the predictors to model the outcome. To do this, we use the formula interface with the formula Class ~ . the classes are stored in the data frame column called class. The most basic function call would be

```
> set.seed(1056)
> svmFit <- train(Class ~ .,
>                 data = GermanCreditTrain,
>                 # The "method" argument indicates the model type.
>                 # See ?train for a list of available models.
>                 method = "svmRadial")
```

However, we would like to tailor the computations by overriding several of the default values. First, we would like to pre-process the predictor data by centering and scaling their values. To do this, the preProc argument can be used:

```
> set.seed(1056)
> svmFit <- train(Class ~ .,
>                 data = GermanCreditTrain,
>                 method = "svmRadial",
>                 preProc = c("center", "scale"))
```

Also, for this function, the user can specify the exact cost values to investigate. In addition, the function has algorithms to determine reasonable values for many models. Using the option tuneLength = 10, the cost values 2^{-2}, 2^{-2} ... 2^7 are evaluated.

```
> set.seed(1056)
> svmFit <- train(Class ~ .,
>                 data = GermanCreditTrain,
>                 method = "svmRadial",
>                 preProc = c("center", "scale"),
>                 tuneLength = 10)
```

By default, the basic bootstrap will be used to calculate performance measures. Repeated 10-fold cross-validation can be specified with the `trainControl` function. The final syntax is then

```
> set.seed(1056)
> svmFit <- train(Class ~ .,
>                   data = GermanCreditTrain,
>                   method = "svmRadial",
>                   preProc = c("center", "scale"),
>                   tuneLength = 10,
>                   trControl = trainControl(method = "repeatedcv",
>                                             repeats = 5,
>                                             classProbs = TRUE))
```

```
> svmFit

  800 samples
   41 predictors
    2 classes: 'Bad', 'Good'

Pre-processing: centered, scaled
Resampling: Cross-Validation (10-fold, repeated 5 times)

Summary of sample sizes: 720, 720, 720, 720, 720, 720, ...

Resampling results across tuning parameters:
```

C	Accuracy	Kappa	Accuracy SD	Kappa SD
0.25	0.7	0	0	0
0.5	0.724	0.141	0.0218	0.0752
1	0.75	0.326	0.0385	0.106
2	0.75	0.363	0.0404	0.0984
4	0.754	0.39	0.0359	0.0857
8	0.738	0.361	0.0404	0.0887
16	0.738	0.361	0.0458	0.1
32	0.732	0.35	0.043	0.0928
64	0.732	0.352	0.0453	0.0961
128	0.731	0.349	0.0451	0.0936

```
Tuning parameter 'sigma' was held constant at a value of 0.0202
Accuracy was used to select the optimal model using  the largest value.
The final values used for the model were C = 4 and sigma = 0.0202.
```

A different random number seed and set of cost values were used in the original analysis, so the results are not exactly the same as those shown in Sect. 4.6. Using a "pick the best" approach, a final model was fit to all 800 training set samples with a σ value of 0.0202 and a cost value of 4. The `plot` method can be used to visualize the performance profile. Figure 4.12 shows an example visualization created from the syntax

```
> # A line plot of the average performance
> plot(svmFit, scales = list(x = list(log = 2)))
```

To predict new samples with this model, the `predict` method is called

```
> predictedClasses <- predict(svmFit, GermanCreditTest)
> str(predictedClasses)
```

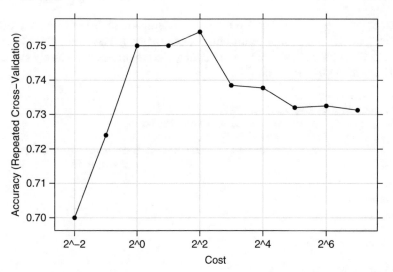

Fig. 4.12: A visualization of the average performance profile of an SVM classification model produced from the `plot` method for the `train` class

```
Factor w/ 2 levels "Bad","Good": 1 1 2 2 1 2 2 2 1 1 ...

> # Use the "type" option to get class probabilities
> predictedProbs <- predict(svmFit, newdata = GermanCreditTest,
+                           type = "prob")
> head(predictedProbs)
        Bad       Good
1 0.5351870 0.4648130
2 0.5084049 0.4915951
3 0.3377344 0.6622656
4 0.1092243 0.8907757
5 0.6024404 0.3975596
6 0.1339467 0.8660533
```

There are other R packages that can estimate performance via resampling. The `validate` function in the Design package and the `errorest` function in the ipred package can be used to estimate performance for a model with a single candidate set of tuning parameters. The `tune` function of the e1071 package can also determine parameter settings using resampling.

Between-Model Comparisons

In Sect. 4.6, the SVM model was contrasted with a logistic regression model. While basic logistic regression has no tuning parameters, resampling can still be used to characterize the performance of the model. The `train` function is once again used, with a different `method` argument of `"glm"` (for generalized linear models). The same resampling specification is used and, since the random number seed is set prior to modeling, the resamples are exactly the same as those in the SVM model.

```
> set.seed(1056)
> logisticReg <- train(Class ~ .,
+                      data = GermanCreditTrain,
+                      method = "glm",
+                      trControl = trainControl(method = "repeatedcv",
+                                               repeats = 5))
```

```
> logisticReg

  800 samples
   41 predictors
    2 classes: 'Bad', 'Good'

No pre-processing
Resampling: Cross-Validation (10-fold, repeated 5 times)

Summary of sample sizes: 720, 720, 720, 720, 720, 720, ...

Resampling results

  Accuracy  Kappa  Accuracy SD  Kappa SD
  0.749     0.365  0.0516       0.122
```

To compare these two models based on their cross-validation statistics, the `resamples` function can be used with models that share a common set of resampled data sets. Since the random number seed was initialized prior to running the SVM and logistic models, paired accuracy measurements exist for each data set. First, we create a `resamples` object from the models:

```
> resamp <- resamples(list(SVM = svmFit, Logistic = logisticReg))
> summary(resamp)

  Call:
  summary.resamples(object = resamp)

  Models: SVM, Logistic
  Number of resamples: 50

  Accuracy
            Min.    1st Qu. Median Mean  3rd Qu. Max.  NA's
  SVM       0.6500  0.7375  0.7500 0.754 0.7625  0.85  0
  Logistic  0.6125  0.7250  0.7562 0.749 0.7844  0.85  0

  Kappa
            Min.     1st Qu. Median Mean   3rd Qu. Max.    NA's
  SVM       0.18920  0.3519  0.3902 0.3897 0.4252  0.5946  0
  Logistic  0.07534  0.2831  0.3750 0.3648 0.4504  0.6250  0
```

The summary indicates that the performance distributions are very similar. The `NA` column corresponds to cases where the resampled models failed (usually due to numerical issues). The `resamples` class has several methods for visualizing the paired values (see `?xyplot.resamples` for a list of plot types). To assess possible differences between the models, the `diff` method is used:

```
> modelDifferences <- diff(resamp)
> summary(modelDifferences)
  Call:
  summary.diff.resamples(object = modelDifferences)

  p-value adjustment: bonferroni
  Upper diagonal: estimates of the difference
  Lower diagonal: p-value for H0: difference = 0

  Accuracy
            SVM     Logistic
  SVM               0.005
  Logistic 0.5921

  Kappa
            SVM     Logistic
  SVM               0.02498
  Logistic 0.2687
```

The p-values for the model comparisons are large (0.592 for accuracy and 0.269 for Kappa), which indicates that the models fail to show any difference in performance.

Exercises

4.1. Consider the music genre data set described in Sect. 1.4. The objective for these data is to use the predictors to classify music samples into the appropriate music genre.

(a) What data splitting method(s) would you use for these data? Explain.
(b) Using tools described in this chapter, provide code for implementing your approach(es).

4.2. Consider the permeability data set described in Sect. 1.4. The objective for these data is to use the predictors to model compounds' permeability.

(a) What data splitting method(s) would you use for these data? Explain.
(b) Using tools described in this chapter, provide code for implementing your approach(es).

4.3. Partial least squares (Sect. 6.3) was used to model the yield of a chemical manufacturing process (Sect. 1.4). The data can be found in the AppliedPredictiveModeling package and can be loaded using

| | Resampled R^2 | |
Components	Mean	Std. Error
1	0.444	0.0272
2	0.500	0.0298
3	0.533	0.0302
4	0.545	0.0308
5	0.542	0.0322
6	0.537	0.0327
7	0.534	0.0333
8	0.534	0.0330
9	0.520	0.0326
10	0.507	0.0324

```
> library(AppliedPredictiveModeling)
> data(ChemicalManufacturingProcess)
```

The objective of this analysis is to find the number of PLS components that yields the optimal R^2 value (Sect. 5.1). PLS models with 1 through 10 components were each evaluated using five repeats of 10-fold cross-validation and the results are presented in the following table:

(a) Using the "one-standard error" method, what number of PLS components provides the most parsimonious model?

(b) Compute the tolerance values for this example. If a 10 % loss in R^2 is acceptable, then what is the optimal number of PLS components?

(c) Several other models (discussed in Part II) with varying degrees of complexity were trained and tuned and the results are presented in Fig. 4.13. If the goal is to select the model that optimizes R^2, then which model(s) would you choose, and why?

(d) Prediction time, as well as model complexity (Sect. 4.8) are other factors to consider when selecting the optimal model(s). Given each model's prediction time, model complexity, and R^2 estimates, which model(s) would you choose, and why?

4.4. Brodnjak-Vonina et al. (2005) develop a methodology for food laboratories to determine the type of oil from a sample. In their procedure, they used a gas chromatograph (an instrument that separate chemicals in a sample) to measure seven different fatty acids in an oil. These measurements would then be used to predict the type of oil in a food samples. To create their model, they used 96 samples[2] of seven types of oils.

These data can be found in the caret package using data(oil). The oil types are contained in a factor variable called oilType. The types are pumpkin

---

[2] The authors state that there are 95 samples of known oils. However, we count 96 in their Table 1 (pp. 33–35 of the article).

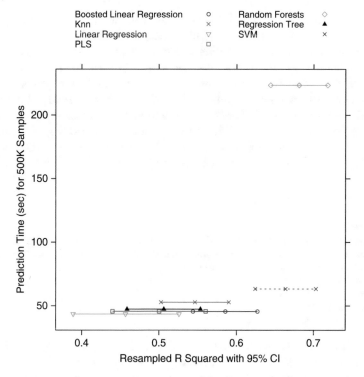

Fig. 4.13: A plot of the estimated model performance against the time to predict 500,000 new samples using the chemical manufacturing data

(coded as A), sunflower (B), peanut (C), olive (D), soybean (E), rapeseed (F) and corn (G). In R,

```
> data(oil)
> str(oilType)
   Factor w/ 7 levels "A","B","C","D",..: 1 1 1 1 1 1 1 1 1 1 ...
> table(oilType)

 oilType
  A  B  C  D  E  F  G
 37 26  3  7 11 10  2
```

(a) Use the sample function in base R to create a completely random sample of 60 oils. How closely do the frequencies of the random sample match the original samples? Repeat this procedure several times of understand the variation in the sampling process.

(b) Use the caret package function createDataPartition to create a stratified random sample. How does this compare to the completely random samples?

(c) With such a small samples size, what are the options for determining performance of the model? Should a test set be used?

(d) One method for understanding the uncertainty of a test set is to use a confidence interval. To obtain a confidence interval for the overall accuracy, the based R function `binom.test` can be used. It requires the user to input the number of samples and the number correctly classified to calculate the interval. For example, suppose a test set sample of 20 oil samples was set aside and 76 were used for model training. For this test set size and a model that is about 80 % accurate (16 out of 20 correct), the confidence interval would be computed using

```
> binom.test(16, 20)
         Exact binomial test

 data:   16 and 20
 number of successes = 16, number of trials = 20, p-value = 0.01182
 alternative hypothesis: true probability of success is not equal to 0.5
 95 percent confidence interval:
  0.563386 0.942666
 sample estimates:
 probability of success
                   0.8
```

In this case, the width of the 95 % confidence interval is 37.9 %. Try different samples sizes and accuracy rates to understand the trade-off between the uncertainty in the results, the model performance, and the test set size.

Part II
Regression Models

Chapter 5
Measuring Performance in Regression Models

For models predicting a numeric outcome, some measure of accuracy is typically used to evaluate the effectiveness of the model. However, there are different ways to measure accuracy, each with its own nuance. To understand the strengths and weaknesses of a particular model, relying solely on a single metric is problematic. Visualizations of the model fit, particularly residual plots, are critical to understanding whether the model is fit for purpose. These techniques are discussed in this chapter.

5.1 Quantitative Measures of Performance

When the outcome is a number, the most common method for characterizing a model's predictive capabilities is to use the root mean squared error (RMSE). This metric is a function of the model residuals, which are the observed values minus the model predictions. The mean squared error (MSE) is calculated by squaring the residuals, summing them and dividing by the number of samples. The RMSE is then calculated by taking the square root of the MSE so that it is in the same units as the original data. The value is usually interpreted as either how far (on average) the residuals are from zero or as the average distance between the observed values and the model predictions.

Another common metric is the coefficient of determination, commonly written as R^2. This value can be interpreted as the proportion of the information in the data that is explained by the model. Thus, an R^2 value of 0.75 implies that the model can explain three-quarters of the variation in the outcome. There are multiple formulas for calculating this quantity (Kvålseth 1985), although the simplest version finds the correlation coefficient between the observed and predicted values (usually denoted by R) and squares it.

M. Kuhn and K. Johnson, *Applied Predictive Modeling*,
DOI 10.1007/978-1-4614-6849-3_5,
© Springer Science+Business Media New York 2013

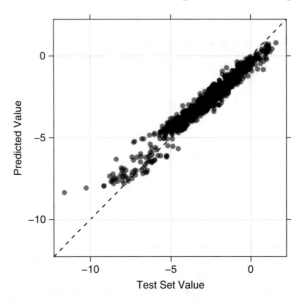

Fig. 5.1: A plot of the observed and predicted outcomes where the R^2 is moderate (51 %), but predictions are not uniformly accurate. The *diagonal grey reference line* indicates where the observed and predicted values would be equal

While this is an easily interpretable statistic, the practitioner must remember that R^2 is a measure of correlation, not accuracy. Figure 5.1 shows an example where the R^2 between the observed and predicted values is high (51 %), but the model has a tendency to overpredict low values and underpredict high ones. This phenomenon can be common to some of the tree-based regression models discussed in Chap. 8. Depending on the context, this systematic bias in the predictions may be acceptable if the model otherwise works well.

It is also important to realize that R^2 is dependent on the variation in the outcome. Using the interpretation that this statistic measures the proportion of variance explained by the model, one must remember that the denominator of that proportion is calculated using the sample variance of the outcome. For example, suppose a test set outcome has a variance of 4.2. If the RMSE of a predictive model were 1, the R^2 would be roughly 76 %. If we had another test set with exactly the same RMSE, but the test outcomes were less variable, the results would look worse. For example, if the test set variance were 3, the R^2 would be 67 %.

Practically speaking, this dependence on the outcome variance can also have a drastic effect on how the model is viewed. For example, suppose we were building a model to predict the sale price of houses using predictors such as house characteristics (e.g., square footage, number of bedrooms, number of bathrooms), as well as lot size and location. If the range of the houses in the test set was large, say from \$60K to \$2M, the variance of the sale price would also be very large. One might view a model with a 90 % R^2 positively, but the RMSE may be in the tens of thousands of dollars—poor predictive accuracy for anyone selling a moderately priced property.

In some cases, the goal of the model is to simply rank new samples. As previously discussed, pharmaceutical scientists may screen large numbers of compounds for their activity in an effort to find "hits." The scientists will then follow up on the compounds predicted to be the most biologically active. Here, the focus is on the ranking ability of the model rather than its predictive accuracy. In this situation, determining the *rank correlation* between the observed and predicted values might be a more appropriate metric. The rank correlation takes the ranks of the observed outcome values (as opposed to their actual numbers) and evaluates how close these are to ranks of the model predictions. To calculate this value, the ranks of the observed and predicted outcomes are obtained and the correlation coefficient between these ranks is calculated. This metric is commonly known as Spearman's rank correlation.

5.2 The Variance-Bias Trade-off

The MSE can be decomposed into more specific pieces. Formally, the MSE of a *model* is

$$\text{MSE} = \frac{1}{n} \sum_{i=1}^{n} (y_i - \hat{y}_i)^2,$$

where y_i is the outcome and $\hat{y}_i$ is the model prediction of that sample's outcome. If we assume that the data points are statistically independent and that the residuals have a theoretical mean of zero and a constant variance of σ^2, then

$$E[\text{MSE}] = \sigma^2 + (\text{Model Bias})^2 + \text{Model Variance}, \tag{5.1}$$

where E is the expected value. The first part (σ^2) is usually called "irreducible noise" and cannot be eliminated by modeling. The second term is the squared *bias* of the model. This reflects how close the functional form of the model can get to the true relationship between the predictors and the outcome. The last term is the model variance. Figure 5.2 shows extreme examples of models that are either high bias or high variance. The data are a simulated *sin* wave. The model fit shown in red splits the data in half and predicts each half with a simple average. This model has low variance since it would not substantially change if another set of data points were generated the same

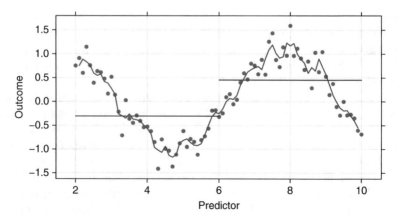

Fig. 5.2: Two model fits to a *sin* wave. The *red line* predicts the data using simple averages of the first and second half of the data. The *blue line* is a three-point moving average

way. However, it is ineffective at modeling the data since, due to its simplicity and for this reason, it has high bias. Conversely, the blue line is a three-point moving average. It is flexible enough to model the *sin* wave (i.e., low bias), but small perturbations in the data will significantly change the model fit. Because of this, it has high variance.

It is generally true that more complex models can have very high variance, which leads to over-fitting. On the other hand, simple models tend not to over-fit, but under-fit if they are not flexible enough to model the true relationship (thus high bias). Also, highly correlated predictors can lead to *collinearity* issues and this can greatly increase the model variance. In subsequent chapters, models will be discussed that can increase the bias in the model to greatly reduce the model variance as a way to mitigate the problem of collinearity. This is referred to as the *variance-bias trade-off*.

5.3 Computing

The following sections will reference functions from the caret package.

To compute model performance, the observed and predicted outcomes should be stored in vectors. For regression, these vectors should be numeric. Here, two example vectors are manually created to illustrate the techniques (in practice, the vector of predictions would be produced by the model function):

```
> # Use the 'c' function to combine numbers into a vector
> observed <- c(0.22,   0.83,  -0.12, 0.89,  -0.23, -1.30,  -0.15, -1.4,
```

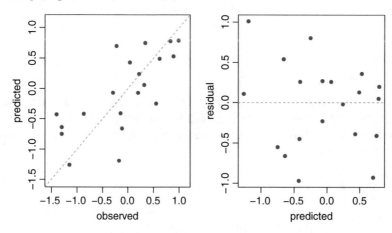

Fig. 5.3: *Left*: a plot of the observed and predicted values. *Right*: the residuals versus the predicted values

```
+                 0.62,   0.99, -0.18, 0.32,  0.34, -0.30,  0.04, -0.87,
+                 0.55, -1.30, -1.15,  0.20)
> predicted <- c(0.24,   0.78, -0.66,  0.53, 0.70, -0.75, -0.41, -0.43,
+                 0.49,   0.79, -1.19,  0.06, 0.75, -0.07,  0.43, -0.42,
+                -0.25, -0.64, -1.26, -0.07)
> residualValues <- observed - predicted
> summary(residualValues)
    Min. 1st Qu.  Median    Mean 3rd Qu.    Max.
 -0.9700 -0.4200  0.0800 -0.0310  0.2625  1.0100
```

An important step in evaluating the quality of the model is to visualize the results. First, a plot of the observed values against the predicted values helps one to understand how well the model fits. Also, a plot of the residuals versus the predicted values can help uncover systematic patterns in the model predictions, such as the trend shown in Fig. 5.1. The following two commands were used to produce the images in Fig. 5.3:

```
> # Observed values versus predicted values
> # It is a good idea to plot the values on a common scale.
> axisRange <- extendrange(c(observed, predicted))
> plot(observed, predicted,
+      ylim = axisRange,
+      xlim = axisRange)
> # Add a 45 degree reference line
> abline(0, 1, col = "darkgrey", lty = 2)

> # Predicted values versus residuals
> plot(predicted, residualValues, ylab = "residual")
> abline(h = 0, col = "darkgrey", lty = 2)
```

The caret package contains functions for calculating the RMSE and the R^2 value:

```
> R2(predicted, observed)
  [1] 0.5170123
> RMSE(predicted, observed)
  [1] 0.5234883
```

There are different formulas for R^2; Kvålseth (1985) provides a survey of these. By default, the R2 function uses the square of the correlation coefficient. Base R contains a function to compute the correlation, including Spearman's rank correlation.

```
> # Simple correlation
> cor(predicted, observed)
  [1] 0.7190357
> # Rank correlation
> cor(predicted, observed, method = "spearman")
  [1] 0.7554552
```

Chapter 6
Linear Regression and Its Cousins

In this chapter we will discuss several models, all of which are akin to linear regression in that each can directly or indirectly be written in the form

$$y_i = b_0 + b_1 x_{i1} + b_2 x_{i2} + \cdots + b_P x_{iP} + e_i, \qquad (6.1)$$

where y_i represents the numeric response for the ith sample, b_0 represents the estimated intercept, b_j represents the estimated coefficient for the jth predictor, x_{ij} represents the value of the jth predictor for the ith sample, and e_i represents random error that cannot be explained by the model. When a model can be written in the form of Eq. 6.1, we say that it is *linear in the parameters*. In addition to ordinary linear regression, these types of models include partial least squares (PLS) and penalized models such as ridge regression, the lasso, and the elastic net.

Each of these models seeks to find estimates of the parameters so that the sum of the squared errors or a function of the sum of the squared errors is minimized. Section 5.2 illustrated that the mean squared error (MSE) can be divided into components of irreducible variation, model bias, and model variance. The objectives of the methods presented in this chapter find parameter estimates that fall along the spectrum of the bias-variance trade-off. Ordinary linear regression, at one extreme, finds parameter estimates that have minimum bias, whereas ridge regression, the lasso, and the elastic net find estimates that have lower variance. The impact of this trade-off on the predictive ability of these models will be illustrated in the sections to follow.

A distinct advantage of models that follow the form of Eq. 6.1 is that they are highly interpretable. For example, if the estimated coefficient of a predictor is 2.5, then a 1 unit increase in that predictor's value would, on average, increase the response by 2.5 units. Furthermore, relationships among predictors can be further interpreted through the estimated coefficients.

Another advantage of these kinds of models is that their mathematical nature enables us to compute standard errors of the coefficients, provided that we make certain assumptions about the distributions of the model residuals.

M. Kuhn and K. Johnson, *Applied Predictive Modeling*,
DOI 10.1007/978-1-4614-6849-3_6,
© Springer Science+Business Media New York 2013

These standard errors can then be used to assess the statistical significance of each predictor in the model. This inferential view can provide a greater degree of understanding of the model, as long as the distributional assumptions are adequately met. Because this work focuses on model prediction, we will not spend much time on the inferential nature of these models.

While linear regression-type models are highly interpretable, they can be limited in their usefulness. First, these models are appropriate when the relationship between the predictors and response falls along a hyperplane. For example, if the data had just one predictor, then the techniques would be appropriate if the relationship between the predictor and response fell along a straight line. With more predictors, the relationship would need to fall close to a flat hyperplane. If there is a curvilinear relationship between the predictors and response (e.g., such as quadratic, cubic, or interactions among predictors), then linear regression models can be augmented with additional predictors that are functions of the original predictors in an attempt to capture these relationships. More discussion about strategies for augmenting the original predictors will follow in the sections below. However, nonlinear relationships between predictors and the response may not be adequately captured with these models. If this is the case for the data, then the methods detailed in Chaps. 7 and 8 will better uncover the predictive relationship between the predictors and the response.

6.1 Case Study: Quantitative Structure-Activity Relationship Modeling

Chemicals, including drugs, can be represented by chemical formulas. For example, Fig. 6.1 shows the structure of aspirin, which contains nine carbon, eight hydrogen, and four oxygen atoms. From this configuration, quantitative measurements can be derived, such as the molecular weight, electrical charge, or surface area. These quantities are referred to as *chemical descriptors*, and there are myriad types of descriptors that can be derived from a chemical equation. Some are simplistic, such as the number of carbon atoms, while others could be described as arcane (e.g., the coefficient sum of the last eigenvector from Barysz matrix weighted by the van der Waals volume).

Some characteristics of molecules cannot be analytically determined from the chemical structure. For example, one way a compound may be of medical value is if it can inhibit production of a specific protein. This is usually called the biological activity of a compound. The relationship between the chemical structure and its activity can be complex. As such, the relationship is usually determined empirically using experiments. One way to do this is to create a biological assay for the target of interest (i.e., the protein). A set of compounds can then be placed into the assay and their activity, or inhibition, is measured. This activity information generates data which can be used as

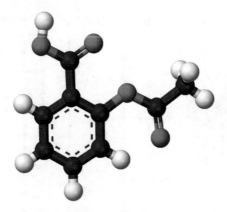

Fig. 6.1: A representation of aspirin, which contains carbon atoms (shown as *black balls*) and hydrogen (*white*) and oxygen atoms (*red*). The chemical formula for this molecule is `O=C(Oc1ccccc1C(=O)O)C`, from which molecular descriptors can be determined, such as a molecular weight of 180.2 g/mol

the training set for predictive modeling so that compounds, which may not yet exist, can be screened for activity. This process is referred to as quantitative structure-activity relationship (QSAR) modeling. Leach and Gillet (2003) provide a high-level introduction to QSAR modeling and molecular descriptors.

While activity is important, other characteristics need to be assessed to determine if a compound is "drug-like" (Lipinski et al. 1997). Physical qualities, such as the solubility or lipophilicity (i.e., "greasiness"), are evaluated as well as other properties, such as toxicity. A compound's solubility is very important if it is to be given orally or by injection. We will demonstrate various regression modeling techniques by predicting solubility using chemical structures.

Tetko et al. (2001) and Huuskonen (2000) investigated a set of compounds with corresponding experimental solubility values using complex sets of descriptors. They used linear regression and neural network models to estimate the relationship between chemical structure and solubility. For our analyses, we will use 1,267 compounds and a set of more understandable descriptors that fall into one of three groups:

- Two hundred and eight binary "fingerprints" that indicate the presence or absence of a particular chemical substructure.
- Sixteen count descriptors, such as the number of bonds or the number of bromine atoms.
- Four continuous descriptors, such as molecular weight or surface area.

On average, the descriptors are uncorrelated. However, there are many pairs that show strong positive correlations; 47 pairs have correlations greater than

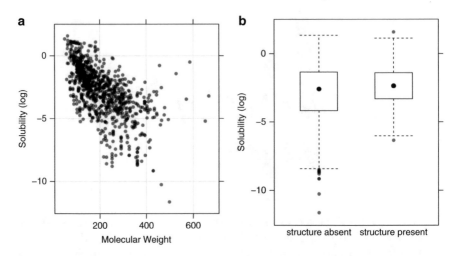

Fig. 6.2: The relationship between solubility and two descriptors. *Left*: As molecular weight of a molecule increases, the solubility generally decreases. The relationship is roughly log-linear, except for several compounds with low solubility and large weight and solubility between 0 and −5. *Right*: For a particular fingerprint descriptor, there is slightly higher solubility when the substructure of interest is absent from the molecule

0.90. In some cases, we should expect correlations between descriptors. In the solubility data, for example, the surface area of a compound is calculated for regions associated with certain atoms (e.g., nitrogen or oxygen). One descriptor in these data measures the surface area associated with two specific elements while another uses the same elements plus two more. Given their definitions, we would expect that the two surface area predictors would be correlated. In fact, the descriptors are identical for 87 % of the compounds. The small differences between surface area predictors may contain some important information for prediction, but the modeler should realize that there are implications of redundancy on the model. Another relevant quality of the solubility predictors is that the count-based descriptors show a significant right skewness, which may have an impact on some models (see Chap. 3 for a discussion of these issues).

The outcome data were measured on the $\log_{10}$ scale and ranged from −11.6 to 1.6 with an average log solubility value of −2.7. Figure 6.2 shows the relationship between the experimentally derived solubility values and two types of descriptors in the example data.

The data were split using random sampling into a training set ($n = 951$) and test set ($n = 316$). The training set will be used to tune and estimate models, as well as to determine initial estimates of performance using repeated 10-fold cross-validation. The test set will be used for a final characterization of the models of interest.

It is useful to explore the training set to understand the characteristics of the data prior to modeling. Recall that 208 of the predictors are binary fingerprints. Since there are only two values of these variables, there is very little that pre-processing will accomplish.

Moving on, we can evaluate the continuous predictors for skewness. The average skewness statistic was 1.6 (with a minimum of 0.7 and a maximum of 3.8), indicating that these predictors have a propensity to be right skewed. To correct for this skewness, a Box–Cox transformation was applied to all predictors (i.e., the transformation parameter was not estimated to be near one for any of the continuous predictors).

Using these transformed predictors, is it safe to assume that the relationship between the predictors and the outcome is linear? Figure 6.3 shows scatter plots of the predictors against the outcome along with a regression line from a flexible "smoother" model called loess (Cleveland 1979). The smoothed regression lines indicate that there are some linear relationships between the predictors and the outcome (e.g., molecular weight) and some nonlinear relationships (e.g., the number of origins or chlorines). Because of this, we might consider augmenting the predictor set with quadratic terms for some variables.

Are there significant between-predictor correlations? To answer this question, principal component analysis (PCA) was used on the full set of transformed predictors, and the percent of variance accounted for by each component is determined. Figure 6.4 is commonly known as a scree plot and displays a profile of the variability accounted for by each component. Notice that the amount of variability summarized by component drops sharply, with no one component accounting for more than 13 % of the variance. This profile indicates that the structure of the data is contained in a much smaller number of dimensions than the number of dimensions of the original space; this is often due to a large number of collinearities among the predictors. Figure 6.5 shows the correlation structure of the transformed continuous predictors; there are many strong positive correlations (indicated by the large, dark blue circles). As previously discussed, this could create problems in developing some models (such as linear regression), and appropriate pre-processing steps will need to be taken to account for this problem.

6.2 Linear Regression

The objective of ordinary least squares linear regression is to find the plane that minimizes the sum-of-squared errors (SSE) between the observed and predicted response:

$$\text{SSE} = \sum_{i=1}^{n}(y_i - \hat{y}_i)^2,$$

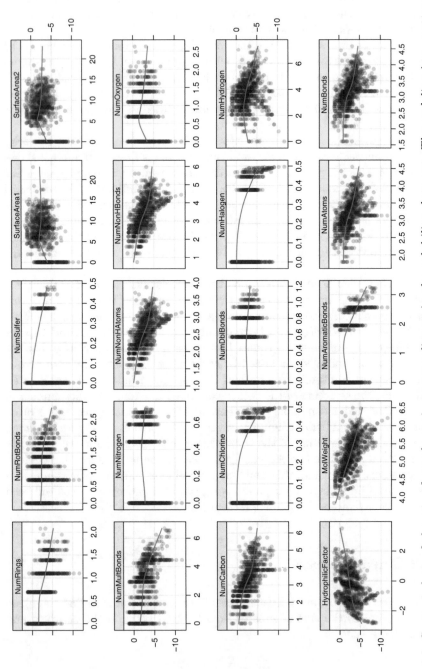

Fig. 6.3: Scatter plots of the transformed continuous predictors in the solubility data set. The *red line* is a scatter plot smoother

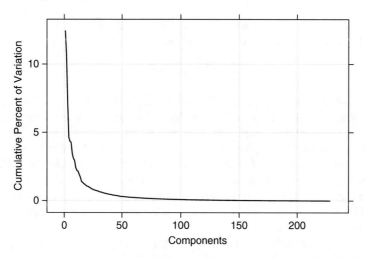

Fig. 6.4: A scree plot from a PCA analysis of the solubility predictors

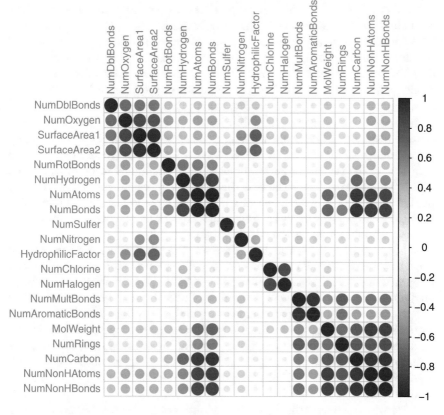

Fig. 6.5: Between-predictor correlations of the transformed continuous solubility predictors

where y_i is the outcome and $\hat{y}_i$ is the model prediction of that sample's outcome. Mathematically, the optimal plane can be shown to be

$$\left(\mathbf{X}^T\mathbf{X}\right)^{-1}\mathbf{X}^T y, \tag{6.2}$$

where $\mathbf{X}$ is the matrix of predictors and y is the response vector. Equation 6.2 is also known as $\hat{\beta}$ ("beta-hat") in statistical texts and is a vector that contains the parameter estimates or coefficients for each predictor. This quantity (6.2) is easy to compute, and the coefficients are directly interpretable. Making some minimal assumptions about the distribution of the residuals, it is straightforward to show that the parameter estimates that minimize SSE are the ones that have the least bias of all possible parameter estimates (Graybill 1976). Hence, these estimates minimize the bias component of the bias-variance trade-off.

The interpretability of coefficients makes it very attractive as a modeling tool. At the same time, the characteristics that make it interpretable also make it prone to potentially fatal flaws. Notice that embedded in Eq. (6.2) is the term $\left(\mathbf{X}^T\mathbf{X}\right)^{-1}$, which is proportional to the covariance matrix of the predictors. A unique inverse of this matrix exists when (1) no predictor can be determined from a combination of one or more of the other predictors and (2) the number of samples is greater than the number of predictors. If the data fall under either of these conditions, then a unique set of regression coefficients does not exist. However, a unique set of predicted values can still be obtained for data that fall under condition (1) by either replacing $\left(\mathbf{X}^T\mathbf{X}\right)^{-1}$ with a conditional inverse (Graybill 1976) or by removing predictors that are collinear. By default, when fitting a linear model with R and collinearity exists among predictors, "...R fits the largest identifiable model by removing variables in the reverse order of appearance in the model formula" (Faraway 2005). The upshot of these facts is that linear regression can still be used for prediction when collinearity exists within the data. But since the regression coefficients to determine these predictions are not unique, we lose our ability to meaningfully interpret the coefficients.

When condition (2) is true for a data set, the practitioner can take several steps to attempt to build a regression model. As a first step we suggest using pre-processing techniques presented in Sect. 3.3 to remove pairwise correlated predictors, which will reduce the number of overall predictors. However, this pre-processing step may not completely eliminate collinearity, since one or more of the predictors may be functions of *two* or more of the other predictors. To diagnose multicollinearity in the context of linear regression, the *variance inflation factor* can be used (Myers 1994). This statistic is computed for each predictor and a function of the correlation between the selected predictor and all of the other predictors.

After pre-processing the data, if the number of predictors still outnumbers the number of observations, then we will need to take other measures to reduce the dimension of the predictor space. PCA pre-processing (Sect. 3.3) is one possible remedy. Other remedies include simultaneous dimension reduction and regression via PLS or employing methods that shrink parameter estimates such as ridge regression, the lasso, or the elastic net.

Another drawback of multiple linear regression is that its solution is linear in the parameters. This means that the solution we obtain is a flat hyperplane. Clearly, if the data have curvature or nonlinear structure, then regression will not be able to identify these characteristics. One visual clue to understanding if the relationship between predictors and the response is not linear is to examine the basic diagnostic plots illustrated in Fig. 5.3. Curvature in the predicted-versus-residual plot is a primary indicator that the underlying relationship is not linear. Quadratic, cubic, or interactions between predictors can be accommodated in regression by adding quadratic, cubic, and interactions of the original predictors. But the larger the number of original predictors, the less practical including some or all of these terms becomes. Taking this approach can cause the data matrix to have more predictors than observations, and we then again cannot invert the matrix.

If easily identifiable nonlinear relationships exist between the predictors and the response, then those additional predictors can be added to the descriptor matrix. If, however, it is not possible to identify these relationships or the relationships between the predictors and the response is highly nonlinear, then more complex methods such as those discussed in Chap. 7 will more effectively and efficiently find this structure.

A third notable problem with multiple linear regression is that it is prone to chasing observations that are away from the overall trend of the majority of the data. Recall that linear regression seeks to find the parameter estimates that minimize SSE; hence, observations that are far from the trend of the majority of the data will have exponentially large residuals. In order to minimize SSE, linear regression will adjust the parameter estimates to better accommodate these unusual observations. Observations that cause significant changes in the parameter estimates are called *influential*, and the field of robust regression has been developed to address these kinds of problems. One common approach is to use an alternative metric to SSE that is less sensitive to large outliers. For example, finding parameter estimates that minimize the sum of the absolute errors is more resistant to outliers, as seen in Fig. 6.6. Also, the Huber function uses the squared residuals when they are "small" and the simple different between the observed and predicted values when the residuals are above a threshold. This approach can effectively minimize the influence of observations that fall away from the overall trend in the data.

There are no tuning parameters for multiple linear regression. This fact, however, does not impugn the practitioner from using rigorous model validation tools, especially when using this model for prediction. In fact, we must use the same training and validation techniques described in Chap. 4 to understand the predictive ability of this model on data which the model has not seen.

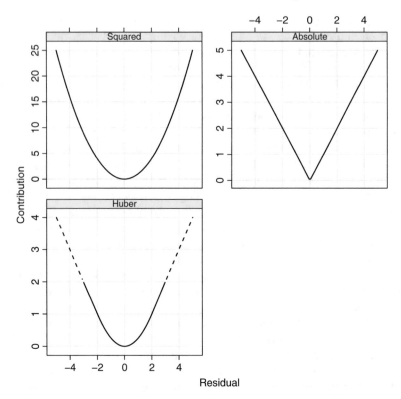

Fig. 6.6: The relationship between a model residual and its contribution to the objective function for several techniques. For the Huber approach, a threshold of 2 was used

When using resampling techniques such as bootstrapping or cross-validation, the practitioner must still be conscious of the problems described above. Consider, for example, a data set where there are 100 samples and 75 predictors. If we use a resampling scheme that uses two-thirds of the data for training, then we will be unable to find a unique set of regression coefficients, since the number of predictors in the training set will be larger than the number of samples. Therefore for multiple linear regression, the practitioner must be aware of its pitfalls not only when working with the original data set but also when working with subsets of data created during model training and evaluation.

To illustrate the problem of correlated predictors, linear models were fit with combinations of descriptors related to the number of non-hydrogen atoms and the number of hydrogen bonds. In the training set, these predictors are highly correlated (correlation: 0.994). Figure 6.3 shows their relationship with the outcome, which is almost identical. First, we fit two separate regression models with the individual terms and then a third model with both

Table 6.1: Regression coefficients for two highly correlated predictors across four separate models

Model	NumNonHAtoms	NumNonHBonds
NumNonHAtoms only	−1.2 (0.1)	
NumNonHBonds only		−1.2 (0.1)
Both	−0.3 (0.5)	−0.9 (0.5)
All predictors	8.2 (1.4)	−9.1 (1.6)

terms. The predictors were centered and scaled prior to modeling so that their units would be the same. Table 6.1 shows the regression coefficients and their standard errors in parentheses. For the individual models, the regression coefficients are almost identical as are their standard errors. However, when fitting a model with both terms, the results differ; the slope related to the number of non-hydrogen atoms is greatly decreased. Also, the standard errors are increased fivefold when compared to the individual models. This reflects the instability in the regression linear caused by the between-predictor relationships and this instability is propagated directly to the model predictions. Table 6.1 also shows the coefficients for these two descriptors when all of the predictors are put into the model. Recall from Fig. 6.5 that there are many collinear predictors in the data and we would expect the effect of collinearity to be exacerbated. In fact, for these two predictors, the values become wildly large in magnitude and their standard errors are 14–16-fold larger than those from the individual models.

In practice, such highly correlated predictors might be managed manually by removing one of the offending predictors. However, if the number of predictors is large, this may be difficult. Also, on many occasions, relationships among predictors can be complex and involve many predictors. In these cases, manual removal of specific predictors may not be possible and models that can tolerate collinearity may be more useful.

Linear Regression for Solubility Data

Recall that in Sect. 6.1 we split the solubility data into training and test sets and that we applied a Box–Cox transformation to the continuous predictors in order to remove skewness. The next step in the model building process for linear regression is to identify predictors that have high pairwise correlations and to remove predictors so that no absolute pairwise correlation is greater than some pre-specified level. In this case we chose to remove predictors that have pairwise correlations greater than 0.9 (see Sect. 3.3). At this level, 38 predictors were identified and removed. Upon removing these predictors, a

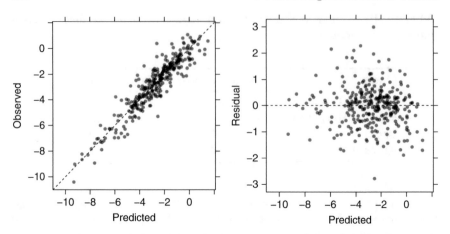

Fig. 6.7: *Left*: Observed versus predicted values for the solubility test set. *Right*: Residuals versus the predicted values. The residuals appear to be randomly scattered about 0 with respect to the predicted values

linear model was fit to the training data.[1] The linear model was resampled using 10-fold cross-validation and the estimated root mean squared error (RMSE) was 0.71 with a corresponding R^2 value of 0.88.

Predictors that were removed from the training data were then also removed from the test data and the model was then applied to the test set. The R^2 value between the observed and predicted values was 0.87, and the basic regression diagnostic plots are displayed in Fig. 6.7. There does not appear to be any bias in the prediction, and the distribution between the predicted values and residuals appears to be random about zero.

6.3 Partial Least Squares

For many real-life data sets, predictors can be correlated and contain similar predictive information like illustrated with the solubility data. If the correlation among predictors is high, then the ordinary least squares solution for multiple linear regression will have high variability and will become unstable.

---

[1] In practice, the correlation threshold would need to be smaller to have a significant effect on collinearity. In these data, it would also remove important variables. Also, one would investigate how the terms fit into the model. For example, there may be interactions between predictors that are important and nonlinear transformations of predictors may also improve the model. For these data, this set of activities is examined more closely in Chap. 19.

For other data sets, the number of predictors may be greater than the number of observations. In this case, too, ordinary least squares in its usual form will be unable to find a unique set of regression coefficients that minimize the SSE.

A couple of common solutions to the regression problem under these conditions include pre-processing the predictors by either (1) removal of the highly correlated predictors using techniques as described in Sect. 3.3 or (2) conducting PCA on the predictors as described in Sect. 3.3. Removing highly correlated predictors ensures that pairwise correlations among predictors are below a pre-specified threshold. However, this process does not necessarily ensure that linear combinations of predictors are uncorrelated with other predictors. If this is the case, then the ordinary least squares solution will still be unstable. Therefore it is important to understand that the removal of highly correlated pairwise predictors may not guarantee a stable least squares solution. Alternatively, using PCA for pre-processing guarantees that the resulting predictors, or combinations thereof, will be uncorrelated. The trade-off in using PCA is that the new predictors are linear combinations of the original predictors, and thus, the practical understanding of the new predictors can become murky.

Pre-processing predictors via PCA prior to performing regression is known as principal component regression (PCR) (Massy 1965); this technique has been widely applied in the context of problems with inherently highly correlated predictors or problems with more predictors than observations. While this two-step regression approach (dimension reduction, then regression) has been successfully used to develop predictive models under these conditions, it can easily be misled. Specifically, dimension reduction via PCA does not necessarily produce new predictors that explain the response. As an example of this scenario, consider the data in Fig. 6.8 which contains two predictors and one response. The two predictors are correlated, and PCA summarizes this relationship using the direction of maximal variability. The right-hand plot of this figure, however, illustrates that the first PCA direction contains no predictive information about the response.

As this simple example illustrates, PCA does not consider any aspects of the response when it selects its components. Instead, it simply chases the variability present throughout the predictor space. If that variability happens to be related to the response variability, then PCR has a good chance to identify a predictive relationship. If, however, the variability in the predictor space is not related to the variability of the response, then PCR can have difficulty identifying a predictive relationship when one might actually exist. Because of this inherent problem with PCR, we recommend using PLS when there are correlated predictors and a linear regression-type solution is desired.

PLS originated with Herman Wold's nonlinear iterative partial least squares (NIPALS) algorithm (Wold 1966, 1982) which linearized models that were nonlinear in the parameters. Subsequently, Wold et al. (1983) adapted the NIPALS method for the regression setting with correlated predictors and

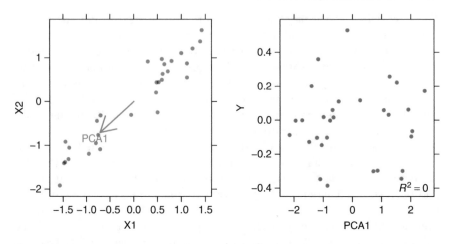

Fig. 6.8: An example of principal component regression for a simple data set with two predictors and one response. *Left*: A scatter plot of the two predictors shows the direction of the first principal component. *Right*: The first PCA direction contains no predictive information for the response

called this adaptation "PLS." Briefly, the NIPALS algorithm iteratively seeks to find underlying, or latent, relationships among the predictors which are highly correlated with the response. For a univariate response, each iteration of the algorithm assesses the relationship between the predictors ($\mathbf{X}$) and response ($\mathbf{y}$) and numerically summarizes this relationship with a vector of weights ($\mathbf{w}$); this vector is also known as a *direction*. The predictor data are then orthogonally projected onto the direction to generate scores ($\mathbf{t}$). The scores are then used to generate loadings ($\mathbf{p}$), which measure the correlation of the score vector to the original predictors. At the end of each iteration, the predictors and the response are "deflated" by subtracting the current estimate of the predictor and response structure, respectively. The new deflated predictor and response information are then used to generate the next set of weights, scores, and loadings. These quantities are sequentially stored in matrices $\mathbf{W}$, $\mathbf{T}$, and $\mathbf{P}$, respectively, and are used for predicting new samples and computing predictor importance. A schematic of the PLS relationship between predictors and the response can be seen in Fig. 6.9, and a thorough explanation of the algorithm can be found in Geladi and Kowalski (1986).

To obtain a better understanding of the algorithm's function, Stone and Brooks (1990) linked it to well-known statistical concepts of covariance and regression. In particular, Stone and Brooks showed that like PCA, PLS finds linear combinations of the predictors. These linear combinations are commonly called *components* or latent variables. While the PCA linear combinations are chosen to maximally summarize predictor space variability, the PLS linear combinations of predictors are chosen to maximally summarize

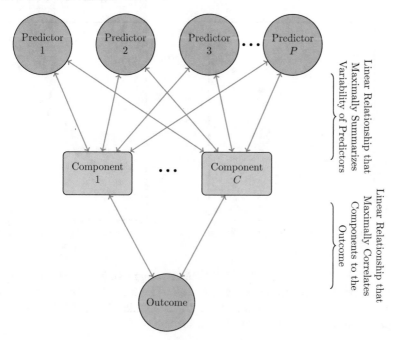

Fig. 6.9: A diagram depicting the structure of a PLS model. PLS finds components that simultaneously summarize variation of the predictors while being optimally correlated with the outcome

covariance with the response. This means that PLS finds components that maximally summarize the variation of the predictors while simultaneously requiring these components to have maximum correlation with the response. PLS therefore strikes a compromise between the objectives of predictor space dimension reduction and a predictive relationship with the response. In other words, PLS can be viewed as a *supervised* dimension reduction procedure; PCR is an *unsupervised* procedure.

To better understand how PLS works and to relate it to PCR, we will revisit the data presented in Fig. 6.8. This time we seek the first PLS component. The left-hand scatter plot in Fig. 6.10 contrasts the first PLS direction with the first PCA direction. For this illustration the two directions are nearly orthogonal, indicating that the optimal dimension reduction direction was not related to maximal variation in the predictor space. Instead, PLS identified the optimal predictor space dimension reduction for the purpose of regression with the response.

Clearly this example is designed to show an important flaw with PCR. In practice, PCR does not fail this drastically; rather, PCR produces models with similar predictive ability to PLS. Based on our experience, the number of components retained via cross-validation using PCR is always equal to

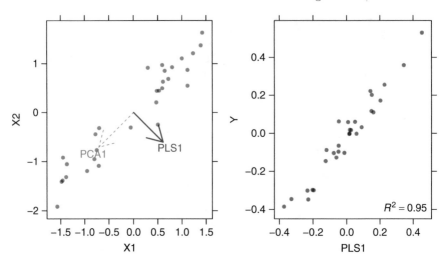

Fig. 6.10: An example of partial least squares regression for a simple data set with two predictors and one response. *Left*: The first PLS direction is nearly orthogonal to the first PCA direction. *Right*: Unlike PCA, the PLS direction contains highly predictive information for the response

or greater than the number of components retained by PLS. This is due to the fact that dimensions retained by PLS have been chosen to be optimally related to the response, while those chosen with PCR are not.

Prior to performing PLS, the predictors should be centered and scaled, especially if the predictors are on scales of differing magnitude. As described above, PLS will seek directions of maximum variation while simultaneously considering correlation with the response. Even with the constraint of correlation with the response, it will be more naturally drawn towards predictors with large variation. Therefore, predictors should be adequately preprocessed prior to performing PLS.

Once the predictors have been preprocessed, the practitioner can model the response with PLS. PLS has one tuning parameter: the number of components to retain. Resampling techniques as described in Sect. 4.4 can be used to determine the optimal number of components.

PCR and PLSR for Solubility Data

To demonstrate the model building process with PLS, let's return to the solubility data from Sect. 6.1. Although there are 228 predictors, Figs. 6.4 and 6.5 show that many predictors are highly correlated and that the overall information within the predictor space is contained in a smaller number of dimensions. These predictor conditions are very favorable for applying PLS.

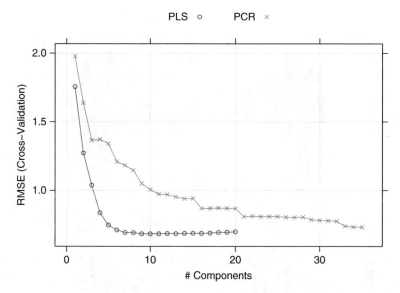

Fig. 6.11: Cross-validated RMSE by component for PLS and PCR. RMSE is minimized with ten PLS components and 35 PCR components

Cross-validation was used to determine the optimal number of PLS components to retain that minimize RMSE. At the same time, PCR was performed using the same cross-validation sets to compare its performance to PLS. Figure 6.11 contains the results, where PLS found a minimum RMSE (0.682) with ten components and PCR found a minimum RMSE (0.731) with 35 components. We see with these data that the supervised dimension reduction finds a minimum RMSE with significantly fewer components than unsupervised dimension reduction. Using the one-standard error rule (Sect. 4.6) would reduce the number of required PLS components to 8.

Figure 6.12 contrasts the relationship between each of the first two PCR and PLS components with the response. Because the RMSE is lower for each of the first two PLS components as compared to the first two PCR components, it is no surprise that the correlation between these components and the response is greater for PLS than PCR. This figure illustrates that PLS is more quickly being steered towards the underlying relationship with the response.

Prediction of the test set using the optimal PCR and PLS models can be seen in Fig. 6.13. The predictive ability of each method is good, and the residuals appear to be randomly scattered about zero. Although the predictive ability of these models is close, PLS finds a simpler model that uses far fewer components than PCR.

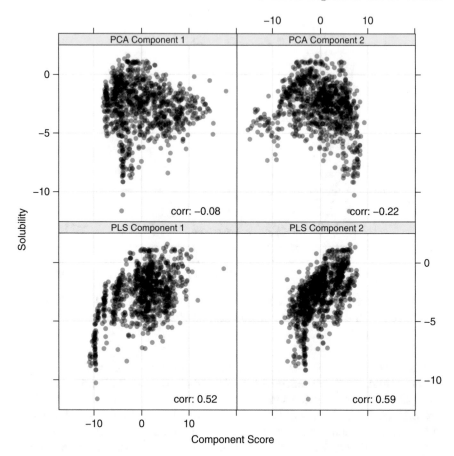

Fig. 6.12: A contrast of the relationship between each of the first two PCR and PLS components with the solubility response. Because the dimension reduction offered by PLS is supervised by the response, it is more quickly steered towards the underlying relationship between the predictors and the response

The PLS regression coefficients for the solubility data are presented in Table 6.2 (page 127), and the magnitudes are similar to the linear regression model that includes only those two predictors.

Because the latent variables from PLS are constructed using linear combinations of the original predictors, it is more difficult to quantify the relative contribution of each predictor to the model. Wold et al. (1993) introduced a heuristic way to assess variable importance when using the NIPALS algorithm and termed this calculation *variable importance in the projection*. In the simple case, suppose that the relationship between the predictors and the response can be adequately summarized by a one-component PLS model. The importance of the jth predictor is then proportional to the value of

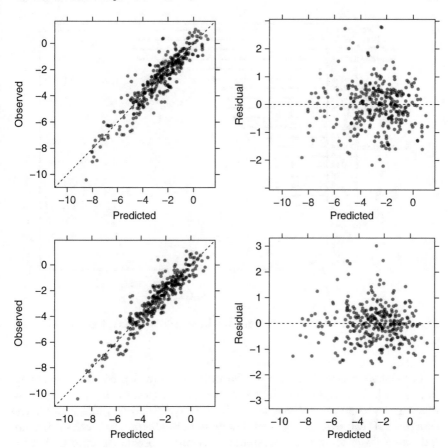

Fig. 6.13: *Left side*: Observed versus predicted values for the solubility test set for PCR (*upper*) and PLS (*lower*). *Right side*: Residuals versus the predicted values for PCR and PLS. The residuals appear to be randomly scattered about 0 with respect to the predicted values. Both methods have similar predictive ability, but PLS does so with far fewer components

the normalized weight vector, w, corresponding to the jth predictor. When the relationship between predictors and the response requires more than one component, the variable importance calculation becomes more involved. In this case, the numerator of the importance of the jth predictor is a weighted sum of the normalized weights corresponding to the jth predictor. The jth normalized weight of the kth component, w_{kj}, is scaled by the amount of variation in the response explained by the kth component. The denominator of the variable importance is the total amount of response variation explained by all k components. Therefore, the larger the normalized weight and amount of response variation explained by the component, the more important predictor is in the PLS model.

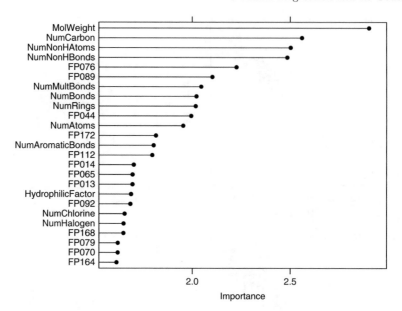

Fig. 6.14: Partial least squares variable importance scores for the solubility data

For the solubility data, the top 25 most important predictors are shown in Fig. 6.14. The larger the VIP value, the more important the predictor is in relating the latent predictor structure to the response. By its construction, the squared VIP values sum to the total number of predictors. As a rule-of-thumb, VIP values exceeding 1 are considered to contain predictive information for the response. Wold (1995) further suggests that predictors with small PLS regression coefficients and small VIP values are likely not important and should be considered as candidates for removal from the model.

Algorithmic Variations of PLS

The NIPALS algorithm works fairly efficiently for data sets of small-to-moderate size (e.g., < 2,500 samples and < 30 predictors) (Alin 2009). But when the number of samples (n) and predictors (P) climbs, the algorithm becomes inefficient. This inefficiency is due to the way the matrix operations on the predictors and the response are performed. Specifically, both the predictor matrix and the response must be deflated (i.e., information must be subtracted from each matrix, thus creating new versions of each matrix) for each latent variable. This implies that different versions of the predictor matrix and response must be kept at each iteration of the algorithm. Therefore an $n \times P$ matrix and an $n \times 1$ vector must be recomputed, operated on, and stored in each iteration. As n and P grow, so do the memory requirements, and operations on these matrices must be performed throughout the iterative process.

In a computational step forward, Lindgren et al. (1993) showed that the constructs of NIPALS could be obtained by working with a "kernel" matrix of dimension $P \times P$, the covariance matrix of the predictors (also of dimension $P \times P$), and the covariance matrix of the predictors and response (of dimension $P \times 1$). This adjustment improved the speed of the algorithm, especially as the number of observations became much larger than the number of predictors.

At nearly the same time as the kernel approach was developed, de Jong (1993) improved upon the NIPALS algorithm by viewing the underlying problem as finding latent orthogonal variables in the predictor space that maximize the covariance with the response. This perspective shift led to a different algorithm that focused on deflating the covariance matrix between the predictors and the response rather than deflating both the predictor matrix and the response. de Jong (1993) termed the new approach "SIMPLS" because it was a simple modification of the PLS algorithm that was framed through statistics. Because the SIMPLS approach deflates the covariance matrix, it requires storing just the deflated covariance matrix at each iteration which has dimension $P \times 1$—a significant computational improvement over the storage requirements of NIPALS. Although the SIMPLS approach solves the optimization in a different way, de Jong (1993) showed that the SIMPLS latent variables are identical to those from NIPALS when there is only one response. (More will be discussed below when modeling a multivariate response.)

Other authors have also proposed computational modifications to the NIPALS algorithm through adjustments to the kernel approach (de Jong and Ter Braak 1994; Dayal and MacGregor 1997). Dayal and MacGregor (1997) developed two efficient modifications, especially when $n >> P$, and, similar to SIMPLS, only require a deflation of the covariance matrix between the predictors and the response at each step of the iterative process. In their first alteration to the inner workings of the algorithm, the original predictor matrix is used in the computations (without deflation). In the second alteration, the covariance matrix of the predictors is used in the computations (also without deflation).

Alin (2009) provided a comprehensive computational efficiency comparison of NIPALS to other algorithmic modifications. In this work, Alin used a varying number of samples (500–10,000), predictors (10–30), responses (1–15), and number of latent variables to derive (3–10). In nearly every scenario, the second kernel algorithm of Dayal and MacGregor was more computationally efficient than all other approaches and provided superior performance when $n > 2,500$ and $P > 30$. And in the cases where the second algorithm did not provide the most computational efficiency, the first algorithm did.

The above approaches to implementing PLS provide clear computational advantages over the original algorithm. However, as the number of predictors grows, each becomes less efficient. To address this scenario when $P > n$,

Rännar et al. (1994) constructed a kernel based on the predictor matrix and response that had dimension $n \times n$. A usual PLS analysis can then be performed using this kernel, the outer products of the predictors, and the outer products of the response (each with dimension $n \times n$). Hence, this algorithm is computationally more efficient when there are more predictors than samples.

As noted in Fig. 6.9, the PLS components summarize the data through linear substructures (i.e., hyperplanes) of the original predictor space that are related to the response. But for many problems, the underlying structure in the predictor space that is optimally related to the response is not linear but curvilinear or nonlinear. Several authors have attempted to address this shortcoming of PLS in order to find this type of predictor space/response relationship. While many methods exist, the most easily adaptable approaches using the algorithms explained above are provided by Berglund and Wold (1997) and Berglund et al. (2001). In Berglund and Wold (1997), the authors show that adding squared predictors (and cubic, if necessary) can be included with the original predictors. PLS is then applied to the augmented data set. The authors also show that there is no need to add cross-product terms, thus greatly reducing the number of new predictors added to the original data. Subsequently, Berglund et al. (2001) employ the use of the GIFI approach (Michailidis and de Leeuw 1998) which splits each predictor into two or more bins for those predictors that are thought to have a nonlinear relationship with the response. Cut points for the bins are selected by the user and are based on either prior knowledge or characteristics of the data. The original predictors that were binned are then excluded from the data set that includes the binned versions of the predictors. PLS is then applied to the new predictor set in usual way.

Both of these approaches have successfully found nonlinear relationships between the predictors and the response. But there can be a considerable amount of effort required in constructing the data sets for input to PLS, especially as the number of predictors becomes large. As we will show in subsequent sections, other predictive modeling techniques can more naturally identify nonlinear structures between predictors and the response without having to modify the predictor space. Therefore, if a more intricate relationship between predictors and response exists, then we suggest employing one of the other techniques rather than trying to improve the performance of PLS through this type of augmentation.

6.4 Penalized Models

Under standard assumptions, the coefficients produced by ordinary least squares regression are unbiased and, of all unbiased linear techniques, this model also has the lowest variance. However, given that the MSE is a combination of variance and bias (Sect. 5.2), it is very possible to produce models with smaller MSEs by allowing the parameter estimates to be biased. It is common that a small increase in bias can produce a substantial drop in the variance and thus a smaller MSE than ordinary least squares regression coefficients. One consequence of large correlations between the predictor variances is that the variance can become very large. Combatting collinearity by using biased models may result in regression models where the overall MSE is competitive.

One method of creating biased regression models is to add a penalty to the sum of the squared errors. Recall that original least squares regression found parameter estimates to minimize the sum of the squared errors:

$$\text{SSE} = \sum_{i=1}^{n}(y_i - \hat{y}_i)^2.$$

When the model over-fits the data, or when there are issues with collinearity (as in Table 6.1), the linear regression parameter estimates may become inflated. As such, we may want to control the magnitude of these estimates to reduce the SSE. Controlling (or *regularizing*) the parameter estimates can be accomplished by adding a penalty to the SSE if the estimates become large. *Ridge regression* (Hoerl 1970) adds a penalty on the sum of the squared regression parameters:

$$\text{SSE}_{L_2} = \sum_{i=1}^{n}(y_i - \hat{y}_i)^2 + \lambda \sum_{j=1}^{P} \beta_j^2.$$

The "L_2" signifies that a second-order penalty (i.e., the square) is being used on the parameter estimates. The effect of this penalty is that the parameter estimates are only allowed to become large if there is a proportional reduction in SSE. In effect, this method *shrinks* the estimates towards 0 as the λ penalty becomes large (these techniques are sometimes called "shrinkage methods").

By adding the penalty, we are making a trade-off between the model variance and bias. By sacrificing some bias, we can often reduce the variance enough to make the overall MSE lower than unbiased models.

For example, Fig. 6.15 shows the *path* of the regression coefficients for the solubility data over different values of λ. Each line corresponds to a model parameter and the predictors were centered and scaled prior to this analysis so that their units are the same. When there is no penalty, many parameters have reasonable values, such as the predictor for the number of multiple bonds (shown in orange). However, some parameter estimates are abnormally large, such as the number of non-hydrogen atoms (in green) and the number of non-hydrogen bonds (purple) previously singled out in Table 6.1. These large values are indicative of collinearity issues. As the penalty is increased, the parameter estimates move closer to 0 at different rates. By the time

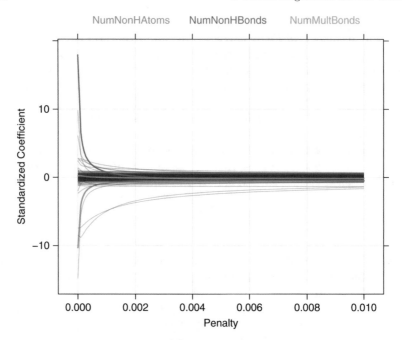

Fig. 6.15: The ridge-regression coefficient path

the penalty has a value of $\lambda = 0.002$, these two predictors are much more well behaved, although other coefficient values are still relatively large in magnitude.

Using cross-validation, the penalty value was optimized. Figure 6.16 shows how the RMSE changes with λ. When there is no penalty, the error is inflated. When the penalty is increased, the error drops from 0.72 to 0.69. As the penalty increases beyond 0.036, the bias becomes to large and the model starts to under-fit, resulting in an increase in MSE.

While ridge regression shrinks the parameter estimates towards 0, the model does not set the values to absolute 0 for any value of the penalty. Even though some parameter estimates become negligibly small, this model does not conduct *feature selection*.

A popular alternative to ridge regression is the *least absolute shrinkage and selection operator* model, frequently called the *lasso* (Tibshirani 1996). This model uses a similar penalty to ridge regression:

$$\text{SSE}_{L_1} = \sum_{i=1}^{n}(y_i - \hat{y}_i)^2 + \lambda \sum_{j=1}^{P} |\beta_j|.$$

While this may seem like a small modification, the practical implications are significant. While the regression coefficients are still shrunk towards 0,

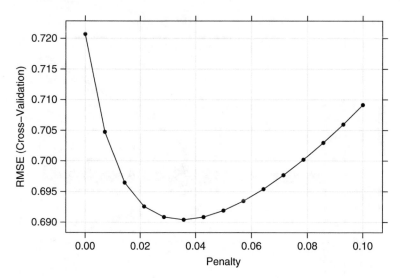

Fig. 6.16: The cross-validation profiles for a ridge regression model

a consequence of penalizing the absolute values is that some parameters are actually set to 0 for some value of λ. Thus the lasso yields models that simultaneously use regularization to improve the model and to conduct feature selection. In comparing, the two types of penalties, Friedman et al. (2010) stated

> "Ridge regression is known to shrink the coefficients of correlated predictors towards each other, allowing them to borrow strength from each other. In the extreme case of k identical predictors, they each get identical coefficients with $1/k$th the size that any single one would get if fit alone.[...]
>
> lasso, on the other hand, is somewhat indifferent to very correlated predictors, and will tend to pick one and ignore the rest."

Figure 6.17 shows the paths of the lasso coefficients over different penalty values. The x-axis is the fraction of the full solution (i.e., ordinary least squares with no penalty). Smaller values on the x-axis indicate that a large penalty has been used. When the penalty is large, many of the regression coefficients are set to 0. As the penalty is reduced, many have nonzero coefficients. Examining the trace for the number of non-hydrogen bonds (in purple), the coefficient is initially 0, has a slight increase, then is shrunken towards 0 again. When the fraction is around 0.4, this predictor is entered back into the model with a nonzero coefficient that consistently increases (most likely due to collinearity). Table 6.2 shows regression coefficients for ordinary least squares, PLS, ridge-regression, and the lasso model. The ridge-regression penalty used in this table is 0.036 and the lasso penalty was 0.15. The ridge-regression model shrinks the coefficients for the non-hydrogen atom and non-hydrogen bond predictors significantly towards 0 in comparison to

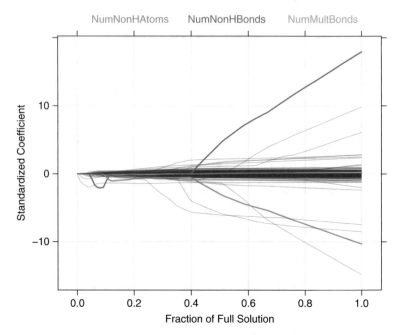

Fig. 6.17: The lasso coefficient path for the solubility data. The x-axis is the fraction of the full least squares solution. As the fraction increases, the lasso penalty (λ) decreases

the ordinary least squares models while the lasso model shrinks the non-hydrogen atom predictor out of the model. Between these models, the lasso model had the smallest cross-validation error of 0.67, slightly better than the PLS model (0.68) and ridge regression (0.69).

This type of regularization has been a very active area of research. The lasso model has been extended to many other techniques, such as linear discriminant analysis (Clemmensen et al. 2011; Witten and Tibshirani 2011), PLS (Chun and Keleş 2010), and PCA (Jolliffe et al. 2003; Zou et al. 2004). A significant advancement for this model was Efron et al. (2004). Their model, least angle regression (LARS), is a broad framework that encompasses the lasso and similar models. The LARS model can be used to fit lasso models more efficiently, especially in high-dimensional problems. Friedman et al. (2010) and Hesterberg et al. (2008) provide a survey of these techniques.

A generalization of the lasso model is the *elastic net* (Zou and Hastie 2005). This model combines the two types of penalties:

$$\text{SSE}_{\text{Enet}} = \sum_{i=1}^{n}(y_i - \hat{y}_i)^2 + \lambda_1 \sum_{j=1}^{P}\beta_j^2 + \lambda_2 \sum_{j=1}^{P}|\beta_j|.$$

Table 6.2: Regression coefficients for two highly correlated predictors for PLS, ridge regression, the elastic net and other models

Model	NumNonHAtoms	NumNonHBonds
NumNonHAtoms only	−1.2 (0.1)	
NumNonHBonds only		−1.2 (0.1)
Both	−0.3 (0.5)	−0.9 (0.5)
All predictors	8.2 (1.4)	−9.1 (1.6)
PLS, all predictors	−0.4	−0.8
Ridge, all predictors	−0.3	−0.3
lasso/elastic net	0.0	−0.8

The ridge penalty used for this table was 0.036 and the lasso penalty was 0.15. The PLS model used ten components.

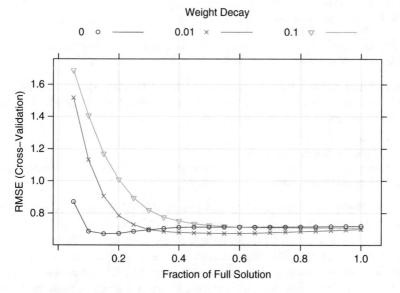

Fig. 6.18: The cross-validation profiles for an elastic net model

The advantage of this model is that it enables effective regularization via the ridge-type penalty with the feature selection quality of the lasso penalty. The Zou and Hastie (2005) suggest that this model will more effectively deal with groups of high correlated predictors.

Both the penalties require tuning to achieve optimal performance. Again, using resampling, this model was tuned for the solubility data. Figure 6.18 shows the performance profiles across three values of the ridge penalty and 20 values of the lasso penalty. The pure lasso model (with $\lambda_1 = 0$) has an initial drop in the error and then an increase when the fraction is greater than 0.2. The two models with nonzero values of the ridge penalty have minimum errors with a larger model. In the end, the optimal performance was associated with the lasso model with a fraction of 0.15, corresponding to 130 predictors out of a possible 228.

6.5 Computing

The R packages elasticnet, caret, lars, MASS, pls and stats will be referenced.

The solubility data can be obtained from the AppliedPredictiveModeling R package. The predictors for the training and test sets are contained in data frames called solTrainX and solTestX, respectively. To obtain the data in R,

```
> library(AppliedPredictiveModeling)
> data(solubility)
> ## The data objects begin with "sol":
> ls(pattern = "^solT")
   [1] "solTestX"      "solTestXtrans" "solTestY"      "solTrainX"
   [5] "solTrainXtrans" "solTrainY"
```

Each column of the data corresponds to a predictor (i.e., chemical descriptor) and the rows correspond to compounds. There are 228 columns in the data. A random sample of column names is

```
> set.seed(2)
> sample(names(solTrainX), 8)
   [1] "FP043"         "FP160"         "FP130"         "FP038"         "NumBonds"
   [6] "NumNonHAtoms"  "FP029"         "FP185"
```

The "FP" columns correspond to the binary 0/1 fingerprint predictors that are associated with the presence or absence of a particular chemical structure. Alternate versions of these data that have been Box–Cox transformed are contained in the data frames solTrainXtrans and solTestXtrans. These modified versions were used in the analyses in this and subsequent chapters.

The solubility values for each compound are contained in numeric vectors named solTrainY and solTestY.

Ordinary Linear Regression

The primary function for creating linear regression models using simple least squares is lm. This function takes a formula and data frame as input. Because of this, the training set predictors and outcome should be contained in the same data frame. We can create a new data frame for this purpose:

```
> trainingData <- solTrainXtrans
> ## Add the solubility outcome
> trainingData$Solubility <- solTrainY
```

To fit a linear model with all the predictors entering in the model as simple, independent linear terms, the formula shortcut Solubility ~ . can be used:

```
> lmFitAllPredictors <- lm(Solubility ~ ., data = trainingData)
```

An intercept term is automatically added to the model. The summary method displays model summary statistics, the parameter estimates, their standard errors, and p-values for testing whether each individual coefficient is different than 0:

```
> summary(lmFitAllPredictors)
```

```
Call:
lm(formula = Solubility ~ ., data = trainingData)

Residuals:
    Min      1Q   Median      3Q     Max
-1.75620 -0.28304  0.01165  0.30030  1.54887

Coefficients:
                    Estimate Std. Error t value Pr(>|t|)
(Intercept)        2.431e+00  2.162e+00   1.124 0.261303
FP001              3.594e-01  3.185e-01   1.128 0.259635
FP002              1.456e-01  2.637e-01   0.552 0.580960
FP003             -3.969e-02  1.314e-01  -0.302 0.762617
FP004             -3.049e-01  1.371e-01  -2.223 0.026520 *
FP005              2.837e+00  9.598e-01   2.956 0.003223 **
FP006             -6.886e-02  2.041e-01  -0.337 0.735917
FP007              4.044e-02  1.152e-01   0.351 0.725643
FP008              1.121e-01  1.636e-01   0.685 0.493331
FP009             -8.242e-01  8.395e-01  -0.982 0.326536
    :                   :          :        :      :
MolWeight         -1.232e+00  2.296e-01  -5.365 1.09e-07 ***
NumAtoms          -1.478e+01  3.473e+00  -4.257 2.35e-05 ***
NumNonHAtoms       1.795e+01  3.166e+00   5.670 2.07e-08 ***
NumBonds           9.843e+00  2.681e+00   3.671 0.000260 ***
NumNonHBonds      -1.030e+01  1.793e+00  -5.746 1.35e-08 ***
NumMultBonds       2.107e-01  1.754e-01   1.201 0.229990
NumRotBonds       -5.213e-01  1.334e-01  -3.908 0.000102 ***
NumDblBonds       -7.492e-01  3.163e-01  -2.369 0.018111 *
NumAromaticBonds  -2.364e+00  6.232e-01  -3.794 0.000161 ***
NumHydrogen        8.347e-01  1.880e-01   4.439 1.04e-05 ***
NumCarbon          1.730e-02  3.763e-01   0.046 0.963335
NumNitrogen        6.125e+00  3.045e+00   2.011 0.044645 *
NumOxygen          2.389e+00  4.523e-01   5.283 1.69e-07 ***
NumSulfer         -8.508e+00  3.619e+00  -2.351 0.018994 *
NumChlorine       -7.449e+00  1.989e+00  -3.744 0.000195 ***
NumHalogen         1.408e+00  2.109e+00   0.668 0.504615
NumRings           1.276e+00  6.716e-01   1.901 0.057731 .
HydrophilicFactor  1.099e-02  1.137e-01   0.097 0.922998
```

```
SurfaceArea1        8.825e-02  6.058e-02   1.457 0.145643
SurfaceArea2        9.555e-02  5.615e-02   1.702 0.089208 .
---
Signif. codes:  0 '***' 0.001 '**' 0.01 '*' 0.05 '.' 0.1 ' ' 1

Residual standard error: 0.5524 on 722 degrees of freedom
Multiple R-squared: 0.9446,        Adjusted R-squared: 0.9271
F-statistic: 54.03 on 228 and 722 DF,  p-value: < 2.2e-16
```

(Since there are 229 predictors in the model, the output is very long and the results have been trimmed.) A more comprehensive discussion of linear models in R can be found in Faraway (2005).

The simple estimates of the RMSE and R^2 were 0.55 and 0.945, respectively. Note that these values are likely to be highly optimistic as they have been derived by re-predicting the training set data.

To compute the model solubility values for new samples, the predict method is used:

```
> lmPred1 <- predict(lmFitAllPredictors, solTestXtrans)
> head(lmPred1)
         20         21         23         25         28         31
 0.99370933 0.06834627 -0.69877632  0.84796356 -0.16578324  1.40815083
```

We can collect the observed and predicted values into a data frame, then use the caret function defaultSummary to estimate the test set performance:

```
> lmValues1 <- data.frame(obs = solTestY, pred = lmPred1)
> defaultSummary(lmValues1)
     RMSE  Rsquared
0.7455802 0.8722236
```

Based on the test set, the summaries produced by the summary function for lm were optimistic.

If we wanted a robust linear regression model, then the robust linear model function (rlm) from the MASS package could be used, which by default employs the Huber approach. Similar to the lm function, rlm is called as follows:

```
> rlmFitAllPredictors <- rlm(Solubility ~ ., data = trainingData)
```

The train function generates a resampling estimate of performance. Because the training set size is not small, 10-fold cross-validation should produce reasonable estimates of model performance. The function trainControl specifies the type of resampling:

```
> ctrl <- trainControl(method = "cv", number = 10)
```

train will accept a model formula or a non-formula interface (see Sect. 4.9 for a summary of different methods for specifying predictor models). The non-formula interface is

```
> set.seed(100)
> lmFit1 <- train(x = solTrainXtrans, y = solTrainY,
+                 method = "lm", trControl = ctrl)
```

The random number seed is set prior to modeling so that the results can be reproduced. The results are:

```
> lmFit1
  951 samples
  228 predictors

  No pre-processing
  Resampling: Cross-Validation (10-fold)

  Summary of sample sizes: 856, 857, 855, 856, 856, 855, ...

  Resampling results

    RMSE   Rsquared  RMSE SD  Rsquared SD
    0.721  0.877     0.07     0.0247
```

For models built to *explain*, it is important to check model assumptions, such as the residual distribution. For predictive models, some of the same diagnostic techniques can shed light on areas where the model is not predicting well. For example, we could plot the residuals versus the predicted values for the model. If the plot shows a random cloud of points, we will feel more comfortable that there are no major terms missing from the model (such as quadratic terms, etc.) or significant outliers. Another important plot is the predicted values versus the observed values to assess how close the predictions are to the actual values. Two methods of doing this (using the training set samples are

```
> xyplot(solTrainY ~ predict(lmFit1),
+        ## plot the points (type = 'p') and a background grid ('g')
+        type = c("p", "g"),
+        xlab = "Predicted", ylab = "Observed")
> xyplot(resid(lmFit1) ~ predict(lmFit1),
+        type = c("p", "g"),
+        xlab = "Predicted", ylab = "Residuals")
```

The results are shown in Fig. 6.19. Note that the resid function generates the model residuals for the training set and that using the predict function without an additional data argument returns the predicted values for the training set. For this model, there are no obvious warning signs in the diagnostic plots.

To build a smaller model without predictors with extremely high correlations, we can use the methods of Sect. 3.3 to reduce the number of predictors such that there are no absolute pairwise correlations above 0.9:

```
> corThresh <- .9
> tooHigh <- findCorrelation(cor(solTrainXtrans), corThresh)
> corrPred <- names(solTrainXtrans)[tooHigh]
> trainXfiltered <- solTrainXtrans[, -tooHigh]
```

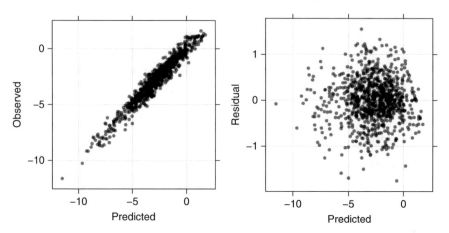

Fig. 6.19: Diagnostic plots for the linear model using the training set. *Left*: A plot of the observed values versus the predicted values. This plot can show outliers or areas where the model is not calibrated. *Right*: A plot of the residuals versus predicted values. If the model has been well specified, this plot should be a random cloud of points with no outliers or patterns (e.g., a funnel shape)

```
> testXfiltered <- solTestXtrans[, -tooHigh]
> set.seed(100)
> lmFiltered <- train(testXfiltered, solTrainY, method = "lm",
+                     trControl = ctrl)
> lmFiltered

 951 samples
 228 predictors

No pre-processing
Resampling: Cross-Validation (10-fold)

Summary of sample sizes: 856, 857, 855, 856, 856, 855, ...

Resampling results

  RMSE   Rsquared  RMSE SD  Rsquared SD
  0.721  0.877     0.07     0.0247
```

Robust linear regression can also be performed using the `train` function which employs the `rlm` function. However, it is important to note that `rlm` does not allow the covariance matrix of the predictors to be singular (unlike the `lm` function). To ensure that predictors are not singular, we will pre-process the predictors using PCA. Using the filtered set of predictors, the robust regression model performance is

```
> set.seed(100)
> rlmPCA <- train(solTrainXtrans, solTrainY,
```

```
+                       method = "rlm",
+                       preProcess = "pca",
+                       trControl = ctrl)
> rlmPCA
  951 samples
  228 predictors

  Pre-processing: principal component signal extraction, scaled, centered
  Resampling: Cross-Validation (10-fold)

  Summary of sample sizes: 856, 857, 855, 856, 856, 855, ...

  Resampling results

    RMSE   Rsquared  RMSE SD  Rsquared SD
    0.782  0.854     0.0372   0.0169
```

Partial Least Squares

The pls package (Mevik and Wehrens 2007) has functions for PLS and PCR. SIMPLS, the first Dayal and MacGregor algorithm, and the algorithm developed by Rännar et al. (1994) are each available. By default, the pls package uses the first Dayal and MacGregor kernel algorithm while the other algorithms can be specified using the method argument using the values "oscorespls", "simpls", or "widekernelpls". The plsr function, like the lm function, requires a model formula:

```
> plsFit <- plsr(Solubility ~ ., data = trainingData)
```

The number of components can be fixed using the ncomp argument or, if left to the default, the maximum number of components will be calculated. Predictions on new samples can be calculated using the predict function. Predictions can be made for a specific number of components or for several values at a time. For example

```
> predict(plsFit, solTestXtrans[1:5,], ncomp = 1:2)
, , 1 comps

     Solubility
20   -1.789335
21   -1.427551
23   -2.268798
25   -2.269782
28   -1.867960


, , 2 comps

     Solubility
```

```
20   0.2520469
21   0.3555028
23  -1.8795338
25  -0.6848584
28  -1.5531552
```

The `plsr` function has options for either K-fold or leave-one-out cross-validation (via the `validation` argument) or the PLS algorithm to use, such as SIMPLS (using the `method` argument).

There are several helper functions to extract the PLS components (in the function `loadings`), the PLS scores (`scores`), and other quantities. The `plot` function has visualizations for many aspects of the model.

`train` can also be used with `method` values of `pls`, such as `"oscorespls"`, `"simpls"`, or `"widekernelpls"`. For example

```
> set.seed(100)
> plsTune <- train(solTrainXtrans, solTrainY,
+                  method = "pls",
+                  ## The default tuning grid evaluates
+                  ## components 1... tuneLength
+                  tuneLength = 20,
+                  trControl = ctrl,
+                  preProc = c("center", "scale"))
```

This code reproduces the PLS model displayed in Fig. 6.11.

Penalized Regression Models

Ridge-regression models can be created using the `lm.ridge` function in the MASS package or the `enet` function in the elasticnet package. When calling the `enet` function, the `lambda` argument specifies the ridge-regression penalty:

```
> ridgeModel <- enet(x = as.matrix(solTrainXtrans), y = solTrainY,
+                    lambda = 0.001)
```

Recall that the elastic net model has both ridge penalties and lasso penalties and, at this point, the R object `ridgeModel` has only fixed the ridge penalty value. The lasso penalty can be computed efficiently for many values of the penalty. The `predict` function for `enet` objects generates predictions for one or more values of the lasso penalty simultaneously using the `s` and `mode` arguments. For ridge regression, we only desire a single lasso penalty of 0, so we want the full solution. To produce a ridge-regression solution we define `s=1` with `mode = "fraction"`. This last option specifies how the amount of penalization is defined; in this case, a value of 1 corresponds to a faction of 1, i.e., the full solution:

```
> ridgePred <- predict(ridgeModel, newx = as.matrix(solTestXtrans),
+                      s = 1, mode = "fraction",
```

```
+                        type = "fit")
> head(ridgePred$fit)
        20          21          23          25          28          31
0.96795590  0.06918538 -0.54365077  0.96072014 -0.03594693  1.59284535
```

To tune over the penalty, `train` can be used with a different method:

```
> ## Define the candidate set of values
> ridgeGrid <- data.frame(.lambda = seq(0, .1, length = 15))
> set.seed(100)
> ridgeRegFit <- train(solTrainXtrans, solTrainY,
+                      method = "ridge",
+                      ## Fir the model over many penalty values
+                      tuneGrid = ridgeGrid,
+                      trControl = ctrl,
+                      ## put the predictors on the same scale
+                      preProc = c("center", "scale"))
```

```
> ridgeRegFit
    951 samples
    228 predictors

Pre-processing: centered, scaled
Resampling: Cross-Validation (10-fold)

Summary of sample sizes: 856, 857, 855, 856, 856, 855, ...

Resampling results across tuning parameters:
```

lambda	RMSE	Rsquared	RMSE SD	Rsquared SD
0	0.721	0.877	0.0699	0.0245
0.00714	0.705	0.882	0.045	0.0199
0.0143	0.696	0.885	0.0405	0.0187
0.0214	0.693	0.886	0.0378	0.018
0.0286	0.691	0.887	0.0359	0.0175
0.0357	0.69	0.887	0.0346	0.0171
0.0429	0.691	0.888	0.0336	0.0168
0.05	0.692	0.888	0.0329	0.0166
0.0571	0.693	0.887	0.0323	0.0164
0.0643	0.695	0.887	0.032	0.0162
0.0714	0.698	0.887	0.0319	0.016
0.0786	0.7	0.887	0.0318	0.0159
0.0857	0.703	0.886	0.0318	0.0158
0.0929	0.706	0.886	0.032	0.0157
0.1	0.709	0.885	0.0321	0.0156

```
RMSE was used to select the optimal model using the smallest value.
The final value used for the model was lambda = 0.0357.
```

The lasso model can be estimated using a number of different functions. The lars package contains the `lars` function, the elasticnet package has `enet`, and the glmnet package has a function of the same name. The syntax for these functions is very similar. For the `enet` function, the usage would be

```
> enetModel <- enet(x = as.matrix(solTrainXtrans), y = solTrainY,
+                   lambda = 0.01, normalize = TRUE)
```

The predictor data must be a matrix object, so the data frame solTrainXtrans needs to be converted for the enet function. The predictors should be centered and scaled prior to modeling. The normalize argument will do this standardization automatically. The parameter lambda controls the ridge-regression penalty and, setting this value to 0, fits the lasso model. The lasso penalty does not need to be specified until the time of prediction:

```
> enetPred <- predict(enetModel, newx = as.matrix(solTestXtrans),
+                     s = .1, mode = "fraction",
+                     type = "fit")
> ## A list is returned with several items:
> names(enetPred)
  [1] "s"        "fraction" "mode"       "fit"
> ## The 'fit' component has the predicted values:
> head(enetPred$fit)
          20          21          23          25          28          31
 -0.60186178 -0.42226814 -1.20465564 -1.23652963 -1.25023517 -0.05587631
```

To determine which predictors are used in the model, the predict method is used with type = "coefficients":

```
> enetCoef<- predict(enetModel, newx = as.matrix(solTestXtrans),
+                    s = .1, mode = "fraction",
+                    type = "coefficients")
> tail(enetCoef$coefficients)
        NumChlorine          NumHalogen          NumRings HydrophilicFactor
         0.00000000          0.00000000        0.00000000        0.12678967
        SurfaceArea1        SurfaceArea2
         0.09035596          0.00000000
```

More than one value of s can be used with the predict function to generate predictions from more than one model simultaneously.

Other packages to fit the lasso model or some alternate version of the model are **biglars** (for large data sets), **FLLat** (for the fused lasso), **grplasso** (the group lasso), **penalized**, **relaxo** (the relaxed lasso), and others. To tune the elastic net model using train, we specify method = "enet". Here, we tune the model over a custom set of penalties:

```
> enetGrid <- expand.grid(.lambda = c(0, 0.01, .1),
+                         .fraction = seq(.05, 1, length = 20))
> set.seed(100)
> enetTune <- train(solTrainXtrans, solTrainY,
+                   method = "enet",
+                   tuneGrid = enetGrid,
+                   trControl = ctrl,
+                   preProc = c("center", "scale"))
```

Figure 6.18 can be created from this object using plot(enetTune).

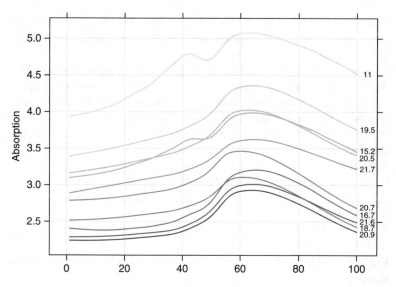

Fig. 6.20: A sample of ten spectra of the Tecator data. The colors of the curves reflect the absorption values, where *yellow* indicates low absorption and *red* is indicative of high absorption

Exercises

6.1. Infrared (IR) spectroscopy technology is used to determine the chemical makeup of a substance. The theory of IR spectroscopy holds that unique molecular structures absorb IR frequencies differently. In practice a spectrometer fires a series of IR frequencies into a sample material, and the device measures the absorbance of the sample at each individual frequency. This series of measurements creates a spectrum profile which can then be used to determine the chemical makeup of the sample material.

   A Tecator Infratec Food and Feed Analyzer instrument was used to analyze 215 samples of meat across 100 frequencies. A sample of these frequency profiles is displayed in Fig. 6.20. In addition to an IR profile, analytical chemistry determined the percent content of water, fat, and protein for each sample. If we can establish a predictive relationship between IR spectrum and fat content, then food scientists could predict a sample's fat content with IR instead of using analytical chemistry. This would provide costs savings, since analytical chemistry is a more expensive, time-consuming process:

(a) Start R and use these commands to load the data:

```
> library(caret)
> data(tecator)
> # use ?tecator to see more details
```

The matrix `absorp` contains the 100 absorbance values for the 215 samples, while matrix `endpoints` contains the percent of moisture, fat, and protein in columns 1–3, respectively.

(b) In this example the predictors are the measurements at the individual frequencies. Because the frequencies lie in a systematic order (850–1,050 nm), the predictors have a high degree of correlation. Hence, the data lie in a smaller dimension than the total number of predictors (100). Use PCA to determine the effective dimension of these data. What is the effective dimension?

(c) Split the data into a training and a test set, pre-process the data, and build each variety of models described in this chapter. For those models with tuning parameters, what are the optimal values of the tuning parameter(s)?

(d) Which model has the best predictive ability? Is any model significantly better or worse than the others?

(e) Explain which model you would use for predicting the fat content of a sample.

6.2. Developing a model to predict permeability (see Sect. 1.4) could save significant resources for a pharmaceutical company, while at the same time more rapidly identifying molecules that have a sufficient permeability to become a drug:

(a) Start R and use these commands to load the data:

```
> library(AppliedPredictiveModeling)
> data(permeability)
```

The matrix `fingerprints` contains the 1,107 binary molecular predictors for the 165 compounds, while `permeability` contains permeability response.

(b) The fingerprint predictors indicate the presence or absence of substructures of a molecule and are often sparse meaning that relatively few of the molecules contain each substructure. Filter out the predictors that have low frequencies using the `nearZeroVar` function from the **caret** package. How many predictors are left for modeling?

(c) Split the data into a training and a test set, pre-process the data, and tune a PLS model. How many latent variables are optimal and what is the corresponding resampled estimate of R^2?

(d) Predict the response for the test set. What is the test set estimate of R^2?

(e) Try building other models discussed in this chapter. Do any have better predictive performance?

(f) Would you recommend any of your models to replace the permeability laboratory experiment?

6.3. A chemical manufacturing process for a pharmaceutical product was discussed in Sect. 1.4. In this problem, the objective is to understand the relationship between biological measurements of the raw materials (predictors), measurements of the manufacturing process (predictors), and the response of product yield. Biological predictors cannot be changed but can be used to assess the quality of the raw material before processing. On the other hand, manufacturing process predictors can be changed in the manufacturing process. Improving product yield by 1 % will boost revenue by approximately one hundred thousand dollars per batch:

(a) Start R and use these commands to load the data:

```
> library(AppliedPredictiveModeling)
> data(chemicalManufacturingProcess)
```

The matrix processPredictors contains the 57 predictors (12 describing the input biological material and 45 describing the process predictors) for the 176 manufacturing runs. yield contains the percent yield for each run.

(b) A small percentage of cells in the predictor set contain missing values. Use an imputation function to fill in these missing values (e.g., see Sect. 3.8).

(c) Split the data into a training and a test set, pre-process the data, and tune a model of your choice from this chapter. What is the optimal value of the performance metric?

(d) Predict the response for the test set. What is the value of the performance metric and how does this compare with the resampled performance metric on the training set?

(e) Which predictors are most important in the model you have trained? Do either the biological or process predictors dominate the list?

(f) Explore the relationships between each of the top predictors and the response. How could this information be helpful in improving yield in future runs of the manufacturing process?

Chapter 7
Nonlinear Regression Models

The previous chapter discussed regression models that were intrinsically linear. Many of these models can be adapted to nonlinear trends in the data by manually adding model terms (e.g., squared terms). However, to do this, one must know the specific nature of the nonlinearity in the data.

There are numerous regression models that are inherently nonlinear in nature. When using these models, the exact form of the nonlinearity does not need to be known explicitly or specified prior to model training. This chapter looks at several models: neural networks, multivariate adaptive regression splines (MARS), support vector machines (SVMs), and K-nearest neighbors (KNNs). Tree-based models are also nonlinear. Due to their popularity and use in ensemble models, we have devoted the next chapter to those methods.

7.1 Neural Networks

Neural networks (Bishop 1995; Ripley 1996; Titterington 2010) are powerful nonlinear regression techniques inspired by theories about how the brain works. Like partial least squares, the outcome is modeled by an intermediary set of unobserved variables (called *hidden variables* or *hidden units* here). These hidden units are linear combinations of the original predictors, but, unlike PLS models, they are not estimated in a hierarchical fashion (Fig. 7.1).

As previously stated, each hidden unit is a linear combination of some or all of the predictor variables. However, this linear combination is typically transformed by a nonlinear function $g(\cdot)$, such as the logistic (i.e., sigmoidal) function:

$$h_k(\mathbf{x}) = g\left(\beta_{0k} + \sum_{i=1}^{P} x_j \beta_{jk}\right), \quad \text{where}$$

$$g(u) = \frac{1}{1 + e^{-u}}.$$

M. Kuhn and K. Johnson, *Applied Predictive Modeling*,
DOI 10.1007/978-1-4614-6849-3_7,
© Springer Science+Business Media New York 2013

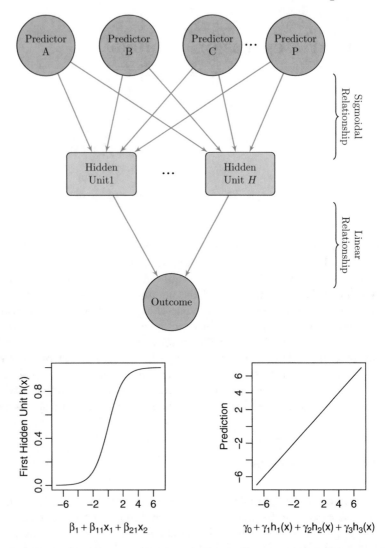

Fig. 7.1: A diagram of a neural network with a single hidden layer. The hidden units are linear combinations of the predictors that have been transformed by a sigmoidal function. The output is modeled by a linear combination of the hidden units

The β coefficients are similar to regression coefficients; coefficient β_{jk} is the effect of the jth predictor on the kth hidden unit. A neural network model usually involves multiple hidden units to model the outcome. Note that, unlike the linear combinations in PLS, there are no constraints that help define these linear combinations. Because of this, there is little likelihood that the coefficients in each unit represent some coherent piece of information.

Once the number of hidden units is defined, each unit must be related to the outcome. Another linear combination connects the hidden units to the outcome:

$$f(\mathbf{x}) = \gamma_0 + \sum_{k=1}^{H} \gamma_k h_k.$$

For this type of network model and P predictors, there are a total of $H(P+1) + H + 1$ total parameters being estimated, which quickly becomes large as P increases. For the solubility data, recall that there are 228 predictors. A neural network model with three hidden units would estimate 691 parameters while a model with five hidden units would have 1,151 coefficients.

Treating this model as a nonlinear regression model, the parameters are usually optimized to minimize the sum of the squared residuals. This can be a challenging numerical optimization problem (recall that there are no constraints on the parameters of this complex nonlinear model). The parameters are usually initialized to random values and then specialized algorithms for solving the equations are used. The back-propagation algorithm (Rumelhart et al. 1986) is a highly efficient methodology that works with derivatives to find the optimal parameters. However, it is common that a solution to this equation is not a *global* solution, meaning that we cannot guarantee that the resulting set of parameters are uniformly better than any other set.

Also, neural networks have a tendency to over-fit the relationship between the predictors and the response due to the large number of regression coefficients. To combat this issue, several different approaches have been proposed. First, the iterative algorithms for solving for the regression equations can be prematurely halted (Wang and Venkatesh 1984). This approach is referred to as *early stopping* and would stop the optimization procedure when some estimate of the error rate starts to increase (instead of some numerical tolerance to indicate that the parameter estimates or error rate are stable). However, there are obvious issues with this procedure. First, how do we estimate the model error? The apparent error rate can be highly optimistic (as discussed in Sect. 4.1) and further splitting of the training set can be problematic. Also, since the measured error rate has some amount of uncertainty associated with it, how can we tell if it is truly increasing?

Another approach to moderating over-fitting is to use *weight decay*, a penalization method to *regularize* the model similar to ridge regression discussed in the last chapter. Here, we add a penalty for large regression coefficients so that any large value must have a significant effect on the model errors to be tolerated. Formally, the optimization produced would try to minimize a alternative version of the sum of the squared errors:

$$\sum_{i=1}^{n} (y_i - f_i(x))^2 + \lambda \sum_{k=1}^{H} \sum_{j=0}^{P} \beta_{jk}^2 + \lambda \sum_{k=0}^{H} \gamma_k^2$$

for a given value of λ. As the regularization value increases, the fitted model becomes more smooth and less likely to over-fit the training set. Of course, the value of this parameter must be specified and, along with the number of hidden units, is a tuning parameter for the model. Reasonable values of λ range between 0 and 0.1. Also note that since the regression coefficients are being summed, they should be on the same scale; hence the predictors should be centered and scaled prior to modeling.

The structure of the model described here is the simplest neural network architecture: a single-layer feed-forward network. There are many other kinds, such as models where there are more than one layer of hidden units (i.e., there is a layer of hidden units that models the other hidden units). Also, other model architectures have loops going both directions between layers. Practitioners of these models may also remove specific connections between objects to further optimize the model. There have also been several Bayesian approaches to neural networks (Neal 1996). The Bayesian framework outlined in Neal (1996) for these models automatically incorporates regularization and automatic feature selection. This approach to neural networks is very powerful, but the computational aspects of the model become even more formidable. A model very similar to neural networks is self-organizing maps (Kohonen 1995). This model can be used as an unsupervised, exploratory technique or in a supervised fashion for prediction (Melssen et al. 2006).

Given the challenge of estimating a large number of parameters, the fitted model finds parameter estimates that are locally optimal; that is, the algorithm converges, but the resulting parameter estimates are unlikely to be the globally optimal estimates. Very often, different locally optimal solutions can produce models that are very different but have nearly equivalent performance. This model instability can sometimes hinder this model. As an alternative, several models can be created using different starting values and averaging the results of these model to produce a more stable prediction (Perrone and Cooper 1993; Ripley 1995; Tumer and Ghosh 1996). Such *model averaging* often has a significantly positive effect on neural networks.

These models are often adversely affected by high correlation among the predictor variables (since they use gradients to optimize the model parameters). Two approaches for mitigating this issue is to pre-filter the predictors to remove the predictors that are associated with high correlations. Alternatively a feature extraction technique, such as principal component analysis, can be used prior to modeling to eliminate correlations. One positive side effect of both these approaches is that fewer model terms need to be optimized, thus improving computation time.

For the solubility data, model averaged neural networks were used. Three different weight decay values were evaluated ($\lambda = 0.00, 0.01, 0.10$) along with a single hidden layer with sizes ranging between 1 and 13 hidden units. The final predictions are the averages of five different neural networks created using different initial parameter values. The cross-validated RMSE profiles of these models are displayed in Fig. 7.2. Increasing the amount of weight decay

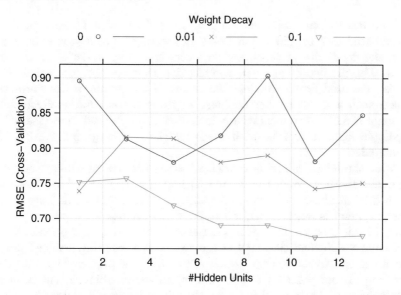

Fig. 7.2: RMSE profiles for the neural network model. The optimal model used $\lambda = 0.1$ and 11 hidden units

clearly improved model performance, while more hidden units also reduce the model error. The optimal model used 11 hidden units with a total of 2,531 coefficients. The performance of the model is fairly stable for a high degree of regularization (i.e., $\lambda = 0.1$), so smaller models could also be effective for these data.

7.2 Multivariate Adaptive Regression Splines

Like neural networks and partial least squares, MARS (Friedman 1991) uses surrogate features instead of the original predictors. However, whereas PLS and neural networks are based on linear combinations of the predictors, MARS creates two contrasted versions of a predictor to enter the model. Also, the surrogate features in MARS are usually a function of only one or two predictors at a time. The nature of the MARS features breaks the predictor into two groups and models linear relationships between the predictor and the outcome in each group. Specifically, given a cut point for a predictor, two new features are "hinge" or "hockey stick" functions of the original (see Fig. 7.3). The "left-hand" feature has values of zero greater than the cut point, while the second feature is zero less than the cut point. The new features are added to a basic linear regression model to estimate the slopes and intercepts. In effect, this scheme creates a *piecewise linear model* where each new feature models an isolated portion of the original data.

How was the cut point determined? Each data point for each predictor is evaluated as a candidate cut point by creating a linear regression model with the candidate features, and the corresponding model error is calculated. The predictor/cut point combination that achieves the smallest error is then used for the model. The nature of the predictor transformation makes such a large number of linear regressions computationally feasible. In some MARS implementations, including the one used here, the utility of simple linear terms for each predictor (i.e., no hinge function) is also evaluated.

After the initial model is created with the first two features, the model conducts another exhaustive search to find the next set of features that, given the initial set, yield the best model fit. This process continues until a stopping point is reached (which can be set by the user).

In the initial search for features in the solubility data, a cut point of 5.9 for molecular weight had the smallest error rate. The resulting artificial predictors are shown in the top two panels of Fig. 7.3. One predictor has all values less than the cut point set to zero and values greater than the cut point are left unchanged. The second feature is the mirror image of the first. Instead of the original data, these two new predictors are used to predict the outcome in a linear regression model. The bottom panel of Fig. 7.3 shows the result of the linear regression with the two new features and the piecewise nature of the relationship. The "left-hand" feature is associated with a negative slope when the molecular weight is less than 5.9 while the "right-hand" feature estimates a positive slope for larger values of the predictor.

Mathematically, the hinge function for new features can be written as

$$h(x) = \begin{cases} x & x > 0 \\ 0 & x \leq 0 \end{cases} \tag{7.1}$$

A pair of hinge functions is usually written as $h(x - a)$ and $h(a - x)$. The first is nonzero when $x > a$, while the second is nonzero when $x < a$. Note that when this is true the value of the function is actually $-x$. For the MARS model shown in Fig. 7.3, the actual model equation would be

$$-5 + 2.1 \times h(MolWeight - 5.94516) + 3 \times h(5.94516 - MolWeight).$$

The first term in this equation (-5) is the intercept. The second term is associated with the right-hand feature shown in Fig. 7.3, while the third term is associated with the left-hand feature.

Table 7.1 shows the first few steps of the feature generation phase (prior to pruning). The features were entered into the linear regression model from top to bottom. Here the binary fingerprint descriptor enters the model as a plain linear term (splitting a binary variable would be nonsensical). The generalized cross-validation (GCV) column shows the estimated RMSE for

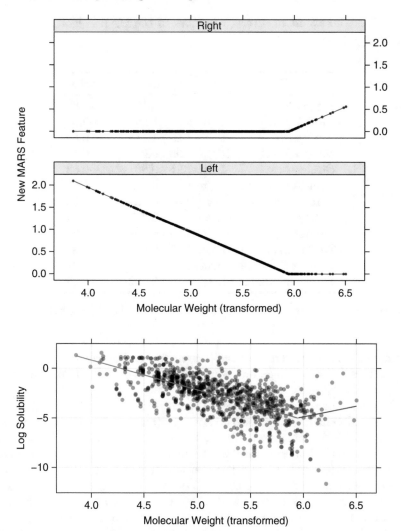

Fig. 7.3: An example of the features used by MARS for the solubility data. After finding a cut point of 5.9 for molecular weight, two new features are created and used in a linear regression model. The *top* two panels show the relationship between the original predictor and the two resulting features. The *bottom* panel shows the predicted relationship when using these two features in a linear regression model. The *red line* indicates the contribution of the "left-hand" hinge function while the *blue line* is associated with the other feature

Table 7.1: The results of several iterations of the MARS algorithm prior to pruning

Predictor	Type	Cut	RMSE	Coefficient
Intercept			4.193	−9.33
MolWeight	Right	5.95	2.351	−3.23
MolWeight	Left	5.95	1.148	0.66
SurfaceArea1	Right	1.96	0.935	0.19
SurfaceArea1	Left	1.96	0.861	−0.66
NumNonHAtoms	Right	3.00	0.803	−7.51
NumNonHAtoms	Left	3.00	0.761	8.53
FP137	Linear		0.727	1.24
NumOxygen	Right	1.39	0.701	2.22
NumOxygen	Left	1.39	0.683	−0.43
NumNonHBonds	Right	2.58	0.670	2.21
NumNonHBonds	Left	2.58	0.662	−3.29

The root mean squared error was estimated using the GCV statistic

the model containing terms on the current row and all rows above. Prior to pruning, each pair of hinge functions is kept in the model despite the slight reduction in the estimated RMSE.

Once the full set of features has been created, the algorithm sequentially removes individual features that do not contribute significantly to the model equation. This "pruning" procedure assesses each predictor variable and estimates how much the error rate was decreased by including it in the model. This process does not proceed backwards along the path that the features were added; some features deemed important at the beginning of the process may be removed while features added towards the end might be retained. To determine the contribution of each feature to the model, the *GCV* statistic is used. This value is a computational shortcut for linear regression models that produces an error value that approximates leave-one-out cross-validation (Golub et al. 1979). GCV produces better estimates than the apparent error rate for determining the importance of each feature in the model. The number of terms to remove can be manually set or treated as a tuning parameter and determined using some other form of resampling.

The process above is a description of an additive MARS model where each surrogate feature involves a single predictor. However, MARS can build models where the features involve multiple predictors at once. With a *second-degree* MARS model, the algorithm would conduct the same search of a single term that improves the model and, after creating the initial pair of features, would instigate another search to create new cuts to couple with each of the original features. Suppose the pair of hinge functions are denoted as A and B.

The search procedure attempts to find hinge functions C and D that, when multiplied by A, result in an improvement in the model; in other words, the model would have terms for A, $A \times B$ and $A \times C$. The same procedure would occur for feature B. Note that the algorithm will not add additional terms if the model is not improved by their addition. Also, the pruning procedure may eliminate the additional terms. For MARS models that can include two or more terms at a time, we have observed occasional instabilities in the model predictions where a few sample predictions are wildly inaccurate (perhaps an order of magnitude off of the true value). This problem has not been observed with additive MARS models.

To summarize, there are two tuning parameters associated with the MARS model: the degree of the features that are added to the model and the number of retained terms. The latter parameter can be automatically determined using the default pruning procedure (using GCV), set by the user or determined using an external resampling technique. For our analysis of the solubility data, we used 10-fold cross-validation to characterize model performance over first- and second-order models and 37 values for the number of model terms, ranging from 2 to 38. The resulting performance profile is shown in Fig. 7.4. There appears to be very little difference in the first- and second-degree models in terms of RMSE.

The cross-validation procedure picked a second-degree model with 38 terms. However, because the profiles of the first- and second-order model are almost identical, the more parsimonious first-order model was chosen as the final model. This model used 38 terms but was a function of only 30 predictors (out of a possible 228).

Cross-validation estimated the RMSE to be 0.7 log units and the R^2 to be 0.887. Recall that the MARS procedure internally uses GCV to estimate model performance. Using GCV, the RMSE was estimated to be 0.4 log units and an R^2 of 0.908. Using the test set of 316 samples, the RMSE was determined to be 0.7 with a corresponding R^2 of 0.879. Clearly, the GCV estimates are more encouraging than those obtained by the cross-validation procedure or the test set. However, note that the internal GCV estimate that MARS employs evaluates an individual model while the external cross-validation procedure is exposed to the variation in the entire model building process, including feature selection. Since the GCV estimate does not reflect the uncertainty from feature selection, it suffers from *selection bias* (Ambroise and McLachlan 2002). This phenomenon will be discussed more in Chap. 19.

There are several advantages to using MARS. First, the model automatically conducts feature selection; the model equation is independent of predictor variables that are not involved with any of the final model features. This point cannot be underrated. Given a large number of predictors seen in many problem domains, MARS potentially thins the predictor set using the same algorithm that builds the model. In this way, the feature selection routine has a direct connection to functional performance. The second advantage is interpretability. Each hinge feature is responsible for modeling a specific

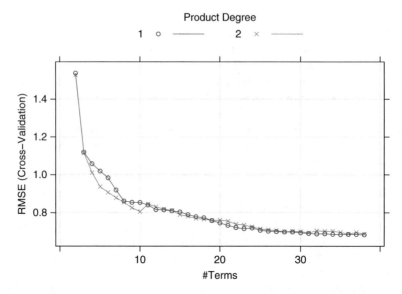

Fig. 7.4: RMSE profiles for the MARS model. The cross-validation procedure picked a second-degree model with 38 terms, although there is little difference between the first- and second-degree models. Given this equivalence, the more simplistic first-order model was chosen as the final model

region in the predictor space using a (piecewise) linear model. When the MARS model is additive, the contribution of each predictor can be isolated without the need to consider the others. This can be used to provide clear interpretations of how each predictor relates to the outcome. For nonadditive models, the interpretive power of the model is not reduced. Consider a second-degree feature involving two predictors. Since each hinge function is split into two regions, three of the four possible regions will be zero and offer no contribution to the model. Because of this, the effect of the two factors can be further isolated, making the interpretation as simple as the additive model. Finally, the MARS model requires very little pre-processing of the data; data transformations and the filtering of predictors are not needed. For example, a zero variance predictor will never be chosen for a split since it offers no possible predictive information. Correlated predictors do not drastically affect model performance, but they can complicate model interpretation. Suppose the training set contained two predictors that were nearly perfectly correlated. Since MARS can select a predictor more than once during the iterations, the choice of which predictor is used in the feature is essentially random. In this case, the model interpretation is hampered by two redundant pieces of information that show up in different parts of the model under different names.

Another method to help understand the nature of how the predictors affect the model is to quantify their *importance* to the model. For MARS, one technique for doing this is to track the reduction in the root mean squared error (as measured using the GCV statistic) that occurs when adding a particular feature to the model. This reduction is attributed to the original predictor(s) associated with the feature. These improvements in the model can be aggregated for each predictor as a relative measure of the impact on the model. As seen in Table 7.1, there is a drop in the RMSE from 4.19 to 1.15 (a reduction of 3.04) after the two molecular weight features were added to the model. After this, adding terms for the first surface area predictor decreases the error by 0.29. Given these numbers, it would appear that the molecular weight predictor is more important to the model than the first surface area predictor. This process is repeated for every predictor used in the model. Predictors that were not used in any feature have an importance of zero. For the solubility model, the predictors MolWeight, NumNonHAtoms, and SurfaceArea2 appear to be have the greatest influence on the MARS model (see the Computing section at the end of the chapter for more details).

Figure 7.5 illustrates the interpretability of the additive MARS model with the continuous predictors. For each panel, the line represents the prediction profile for that variable when all the others are held constant at their mean level. The additive nature of the model allows each predictor to be viewed in isolation; changing the values of the other predictor variables will not alter the shape of the profile, only the location on the y-axis where the profile starts.

7.3 Support Vector Machines

SVMs are a class of powerful, highly flexible modeling techniques. The theory behind SVMs was originally developed in the context of classification models. Later, in Chap. 13, the motivation for this technique is discussed in its more natural form. For regression, we follow Smola (1996) and Drucker et al. (1997) and motivate this technique in the framework of *robust regression* where we seek to minimize the effect of outliers on the regression equations. Also, there are several flavors of support vector regression and we focus on one particular technique called ϵ-*insensitive regression*.

Recall that linear regression seeks to find parameter estimates that minimize SSE (Sect. 6.2). One drawback of minimizing SSE is that the parameter estimates can be influenced by just one observation that falls far from the overall trend in the data. When data may contain influential observations, an alternative minimization metric that is less sensitive, such as the Huber function, can be used to find the best parameter estimates. This function uses the squared residuals when they are "small" and uses the absolute residuals when the residuals are large. See Fig. 6.6 on p. 110 for an illustration.

SVMs for regression use a function similar to the Huber function, with an important difference. Given a threshold set by the user (denoted as ϵ),

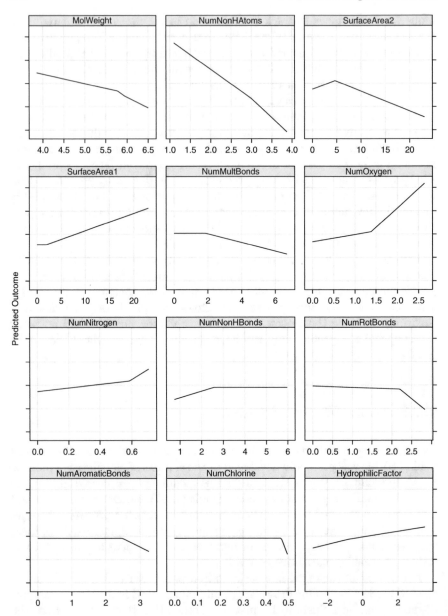

Fig. 7.5: The predicted relationship between the outcome and the continuous predictors using the MARS model (holding all other predictors at their mean value). The additive nature of the model allows each predictor to be viewed in isolation. Note that the final predicted values are the summation of each individual profile. The panels are ordered from top to bottom by their importance to the model

data points with residuals within the threshold do not contribute to the regression fit while data points with an absolute difference greater than the threshold contribute a linear-scale amount. There are several consequences to this approach. First, since the squared residuals are not used, large outliers have a limited effect on the regression equation. Second, samples that the model fits well (i.e., the residuals are small) have *no* effect on the regression equation. In fact, if the threshold is set to a relatively large value, then the outliers are the only points that define the regression line! This is somewhat counterintuitive: the poorly predicted points define the line. However, this approach has been shown to be very effective in defining the model.

To estimate the model parameters, SVM uses the ϵ loss function shown in Fig. 7.6 but also adds a penalty. The SVM regression coefficients minimize

$$Cost \sum_{i=1}^{n} L_\epsilon(y_i - \hat{y}_i) + \sum_{j=1}^{P} \beta_j^2,$$

where $L_\epsilon(\cdot)$ is the ϵ-insensitive function. The *Cost* parameter is the *cost* penalty that is set by the user, which penalizes large residuals.[1]

Recall that the simple linear regression model predicted new samples using linear combinations of the data and parameters. For a new sample, u, the prediction equation is

$$\hat{y} = \beta_0 + \beta_1 u_1 + \ldots + \beta_P u_P$$

$$= \beta_0 + \sum_{j=1}^{P} \beta_j u_j$$

The linear support vector machine prediction function is very similar. The parameter estimates can be written as functions of a set of unknown parameters (α_i) and the training set data points so that

$$\hat{y} = \beta_0 + \beta_1 u_1 + \ldots + \beta_P u_P$$

$$= \beta_0 + \sum_{j=1}^{P} \beta_j u_j$$

$$= \beta_0 + \sum_{j=1}^{P} \sum_{i=1}^{n} \alpha_i x_{ij} u_j$$

$$= \beta_0 + \sum_{i=1}^{n} \alpha_i \left(\sum_{j=1}^{P} x_{ij} u_j \right). \qquad (7.2)$$

---

[1] The penalty here is written as the reverse of ridge regression or weight decay in neural networks since it is attached to residuals and not the parameters.

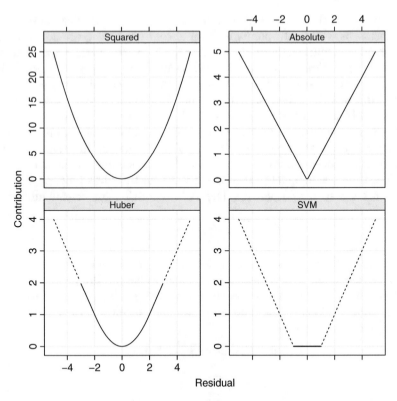

Fig. 7.6: The relationship between a model residual and its contribution to the regression line for several techniques. For the Huber approach, a threshold of 2 was used while for the support vector machine, a value of $\epsilon = 1$ was used. Note that the y-axis scales are different to make the figures easier to read

There are several aspects of this equation worth pointing out. First, there are as many α parameters as there are data points. From the standpoint of classical regression modeling, this model would be considered *overparameterized*; typically, it is better to estimate fewer parameters than data points. However, the use of the cost value effectively regularizes the model to help alleviate this problem.

Second, the individual training set data points (i.e., the x_{ij}) are required for new predictions. When the training set is large, this makes the prediction equations less compact than other techniques. However, for some percentage of the training set samples, the α_i parameters will be exactly zero, indicating that they have no impact on the prediction equation. The data points associated with an α_i parameter of zero are the training set samples that are within $\pm\epsilon$ of the regression line (i.e., are within the "funnel" or "tube" around the regression line). As a consequence, only a subset of training set data points, where $\alpha \neq 0$, are needed for prediction. Since the regression line is determined using these samples, they are called the *support vectors* as they support the regression line.

Figure 7.7 illustrates the robustness of this model. A simple linear model was simulated with a slope of 4 and an intercept of 1; one extreme outlier was added to the data. The top panel shows the model fit for a linear regression model (black solid line) and a support vector machine regression model (blue dashed line) with $\epsilon = 0.01$. The linear regression line is pulled towards this point, resulting in estimates of the slope and intercept of 3.5 and 1.2, respectively. The support vector regression fit is shown in blue and is much closer to the true regression line with a slope of 3.9 and an intercept of 0.9. The middle panel again shows the SVM model, but the support vectors are solid black circles and the other points are shown in red. The horizontal grey reference lines indicate zero $\pm \epsilon$. Out of 100 data points, 70 of these were support vectors.

Finally, note that in the last form of Eq. 7.2, the new samples enter into the prediction function as sum of cross products with the new sample values. In matrix algebra terms, this corresponds to a *dot product* (i.e., $\mathbf{x}'\mathbf{u}$). This is important because this regression equation can be rewritten more generally as

$$f(\mathbf{u}) = \beta_0 + \sum_{i=1}^{n} \alpha_i K(\mathbf{x}_i, \mathbf{u}),$$

where $K(\cdot)$ is called the *kernel function*. When predictors enter the model linearly, the kernel function reduces to a simple sum of cross products shown above:

$$K(\mathbf{x}_i, \mathbf{u}) = \sum_{j=1}^{P} x_{ij} u_j = \mathbf{x}_i'\mathbf{u}.$$

However, there are other types of kernel functions that can be used to generalize the regression model and encompass *nonlinear* functions of the predictors:

$$\text{polynomial} = \left(\phi\left(\mathbf{x}'\mathbf{u}\right) + 1\right)^{degree}$$
$$\text{radial basis function} = \exp(-\sigma\|\mathbf{x} - \mathbf{u}\|^2)$$
$$\text{hyperbolic tangent} = \tanh\left(\phi\left(\mathbf{x}'\mathbf{u}\right) + 1\right),$$

where ϕ and σ are scaling parameters. Since these functions of the predictors lead to nonlinear models, this generalization is often called the "kernel trick."

To illustrate the ability of this model to adapt to nonlinear relationships, we simulated data that follow a sin wave in the bottom of Fig. 7.7. Outliers were also added to these data. A linear regression model with an intercept and a term for $sin(x)$ was fit to the model (solid black line). Again, the regression line is pulled towards the outlying points. An SVM model with a radial basis kernel function is represented by the blue dashed line (without specifying the *sin* functional form). This line better describes the overall structure of the data.

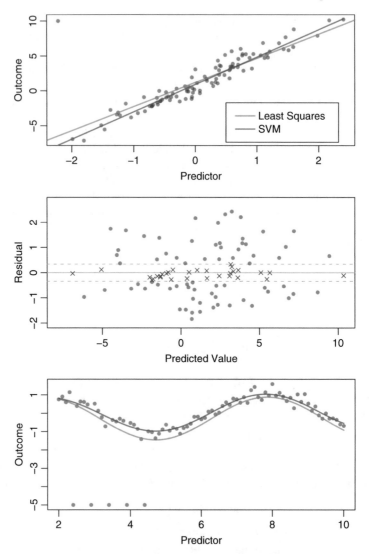

Fig. 7.7: The robustness qualities of SVM models. *Top*: a small simulated data set with a single large outlier is used to show the difference between an ordinary regression line (*red*) and the linear SVM model (*blue*). *Middle*: the SVM residuals versus the predicted values (the upper end of the y-axis scale was reduced to make the plot more readable). The plot symbols indicate the support vectors (shown as *grey colored circles*) and the other samples (*red crosses*). The *horizontal lines* are $\pm\epsilon = 0.01$. *Bottom*: A simulated sin wave with several outliers. The *red line* is an ordinary regression line (intercept and a term for $sin(x)$) and the *blue line* is a radial basis function SVM model

Which kernel function should be used? This depends on the problem. The radial basis function has been shown to be very effective. However, when the regression line is truly linear, the linear kernel function will be a better choice.

Note that some of the kernel functions have extra parameters. For example, the polynomial degree in the polynomial kernel must be specified. Similarly, the radial basis function has a parameter (σ) that controls the scale. These parameters, along with the cost value, constitute the tuning parameters for the model. In the case of the radial basis function, there is a possible computational shortcut to estimating the kernel parameter. Caputo et al. (2002) suggested that the parameter can be estimated using combinations of the training set points to calculate the distribution of $||x - x'||^2$, then use the 10th and 90th percentiles as a range for σ. Instead of tuning this parameter over a grid of candidate values, we can use the midpoint of these two percentiles.

The cost parameter is the main tool for adjusting the complexity of the model. When the cost is large, the model becomes very flexible since the effect of errors is amplified. When the cost is small, the model will "stiffen" and become less likely to over-fit (but more likely to underfit) because the contribution of the squared parameters is proportionally large in the modified error function. One could also tune the model over the size of the funnel (e.g., over ϵ). However, there is a relationship between ϵ and the cost parameter. In our experience, we have found that the cost parameter provides more flexibility for tuning the model. So we suggest fixing a value for ϵ and tuning over the other kernel parameters.

Since the predictors enter into the model as the sum of cross products, differences in the predictor scales can affect the model. Therefore, we recommend centering and scaling the predictors prior to building an SVM model.

SVMs were applied to the solubility data. First, a radial basis function kernel was used. The kernel parameter was estimated analytically to be $\sigma = 0.0039$ and the model was tuned over 14 cost values between 0.25 and 2048 on the $\log_2$ scale (Fig. 7.8). When the cost values are small, the model *under*-fits the data, but, as the error starts to increase when the cost approaches 2^{10}, over-fitting begins. The cost value associated with the smallest RMSE was 128. A polynomial model was also evaluated. Here, we tuned over the cost, the polynomial degree, and a scale factor. In general, quadratic models have smaller error rates than the linear models. Also, models associated with larger-scale factors have better performance. The optimal model was quadratic with a scale factor of 0.01 and a cost value of 2 (Fig. 7.9).

As a comparison, both the optimal radial basis and the polynomial SVM models use a similar number of support vectors, 623 and 627, respectively (out of 951 training samples). Also it is important to point out that tuning the radial basis function kernel parameter was easier than tuning the polynomial model (which has three tuning parameters).

The literature on SVM models and other kernel methods has been vibrant and many alternate methodologies have been proposed. One method,

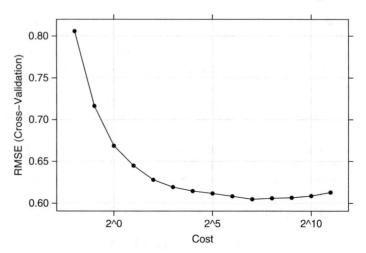

Fig. 7.8: The cross-validation profiles for a radial basis function SVM model applied to the solubility data. The kernel parameter was estimated analytically to be $\sigma = 0.0039$

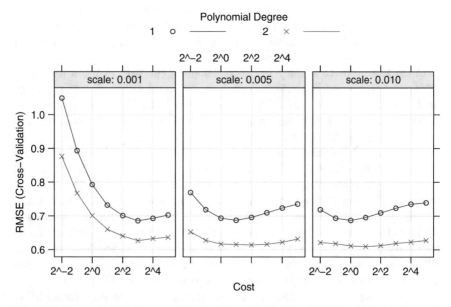

Fig. 7.9: Cross-validation results for the polynomial SVM model for the solubility data. The final model was fit using a quadratic model with a scale factor of 0.01 and a cost value of 2

the *relevance vector machine* (Tipping 2001), is a Bayesian analog to the SVM model. In this case, the α parameters described above have associated prior distributions and the selection of *relevance vectors* is determined using their posterior distribution. If the posterior distribution is highly concentrated around zero, the sample is not used in the prediction equation. There are usually less relevance vectors in this model than support vectors in an SVM model.

7.4 *K*-Nearest Neighbors

The *K*NN approach simply predicts a new sample using the *K*-closest samples from the training set (similar to Fig. 4.3). Unlike other methods in this chapter, *K*NN cannot be cleanly summarized by a model like the one presented in Eq. 7.2. Instead, its construction is solely based on the individual samples from the training data. To predict a new sample for regression, *K*NN identifies that sample's *K*NNs in the predictor space. The predicted response for the new sample is then the mean of the *K* neighbors' responses. Other summary statistics, such as the median, can also be used in place of the mean to predict the new sample.

The basic *K*NN method as described above depends on how the user defines distance between samples. Euclidean distance (i.e., the straight-line distance between two samples) is the most commonly used metric and is defined as follows:

$$\left(\sum_{j=1}^{P} (x_{aj} - x_{bj})^2 \right)^{\frac{1}{2}},$$

where $\mathbf{x_a}$ and $\mathbf{x_b}$ are two individual samples. Minkowski distance is a generalization of Euclidean distance and is defined as

$$\left(\sum_{j=1}^{P} |x_{aj} - x_{bj}|^q \right)^{\frac{1}{q}},$$

where $q > 0$ (Liu 2007). It is easy to see that when $q = 2$, then Minkowski distance is the same as Euclidean distance. When $q = 1$, then Minkowski distance is equivalent to Manhattan (or city-block) distance, which is a common metric used for samples with binary predictors. Many other distance metrics exist, such as Tanimoto, Hamming, and cosine, and are more appropriate for specific types of predictors and in specific scientific contexts. Tanimoto distance, for example, is regularly used in computational chemistry problems when molecules are described using binary fingerprints (McCarren et al. 2011).

Because the KNN method fundamentally depends on distance between samples, the scale of the predictors can have a dramatic influence on the distances among samples. Data with predictors that are on vastly different scales will generate distances that are weighted towards predictors that have the largest scales. That is, predictors with the largest scales will contribute most to the distance between samples. To avoid this potential bias and to enable each predictor to contribute equally to the distance calculation, we recommend that all predictors be centered and scaled prior to performing KNN.

In addition to the issue of scaling, using distances between samples can be problematic if one or more of the predictor values for a sample is missing, since it is then not possible to compute the distance between samples. If this is the case, then the analyst has a couple of options. First, either the samples or the predictors can be excluded from the analysis. This is the least desirable option; however, it may be the only practical choice if the sample(s) or predictor(s) are sparse. If a predictor contains a sufficient amount of information across the samples, then an alternative approach is to impute the missing data using a naïve estimator such as the mean of the predictor, or a nearest neighbor approach that uses only the predictors with complete information (see Sect. 3.4).

Upon pre-processing the data and selecting the distance metric, the next step is to find the optimal number of neighbors. Like tuning parameters from other models, K can be determined by resampling. For the solubility data, 20 values of K ranging between 1 and 20 were evaluated. As illustrated in Fig. 7.10, the RMSE profile rapidly decreases across the first four values of K, then levels off through $K = 8$, followed by a steady increase in RMSE as K increases. This performance profile is typical for KNN, since small values of K usually over-fit and large values of K underfit the data. RMSE ranged from 1.041 to 1.23 across the candidate values, with the minimum occurring at $K = 4$; cross-validated R^2 at the optimum K is 0.747.

The elementary version of KNN is intuitive and straightforward and can produce decent predictions, especially when the response is dependent on the local predictor structure. However, this version does have some notable problems, of which researchers have sought solutions. Two commonly noted problems are computational time and the disconnect between local structure and the predictive ability of KNN.

First, to predict a sample, distances between the sample and all other samples must be computed. Computation time therefore increases with n because the training data must be loaded into memory and because distances between the new sample and all of the training samples must be computed. To mitigate this problem, one can replace the original data with a less memory-intensive representation of the data that describes the locations of the original data. One specific example of this representation is a k-dimensional tree (or k-d tree) (Bentley 1975). A k-d tree orthogonally partitions the predictor space using a tree approach but with different rules than the kinds of trees described

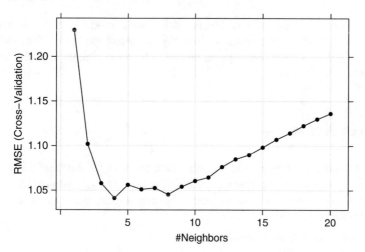

Fig. 7.10: The RMSE cross-validation profile for a KNN model applied to the solubility data. The optimal number of neighbors is 4

in Chap. 8. After the tree has been grown, a new sample is placed through the structure. Distances are only computed for those training observations in the tree that are close to the new sample. This approach provides significant computational improvements, especially when the number of training samples is much larger than the number of predictors.

The KNN method can have poor predictive performance when local predictor structure is not relevant to the response. Irrelevant or noisy predictors are one culprit, since these can cause similar samples to be driven away from each other in the predictor space. Hence, removing irrelevant, noise-laden predictors is a key pre-processing step for KNN. Another approach to enhancing KNN predictivity is to weight the neighbors' contribution to the prediction of a new sample based on their distance to the new sample. In this variation, training samples that are closer to the new sample contribute more to the predicted response, while those that are farther away contribute less to the predicted response.

7.5 Computing

This section will reference functions from the caret, earth, kernlab, and nnet packages.

R has a number of packages and functions for creating neural networks. Relevant packages include nnet, neural, and RSNNS. The nnet package is the focus here since it supports the basic neural network models outlined in this chapter (i.e., a single layer of hidden units) and weight decay and has simple syntax. RSNNS supports a wide array of neural networks. Bergmeir and Benitez (2012) outline the various neural network packages in R and contain a tutorial on RSNNS.

Neural Networks

To fit a regression model, the nnet function takes both the formula and non-formula interfaces. For regression, the linear relationship between the hidden units and the prediction can be used with the option linout = TRUE. A basic neural network function call would be

```
> nnetFit <- nnet(predictors, outcome,
+               size = 5,
+               decay = 0.01,
+               linout = TRUE,
+               ## Reduce the amount of printed output
+               trace = FALSE,
+               ## Expand the number of iterations to find
+               ## parameter estimates..
+               maxit = 500,
+               ## and the number of parameters used by the model
+               MaxNWts = 5 * (ncol(predictors) + 1) + 5 + 1)
```

This would create a single model with 5 hidden units. Note, this assumes that the data in predictors have been standardized to be on the same scale.

To use model averaging, the avNNet function in the caret package has nearly identical syntax:

```
> nnetAvg <- avNNet(predictors, outcome,
+               size = 5,
+               decay = 0.01,
+               ## Specify how many models to average
+               repeats = 5,
+               linout = TRUE,
+               ## Reduce the amount of printed output
+               trace = FALSE,
+               ## Expand the number of iterations to find
+               ## parameter estimates..
+               maxit = 500,
+               ## and the number of parameters used by the model
+               MaxNWts = 5 * (ncol(predictors) + 1) + 5 + 1)
```

Again, new samples are processed using

```
> predict(nnetFit, newData)
> ## or
> predict(nnetAvg, newData)
```

To mimic the earlier approach of choosing the number of hidden units and the amount of weight decay via resampling, the train function can be applied using either method = "nnet" or method = "avNNet". First, we remove predictors to ensure that the maximum absolute pairwise correlation between the predictors is less than 0.75.

```
> ## The findCorrelation takes a correlation matrix and determines the
> ## column numbers that should be removed to keep all pair-wise
> ## correlations below a threshold
> tooHigh <- findCorrelation(cor(solTrainXtrans), cutoff = .75)
> trainXnnet <- solTrainXtrans[, -tooHigh]
> testXnnet <- solTestXtrans[, -tooHigh]
> ## Create a specific candidate set of models to evaluate:
> nnetGrid <- expand.grid(.decay = c(0, 0.01, .1),
+                         .size = c(1:10),
+                         ## The next option is to use bagging (see the
+                         ## next chapter) instead of different random
+                         ## seeds.
+                         .bag = FALSE)
> set.seed(100)
> nnetTune <- train(solTrainXtrans, solTrainY,
+                   method = "avNNet",
+                   tuneGrid = nnetGrid,
+                   trControl = ctrl,
+                   ## Automatically standardize data prior to modeling
+                   ## and prediction
+                   preProc = c("center", "scale"),
+                   linout = TRUE,
+                   trace = FALSE,
+                   MaxNWts = 10 * (ncol(trainXnnet) + 1) + 10 + 1,
+                   maxit = 500)
```

Multivariate Adaptive Regression Splines

MARS models are in several packages, but the most extensive implementation is in the earth package. The MARS model using the nominal forward pass and pruning step can be called simply

```
> marsFit <- earth(solTrainXtrans, solTrainY)

> marsFit
  Selected 38 of 47 terms, and 30 of 228 predictors
  Importance: NumNonHAtoms, MolWeight, SurfaceArea2, SurfaceArea1, FP142, ...
  Number of terms at each degree of interaction: 1 37 (additive model)
  GCV 0.3877448    RSS 312.877    GRSq 0.907529    RSq 0.9213739
```

Note that since this model used the internal GCV technique for model selection, the details of this model are different than the one used previously in the chapter. The summary method generates more extensive output:

```
> summary(marsFit)
```

```
Call: earth(x=solTrainXtrans, y=solTrainY)

                                        coefficients
(Intercept)                               -3.223749
FP002                                      0.517848
FP003                                     -0.228759
FP059                                     -0.582140
FP065                                     -0.273844
FP075                                      0.285520
FP083                                     -0.629746
FP085                                     -0.235622
FP099                                      0.325018
FP111                                     -0.403920
FP135                                      0.394901
FP142                                      0.407264
FP154                                     -0.620757
FP172                                     -0.514016
FP176                                      0.308482
FP188                                      0.425123
FP202                                      0.302688
FP204                                     -0.311739
FP207                                      0.457080
h(MolWeight-5.77508)                      -1.801853
h(5.94516-MolWeight)                       0.813322
h(NumNonHAtoms-2.99573)                   -3.247622
h(2.99573-NumNonHAtoms)                    2.520305
h(2.57858-NumNonHBonds)                   -0.564690
h(NumMultBonds-1.85275)                   -0.370480
h(NumRotBonds-2.19722)                    -2.753687
h(2.19722-NumRotBonds)                     0.123978
h(NumAromaticBonds-2.48491)               -1.453716
h(NumNitrogen-0.584815)                    8.239716
h(0.584815-NumNitrogen)                   -1.542868
h(NumOxygen-1.38629)                       3.304643
h(1.38629-NumOxygen)                      -0.620413
h(NumChlorine-0.46875)                   -50.431489
h(HydrophilicFactor- -0.816625)            0.237565
h(-0.816625-HydrophilicFactor)            -0.370998
h(SurfaceArea1-1.9554)                     0.149166
h(SurfaceArea2-4.66178)                   -0.169960
h(4.66178-SurfaceArea2)                   -0.157970

Selected 38 of 47 terms, and 30 of 228 predictors
Importance: NumNonHAtoms, MolWeight, SurfaceArea2, SurfaceArea1, FP142, ...
Number of terms at each degree of interaction: 1 37 (additive model)
GCV 0.3877448    RSS 312.877    GRSq 0.907529    RSq 0.9213739
```

In this output, $h(\cdot)$ is the hinge function. In the output above, the term
h(MolWeight-5.77508) is zero when the molecular weight is less than 5.77508
(i.e., similar to the top panel of Fig. 7.3). The reflected hinge function would
be shown as h(5.77508 - MolWeight).

The `plotmo` function in the **earth** package can be used to produce plots similar to Fig. 7.5. To tune the model using external resampling, the `train` function can be used. The following code reproduces the results in Fig. 7.4:

```
> # Define the candidate models to test
> marsGrid <- expand.grid(.degree = 1:2, .nprune = 2:38)
> # Fix the seed so that the results can be reproduced
> set.seed(100)
> marsTuned <- train(solTrainXtrans, solTrainY,
+                    method = "earth",
+                    # Explicitly declare the candidate models to test
+                    tuneGrid = marsGrid,
+                    trControl = trainControl(method = "cv"))

> marsTuned


951 samples
228 predictors

No pre-processing
Resampling: Cross-Validation (10-fold)

Summary of sample sizes: 856, 857, 855, 856, 856, 855, ...

Resampling results across tuning parameters:
```

degree	nprune	RMSE	Rsquared	RMSE SD	Rsquared SD
1	2	1.54	0.438	0.128	0.0802
1	3	1.12	0.7	0.0968	0.0647
1	4	1.06	0.73	0.0849	0.0594
1	5	1.02	0.75	0.102	0.0551
1	6	0.984	0.768	0.0733	0.042
1	7	0.919	0.796	0.0657	0.0432
1	8	0.862	0.821	0.0418	0.0237
:	:	:	:	:	:
2	33	0.701	0.883	0.068	0.0307
2	34	0.702	0.883	0.0699	0.0307
2	35	0.696	0.885	0.0746	0.0315
2	36	0.687	0.887	0.0604	0.0281
2	37	0.696	0.885	0.0689	0.0291
2	38	0.686	0.887	0.0626	0.029

```
RMSE was used to select the optimal model using  the smallest value.
The final values used for the model were degree = 1 and nprune = 38.

> head(predict(marsTuned, solTestXtrans))
 [1]   0.3677522 -0.1503220 -0.5051844  0.5398116 -0.4792718  0.7377222
```

There are two functions that estimate the importance of each predictor in the MARS model: `evimp` in the **earth** package and `varImp` in the **caret** package (although the latter calls the former):

```
> varImp(marsTuned)
  earth variable importance

    only 20 most important variables shown (out of 228)

               Overall
MolWeight      100.00
NumNonHAtoms    89.96
SurfaceArea2    89.51
SurfaceArea1    57.34
FP142           44.31
FP002           39.23
NumMultBonds    39.23
FP204           37.10
FP172           34.96
NumOxygen       30.70
NumNitrogen     29.12
FP083           28.21
NumNonHBonds    26.58
FP059           24.76
FP135           23.51
FP154           21.20
FP207           19.05
FP202           17.92
NumRotBonds     16.94
FP085           16.02
```

These results are scaled to be between 0 and 100 and are different than those shown in Table 7.1 (since the model in Table 7.1 did not undergo the full model growing and pruning process). Note that after the first few variables, the remainder have much smaller importance to the model.

Support Vector Machines

There are a number of R packages with implementations of support vector machine models. The svm function in the e1071 package has an interface to the LIBSVM library (Chang and Lin 2011) for regression. A more comprehensive implementation of SVM models for regression is the kernlab package (Karatzoglou et al. 2004). In that package, the ksvm function is available for regression models and a large number of kernel functions. The radial basis function is the default kernel function. If appropriate values of the cost and kernel parameters are known, this model can be fit as

```
> svmFit <- ksvm(x = solTrainXtrans, y = solTrainY,
+                kernel ="rbfdot", kpar = "automatic",
+                C = 1, epsilon = 0.1)
```

The function automatically uses the analytical approach to estimate σ. Since y is a numeric vector, the function knows to fit a regression model (instead of a classification model). Other kernel functions can be used, including the polynomial (using kernel = "polydot") and linear (kernel = "vanilladot").

If the values are unknown, they can be estimated through resampling. In train, the method values of "svmRadial", "svmLinear", or "svmPoly" fit different kernels:

```
> svmRTuned <- train(solTrainXtrans, solTrainY,
+                    method = "svmRadial",
+                    preProc = c("center", "scale"),
+                    tuneLength = 14,
+                    trControl = trainControl(method = "cv"))
```

The tuneLength argument will use the default grid search of 14 cost values between $2^{-2}, 2^{-1}, \ldots, 2^{11}$. Again, σ is estimated analytically by default.

```
> svmRTuned
  951 samples
  228 predictors

  Pre-processing: centered, scaled
  Resampling: Cross-Validation (10-fold)

  Summary of sample sizes: 855, 858, 856, 855, 855, 856, ...

  Resampling results across tuning parameters:
```

C	RMSE	Rsquared	RMSE SD	Rsquared SD
0.25	0.793	0.87	0.105	0.0396
0.5	0.708	0.889	0.0936	0.0345
1	0.664	0.898	0.0834	0.0306
2	0.642	0.903	0.0725	0.0277
4	0.629	0.906	0.067	0.0253
8	0.621	0.908	0.0634	0.0238
16	0.617	0.909	0.0602	0.0232
32	0.613	0.91	0.06	0.0234
64	0.611	0.911	0.0586	0.0231
128	0.609	0.911	0.0561	0.0223
256	0.609	0.911	0.056	0.0224
512	0.61	0.911	0.0563	0.0226
1020	0.613	0.91	0.0563	0.023
2050	0.618	0.909	0.0541	0.023

```
  Tuning parameter 'sigma' was held constant at a value of 0.00387
  RMSE was used to select the optimal model using  the smallest value.
  The final values used for the model were C = 256 and sigma = 0.00387.
```

The subobject named finalModel contains the model created by the ksvm function:

```
> svmRTuned$finalModel
  Support Vector Machine object of class "ksvm"

  SV type: eps-svr  (regression)
   parameter : epsilon = 0.1  cost C = 256
```

```
Gaussian Radial Basis kernel function.
 Hyperparameter : sigma =  0.00387037424967707

Number of Support Vectors : 625

Objective Function Value : -1020.558
Training error : 0.009163
```

Here, we see that the model used 625 training set data points as support vectors (66 % of the training set).

kernlab has an implementation of the RVM model for regression in the function rvm. The syntax is very similar to the example shown for ksvm.

K-Nearest Neighbors

The knnreg function in the caret package fits the KNN regression model; train tunes the model over K:

```
> # Remove a few sparse and unbalanced fingerprints first
> knnDescr <- solTrainXtrans[, -nearZeroVar(solTrainXtrans)]
> set.seed(100)
> knnTune <- train(knnDescr,
+                  solTrainY,
+                  method = "knn",
+                  # Center and scaling will occur for new predictions too
+                  preProc = c("center", "scale"),
+                  tuneGrid = data.frame(.k = 1:20),
+                  trControl = trainControl(method = "cv"))
```

When predicting new samples using this object, the new samples are automatically centered and scaled using the values determined by the training set.

Exercises

7.1. Simulate a single predictor and a nonlinear relationship, such as a *sin* wave shown in Fig. 7.7, and investigate the relationship between the cost, ϵ, and kernel parameters for a support vector machine model:

```
> set.seed(100)
> x <- runif(100, min = 2, max = 10)
> y <-  sin(x) + rnorm(length(x)) * .25
> sinData <- data.frame(x = x, y = y)
> plot(x, y)
> ## Create a grid of x values to use for prediction
> dataGrid <- data.frame(x = seq(2, 10, length = 100))
```

(a) Fit different models using a radial basis function and different values of
the cost (the C parameter) and ϵ. Plot the fitted curve. For example:

```
> library(kernlab)
> rbfSVM <- ksvm(x = x, y = y, data = sinData,
+                kernel ="rbfdot", kpar = "automatic",
+                C = 1, epsilon = 0.1)
> modelPrediction <- predict(rbfSVM, newdata = dataGrid)
> ## This is a matrix with one column. We can plot the
> ## model predictions by adding points to the previous plot
> points(x = dataGrid$x, y = modelPrediction[,1],
+        type = "l", col = "blue")
> ## Try other parameters
```

(b) The σ parameter can be adjusted using the kpar argument, such as
kpar = list(sigma = 1). Try different values of σ to understand how this
parameter changes the model fit. How do the cost, ϵ, and σ values affect
the model?

7.2. Friedman (1991) introduced several benchmark data sets create by simulation. One of these simulations used the following nonlinear equation to
create data:

$$y = 10\sin(\pi x_1 x_2) + 20(x_3 - 0.5)^2 + 10x_4 + 5x_5 + N(0, \sigma^2)$$

where the x values are random variables uniformly distributed between [0, 1]
(there are also 5 other non-informative variables also created in the simulation). The package mlbench contains a function called mlbench.friedman1 that
simulates these data:

```
> library(mlbench)
> set.seed(200)
> trainingData <- mlbench.friedman1(200, sd = 1)
> ## We convert the 'x' data from a matrix to a data frame
> ## One reason is that this will give the columns names.
> trainingData$x <- data.frame(trainingData$x)
> ## Look at the data using
> featurePlot(trainingData$x, trainingData$y)
> ## or other methods.
>
> ## This creates a list with a vector 'y' and a matrix
> ## of predictors 'x'. Also simulate a large test set to
> ## estimate the true error rate with good precision:
> testData <- mlbench.friedman1(5000, sd = 1)
> testData$x <- data.frame(testData$x)
>
```

Tune several models on these data. For example:

```
> library(caret)
> knnModel <- train(x = trainingData$x,
+                   y = trainingData$y,
+                   method = "knn",
```

```
+                           preProc = c("center", "scale"),
+                           tuneLength = 10)
> knnModel

  200 samples
   10 predictors

Pre-processing: centered, scaled
Resampling: Bootstrap (25 reps)

Summary of sample sizes: 200, 200, 200, 200, 200, 200, ...

Resampling results across tuning parameters:

  k    RMSE   Rsquared   RMSE SD   Rsquared SD
  5    3.51   0.496      0.238     0.0641
  7    3.36   0.536      0.24      0.0617
  9    3.3    0.559      0.251     0.0546
  11   3.24   0.586      0.252     0.0501
  13   3.2    0.61       0.234     0.0465
  15   3.19   0.623      0.264     0.0496
  17   3.19   0.63       0.286     0.0528
  19   3.18   0.643      0.274     0.048
  21   3.2    0.646      0.269     0.0464
  23   3.2    0.652      0.267     0.0465

RMSE was used to select the optimal model using  the smallest value.
The final value used for the model was k = 19.
> knnPred <- predict(knnModel, newdata = testData$x)
> ## The function 'postResample' can be used to get the test set
> ## perforamnce values
> postResample(pred = knnPred, obs = testData$y)

      RMSE   Rsquared
 3.2286834  0.6871735
```

Which models appear to give the best performance? Does MARS select the informative predictors (those named X1–X5)?

7.3. For the Tecator data described in the last chapter, build SVM, neural network, MARS, and KNN models. Since neural networks are especially sensitive to highly correlated predictors, does pre-processing using PCA help the model?

7.4. Return to the permeability problem outlined in Exercise 6.2. Train several nonlinear regression models and evaluate the resampling and test set performance.

(a) Which nonlinear regression model gives the optimal resampling and test set performance?
(b) Do any of the nonlinear models outperform the optimal linear model you previously developed in Exercise 6.2? If so, what might this tell you about the underlying relationship between the predictors and the response?

(c) Would you recommend any of the models you have developed to replace the permeability laboratory experiment?

7.5. Exercise 6.3 describes data for a chemical manufacturing process. Use the same data imputation, data splitting, and pre-processing steps as before and train several nonlinear regression models.

(a) Which nonlinear regression model gives the optimal resampling and test set performance?
(b) Which predictors are most important in the optimal nonlinear regression model? Do either the biological or process variables dominate the list? How do the top ten important predictors compare to the top ten predictors from the optimal linear model?
(c) Explore the relationships between the top predictors and the response for the predictors that are unique to the optimal nonlinear regression model. Do these plots reveal intuition about the biological or process predictors and their relationship with yield?

Chapter 8
Regression Trees and Rule-Based Models

Tree-based models consist of one or more nested `if-then` statements for the predictors that partition the data. Within these partitions, a model is used to predict the outcome. For example, a very simple tree could be defined as

```
if Predictor A >= 1.7 then
|    if Predictor B >= 202.1 then Outcome = 1.3
|    else Outcome = 5.6
else Outcome = 2.5
```

In this case, two-dimensional predictor space is cut into three regions, and, within each region, the outcome is predicted by a single number (either 1.3, 2.5, or 5.6). Figure 8.1 presents these rules in the predictor space.

In the terminology of tree models, there are two *splits* of the data into three *terminal nodes* or *leaves* of the tree. To obtain a prediction for a new sample, we would follow the `if-then` statements defined by the tree using values of that sample's predictors until we come to a terminal node. The model formula in the terminal node would then be used to generate the prediction. In the illustration above, the model is a simple numeric value. In other cases, the terminal node may be defined by a more complex function of the predictors. Trees for regression will be discussed in Sects. 8.1 and 8.2.

Notice that the `if-then` statements generated by a tree define a unique route to one terminal node for any sample. A *rule* is a set of `if-then` conditions (possibly created by a tree) that have been collapsed into independent conditions. For the example above, there would be three rules:

```
if Predictor A >= 1.7 and Predictor B >= 202.1 then Outcome = 1.3
if Predictor A >= 1.7 and Predictor B <  202.1 then Outcome = 5.6
if Predictor A <  1.7 then Outcome = 2.5
```

Rules can be simplified or pruned in a way that samples are covered by multiple rules. This approach can have some advantages over simple tree-based models; rule-based models will be discussed in Sects. 8.3 and 8.7.

M. Kuhn and K. Johnson, *Applied Predictive Modeling*,
DOI 10.1007/978-1-4614-6849-3_8,
© Springer Science+Business Media New York 2013

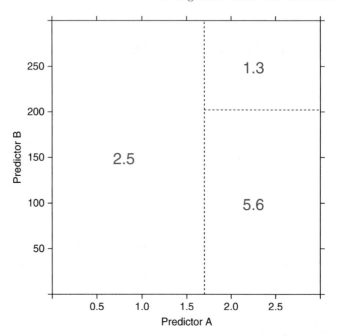

Fig. 8.1: An example of the predicted values within regions defined by a tree-based model

Tree-based and rule-based models are popular modeling tools for a number of reasons. First, they generate a set of conditions that are highly interpretable and are easy to implement. Because of the logic of their construction, they can effectively handle many types of predictors (sparse, skewed, continuous, categorical, etc.) without the need to pre-process them. In addition, these models do not require the user to specify the form of the predictors' relationship to the response like, for example, a linear regression model requires. Furthermore, these models can effectively handle missing data and implicitly conduct feature selection, characteristics that are desirable for many real-life modeling problems.

Models based on single trees or rules, however, do have particular weaknesses. Two well-known weaknesses are (1) model instability (i.e., slight changes in the data can drastically change the structure of the tree or rules and, hence, the interpretation) and (2) less-than-optimal predictive performance. The latter is due to the fact that these models define rectangular regions that contain more homogeneous outcome values. If the relationship between predictors and the response cannot be adequately defined by rectangular subspaces of the predictors, then tree-based or rule-based models will have larger prediction error than other kinds of models.

To combat these problems, researchers developed ensemble methods that combine many trees (or rule-based models) into one model. Ensembles tend to have much better predictive performance than single trees (and this is generally true for rule-based models, too). Ensembles will be discussed in Sects. 8.4–8.7.

8.1 Basic Regression Trees

Basic regression trees partition the data into smaller groups that are more homogenous with respect to the response. To achieve outcome homogeneity, regression trees determine:

- The predictor to split on and value of the split
- The depth or complexity of the tree
- The prediction equation in the terminal nodes

In this section, we focus on techniques where the model in the terminal nodes are simple constants.

There are many techniques for constructing regression trees. One of the oldest and most utilized is the classification and regression tree (CART) methodology of Breiman et al. (1984). For regression, the model begins with the entire data set, S, and searches every distinct value of every predictor to find the predictor and split value that partitions the data into two groups (S_1 and S_2) such that the overall sums of squares error are minimized:

$$\text{SSE} = \sum_{i \in S_1} (y_i - \bar{y}_1)^2 + \sum_{i \in S_2} (y_i - \bar{y}_2)^2, \tag{8.1}$$

where $\bar{y}_1$ and $\bar{y}_2$ are the averages of the training set outcomes within groups S_1 and S_2, respectively. Then within each of groups S_1 and S_2, this method searches for the predictor and split value that best reduces SSE. Because of the recursive splitting nature of regression trees, this method is also known as recursive partitioning.

Returning to the solubility data, Fig. 8.2 shows the SSE for the continuum of splits for the number of carbon atoms (on a transformed scale). Using the regression tree approach, the optimal split point for this variable is 3.78. The reduction in the SSE associated with this split is compared to the optimal values for all of the other predictors and the split corresponding to the absolute minimum error is used to form subsets S_1 and S_2. After considering all other variables, this variable was chosen to be the best (see Fig. 8.3). If the process were stopped at this point, all sample with values for this predictor less than 3.78 would be predicted to be -1.84 (the average of the solubility results for these samples) and samples above the splits all have a predicted value of -4.49:

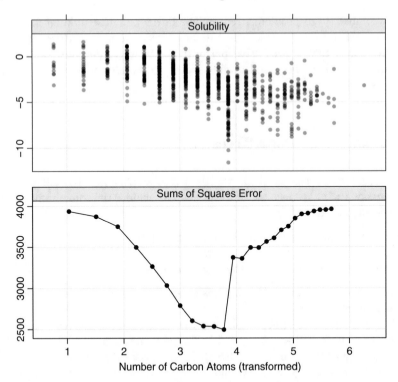

Fig. 8.2: *Top*: A scatter plot of the solubility values (y-axis) versus the number of carbon atoms (on a transformed scale). *Bottom*: The SSE profile across all possible splits for this predictor. The splits used here are the midpoints between two distinct data points

```
if the number of carbon atoms >= 3.78 then  Solubility = -4.49
else Solubility = -1.84
```

In practice, the process then continues within sets S_1 and S_2 until the number of samples in the splits falls below some threshold (such as 20 samples). This would conclude the *tree growing step*. Figure 8.4 shows the second set of splits for the example data.

When the predictor is continuous, the process for finding the optimal split-point is straightforward since the data can be ordered in a natural way. Binary predictors are also easy to split, because there is only one possible split point. However, when a predictor has more than two categories, the process for finding the optimal split point can take a couple of justifiable paths. For a detailed discussion on this topic, see Sect. 14.1.

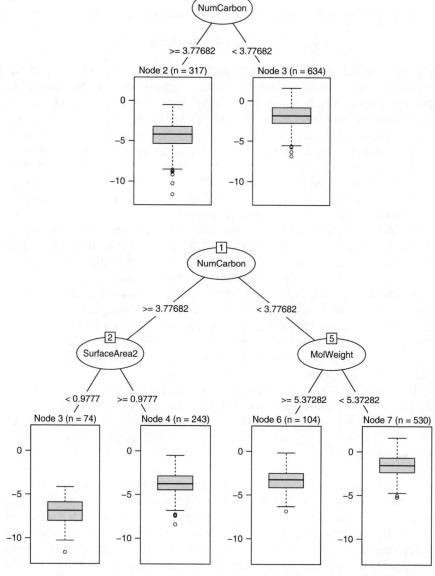

Fig. 8.3: *Top*: The initial splits of the solubility data. *Bottom*: After the first split, the two groups are split further into four partitions

Once the full tree has been grown, the tree may be very large and is likely to over-fit the training set. The tree is then *pruned* back to a potentially smaller depth. The processed used by Breiman et al. (1984) is *cost–complexity tuning*.

The goal of this process is to find a "right-sized tree" that has the smallest error rate. To do this, we penalize the error rate using the size of the tree:

$$\text{SSE}_{c_p} = \text{SSE} + c_p \times (\# \text{ Terminal Nodes}),$$

where c_p is called the *complexity parameter*. For a specific value of the complexity parameter, we find the smallest pruned tree that has the lowest penalized error rate. Breiman et al. (1984) show the theory and algorithms for finding the best tree for a particular value of c_p. As with other regularization methods previously discussed, smaller penalties tend to produce more complex models, which, in this case, result in larger trees. Larger values of the complexity parameter may result in a tree with one split (i.e., a stump) or, perhaps, even a tree with no splits. The latter result would indicate that no predictor adequately explains enough of the variation in the outcome at the chosen value of the complexity parameter.

To find the best pruned tree, we evaluate the data across a sequence of c_p values. This process generates one *SSE* for each chosen c_p value. But we know that these *SSE* values will vary if we select a different sample of observations. To understand variation in *SSE*s at each c_p value, Breiman et al. (1984) suggest using a cross-validation approach similar to the method discussed in Chap. 4. They also propose using the *one-standard-error rule* on the optimization criteria for identifying the simplest tree: find the smallest tree that is within one standard error of the tree with smallest absolute error (see Sect. 4.6, page 74). Another approach selects the tree size associated with the numerically smallest error (Hastie et al. 2008).

Using the one-standard-error rule, the regression tree built on the solubility data had 11 terminal nodes ($c_p = 0.01$) and the cross-validation estimate of the RMSE was 1.05. Figure 8.4 shows the regression tree for the model. All of the splits retained in the model involve the continuous or count predictors and several paths through the tree use some of the same predictors more than once.

On the surface, the tree in Fig. 8.4 appears to be fairly interpretable. For example, one could say that if a compound has a moderately large number of carbon atoms, has very lower surface area, and has a large number of non-hydrogen atoms, then it has the lowest solubility. However, there are many partitions in the data that overlap. For example, nodes 12 and 16 have roughly the same distribution of solubility values, although one of these paths has low surface area and another has high surface area.

Alternatively, the model can be tuned by choosing the value of the complexity parameter associated with the smallest possible RMSE value. The cross-validation profile is shown in Fig. 8.5. In this case, the tuning process chose a larger tree with a c_p value of 0.003 and 25 terminal nodes. The estimated RMSE from this model was 0.97. Although this model more accurately fits the data, it is much deeper than the tree shown in Fig. 8.4. Interpreting this model will be much more difficult.

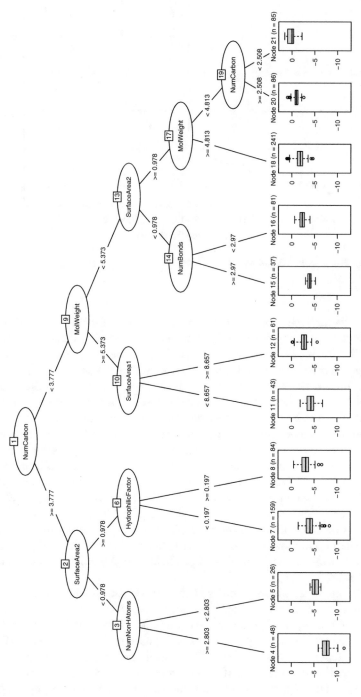

Fig. 8.4: The final CART model for the solubility data. The *box plots* in the terminal nodes show the distribution of the training set solubility values. The final prediction is based on the average of the samples in the box plots

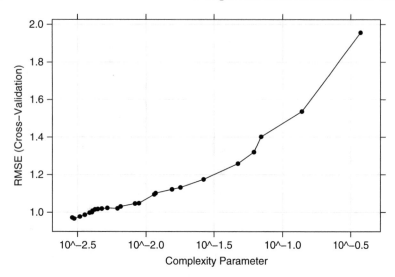

Fig. 8.5: Cross-validated RMSE profile for the regression tree

This particular tree methodology can also handle missing data. When building the tree, missing data are ignored. For each split, a variety of alternatives (called *surrogate splits*) are evaluated. A surrogate split is one whose results are similar to the original split actually used in the tree. If a surrogate split approximates the original split well, it can be used when the predictor data associated with the original split are not available. In practice, several surrogate splits may be saved for any particular split in the tree.

Once the tree has been finalized, we begin to assess the relative importance of the predictors to the outcome. One way to compute an aggregate measure of importance is to keep track of the overall reduction in the optimization criteria for each predictor (Breiman et al. 1984). If SSE is the optimization criteria, then the reduction in the SSE for the training set is aggregated for each predictor. Intuitively, predictors that appear higher in the tree (i.e., earlier splits) or those that appear multiple times in the tree will be more important than predictors that occur lower in the tree or not at all. Figure 8.6 shows the importance values for the 16 predictors in the more complex final solubility model.

An advantage of tree-based models is that, when the tree is not large, the model is simple and interpretable. Also, this type of tree can be computed quickly (despite using multiple exhaustive searches). Tree models intrinsically conduct feature selection; if a predictor is never used in a split, the prediction equation is independent of these data. This advantage is weakened when there are highly correlated predictors. If two predictors are extremely correlated, the choice of which to use in a split is somewhat random. For example, the two surface area predictors have an extremely high correlation (0.96) and each

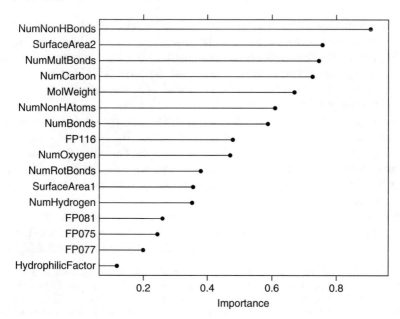

Fig. 8.6: Variable importance scores for the 16 predictors used in the regression tree model for solubility

is used in the tree shown in Fig. 8.4. It is possible that the small difference between these predictors is strongly driving the choice between the two, but it is more likely to be due to small, random differences in the variables. Because of this, more predictors may be selected than actually needed. In addition, the variable importance values are affected. If the solubility data only contained one of the surface area predictors, then this predictor would have likely been used twice in the tree, therefore inflating its importance value. Instead, including both surface area predictors in the data causes their importance to have only moderate values.

While trees are highly interpretable and easy to compute, they do have some noteworthy disadvantages. First, single regression trees are more likely to have sub-optimal predictive performance compared to other modeling approaches. This is partly due to the simplicity of the model. By construction, tree models partition the data into rectangular regions of the predictor space. If the relationship between predictors and the outcome is not adequately described by these rectangles, then the predictive performance of a tree will not be optimal. Also, the number of possible predicted outcomes from a tree is finite and is determined by the number of terminal nodes. For the solubility data, the optimal tree has 11 terminal nodes and consequently can only produce 11 possible predicted values. This limitation is unlikely to capture all of the nuances of the data. For example, in Fig. 8.4, Node 21 corresponds to the highest solubility prediction. Note, however, that the training set data falling within this path of the tree vary across several log units of data. If new data points are consistent with the training data, many of the new samples falling along this path will not be predicted with a high degree of accuracy. The two regression tree models shown thus far have RMSE values that are appreciably larger than the RMSE produced by the simple linear regression model shown in Chap. 6.

An additional disadvantage is that an individual tree tends to be *unstable* [see Breiman (1996b) and Hastie et al. (2008, Chap. 8)]. If the data are slightly altered, a completely different set of splits might be found (i.e., the model variance is high). While this is a disadvantage, ensemble methods (discussed later in this chapter) exploit this characteristic to create models that tend to have extremely good performance.

Finally, these trees suffer from *selection bias*: predictors with a higher number of distinct values are favored over more granular predictors (Loh and Shih 1997; Carolin et al. 2007; Loh 2010). Loh and Shih (1997) remarked that

> "The danger occurs when a data set consists of a mix of informative and noise variables, and the noise variables have many more splits than the informative variables. Then there is a high probability that the noise variables will be chosen to split the top nodes of the tree. Pruning will produce either a tree with misleading structure or no tree at all."

Also, as the number of missing values increases, the selection of predictors becomes more biased (Carolin et al. 2007).

It is worth noting that the variable importance scores for the solubility regression tree (Fig. 8.6) show that the model tends to rely more on continuous (i.e., less granular) predictors than the binary fingerprints. This could be due to the selection bias or the content of the variables.

There are several *unbiased* regression tree techniques. For example, Loh (2002) proposed the generalized, unbiased, interaction detection and estimation (GUIDE) algorithm which solves the problem by decoupling the process of selecting the split variable and the split value. This algorithm ranks the predictors using statistical hypothesis testing and then finds the appropriate split value associated with the most important factor.

Another approach is *conditional inference trees* of Hothorn et al. (2006). They describe a unified framework for unbiased tree-based models for regression, classification, and other scenarios. In this model, statistical hypothesis tests are used to do an exhaustive search across the predictors and their possible split points. For a candidate split, a statistical test is used to evaluate the difference between the means of the two groups created by the split and a p-value can be computed for the test.

Utilizing the test statistic p-value has several advantages. First, predictors that are on disparate scales can be compared since the p-values are on the same scale. Second, multiple comparison corrections (Westfall and Young 1993) can be applied to the raw p-values within a predictor to reduce the bias resulting from a large number of split candidates. These corrections attempt to reduce the number of false-positive test results that are incurred by

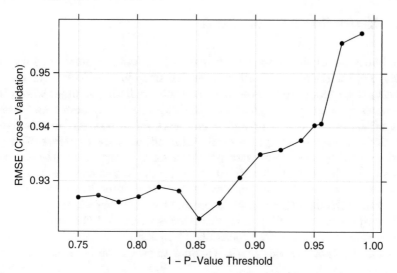

Fig. 8.7: Cross-validated RMSE profile for the conditional inference regression trees

conducting a large number of statistical hypothesis tests. Thus, predictors are increasingly penalized by multiple comparison procedures as the number of splits (and associated p-values) increases. For this reason, the bias is reduced for highly granular data. A threshold for statistical significance is used to determine whether additional splits should be created [Hothorn et al. (2006) use one minus the p-value].

By default, this algorithm does not use pruning; as the data sets are further split, the decrease in the number of samples reduces the power of the hypothesis tests. This results in higher p-values and a lower likelihood of a new split (and over-fitting). However, statistical hypothesis tests are not directly related to predictive performance, and, because of this, it is still advisable to choose the complexity of the tree on the basis of performance (via resampling or some other means).

With a significance threshold of 0.05 (i.e., a 5 % false-positive rate for statistical significance), a conditional inference tree for the solubility data had 32 terminal nodes. This tree is much larger than the basic regression tree shown in Fig. 8.4. We also treated the significance threshold as a tuning parameter and evaluated 16 values between 0.75 and 0.99 (see Fig. 8.7 for the cross-validation profile). The tree size associated with the smallest error had 36 terminal nodes (using a threshold of 0.853). Tuning the threshold improved the estimated RMSE to a value of 0.92 compared to an RMSE of 0.94 associated with a significance threshold of 0.05.

8.2 Regression Model Trees

One limitation of simple regression trees is that each terminal node uses the average of the training set outcomes in that node for prediction. As a consequence, these models may not do a good job predicting samples whose true outcomes are extremely high or low. In Chap. 5, Fig. 5.1 showed an example plot of the observed and predicted outcomes for a data set. In this figure, the model tends to underpredict samples in either of the extremes. The predictions used in this figure were produced using a regression tree ensemble technique called random forests (described later in this chapter) which also uses the average of the training data in the terminal nodes and suffers from the same problem, although not as severe as with a single tree.

One approach to dealing with this issue is to use a different estimator in the terminal nodes. Here we focus on the *model tree* approach described in Quinlan (1992) called M5, which is similar to regression trees except:

- The splitting criterion is different.
- The terminal nodes predict the outcome using a linear model (as opposed to the simple average).
- When a sample is predicted, it is often a combination of the predictions from different models along the same path through the tree.

The main implementation of this technique is a "rational reconstruction" of this model called M5, which is described by Wang and Witten (1997) and is included in the Weka software package. There are other approaches to trees with models in the leaves, such as Loh (2002) and Zeileis et al. (2008).

Like simple regression trees, the initial split is found using an exhaustive search over the predictors and training set samples, but, unlike those models, the expected reduction in the node's error rate is used. Let S denote the entire set of data and let $S_1, \ldots, S_P$ represent the P subsets of the data after splitting. The split criterion would be

$$\text{reduction} = \text{SD}(S) - \sum_{i=1}^{P} \frac{n_i}{n} \times \text{SD}(S_i), \tag{8.2}$$

where SD is the standard deviation and n_i is the number of samples in partition i. This metric determines if the total variation in the splits, weighted by sample size, is lower than in the presplit data. This scheme is similar to the methodology for classification trees discussed in Quinlan (1993b). The split that is associated with the largest reduction in error is chosen and a linear model is created within the partitions using the split variable in the model. For subsequent splitting iterations, this process is repeated: an initial split is determined and a linear model is created for the partition using the current split variable and all others that preceded it. The error associated with each linear model is used in place of $\text{SD}(S)$ in Eq. 8.2 to determine the expected reduction in the error rate for the next split. The tree growing process continues along the branches of the tree until there are no further improvements in the error rate or there are not enough samples to continue the process. Once the tree is fully grown, there is a linear model for every node in the tree.

Figure 8.8 shows an example of a model tree with four splits and eight linear regression models. Model 5, for instance, would be created using all the predictors that were in splits 1–3 and with the training set data points satisfying conditions 1a, 2b, and 3b.

Once the complete set of linear models have been created, each undergoes a simplification procedure to potentially drop some of the terms. For a given model, an adjusted error rate is computed. First, the absolute differences between the observed and predicted data are calculated then multiplied by a term that penalizes models with large numbers of parameters:

$$\text{Adjusted Error Rate} = \frac{n^* + p}{n^* - p} \sum_{i=1}^{n^*} |y_i - \hat{y}_i|, \tag{8.3}$$

where n^* is the number of training set data points that were used to build the model and p is the number of parameters. Each model term is dropped and the adjusted error rate is computed. Terms are dropped from the model as long as the adjusted error rate decreases. In some cases, the linear model may be simplified to having only an intercept. This procedure is independently applied to each linear model.

Model trees also incorporate a type of *smoothing* to decrease the potential for over-fitting. The technique is based on the "recursive shrinking" methodology of Hastie and Pregibon (1990). When predicting, the new sample goes down the appropriate path of the tree, and moving from the bottom up, the linear models along that path are combined. Using Fig. 8.8 as a reference, suppose a new sample goes down the path associated with Model 5. The tree generates a prediction for this sample using Model 5 as well as the linear model in the parent node (Model 3 in this case). These two predictions are combined using

$$\hat{y}_{(p)} = \frac{n_{(k)}\, \hat{y}_{(k)} + c\, \hat{y}_{(p)}}{n_{(k)} + c},$$

where $\hat{y}_{(k)}$ is the prediction from the child node (Model 5), $n_{(k)}$ is the number of training set data points in the child node, $\hat{y}_{(p)}$ is the prediction from the parent node, and c is a constant with a default value of 15. Once this combined prediction is calculated, it is similarly combined with the next model along the tree (Model 1) and so on. For our example, the new sample falling under conditions 1a, 2b, and 3b would use a combination of three linear models. Note that the smoothing equation is a relatively simple linear combination of models.

This type of smoothing can have a significant positive effect on the model tree when the linear models across nodes are very different. There are several possible reasons that the linear models may produce very different predic-

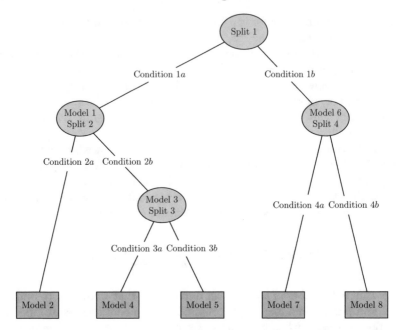

Fig. 8.8: An example of a regression model tree

tions. Firstly, the number of training set samples that are available in a node will decrease as new splits are added. This can lead to nodes which model very different regions of the training set and, thus, produce very different linear models. This is especially true for small training sets. Secondly, the linear models derived by the splitting process may suffer from significant collinearity. Suppose two predictors in the training set have an extremely high correlation with one another. In this case, the algorithm may choose between the two predictors randomly. If both predictors are eventually used in splits and become candidates for the linear models, there would be two terms in the linear model for effectively one piece of information. As discussed in previous chapters, this can lead to substantial instability in the model coefficients. Smoothing using several models can help reduce the impact of any unstable linear models.

Once the tree is fully grown, it is pruned back by finding inadequate subtrees and removing them. Starting at the terminal nodes, the adjusted error rate with and without the sub-tree is computed. If the sub-tree does not decrease the adjusted error rate, it is pruned from the model. This process is continued until no more sub-trees can be removed.

Model trees were built on the solubility data under the conditions of with and without pruning and with and without smoothing. Figure 8.9 shows a plot of the cross-validation profiles for these data. The unpruned tree has 159 paths through the tree, which may over-fit the training data. When the

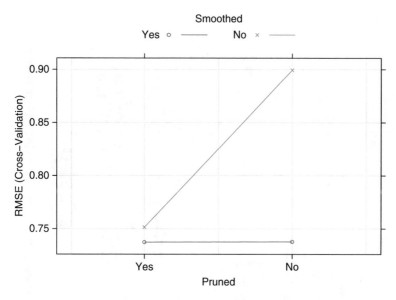

Fig. 8.9: Cross-validated RMSE profiles for the model tree

tree is not pruned, model smoothing significantly improves the error rate. For these data, the effect of pruning on the model was also substantial: the number of paths through the tree dropped from 159 to 18. For the pruned trees, smoothing produced a slight gain in performance, and, as a result, the optimal model used pruning and smoothing.

The resulting model tree (Fig. 8.10) shows that many of the splits involve the same predictors, such as the number of carbons. Also, for these data, the splits tend to favor the continuous predictors instead of the fingerprints.[1] For these data, splits based on the SSE and the error rate reduction produce almost identical results. The details of the linear models are shown in Fig. 8.11 (the model coefficients have been normalized to be on the same scale). We can see from this figure that the majority of models use many predictors, including a large number of the fingerprints. However, the coefficients of the fingerprints are small relative to the continuous predictors.

Additionally, this model can be used to demonstrate issues with collinearity. In the figure, linear model 5 (in the lower left of the tree) is associated with the following conditions:

```
NumCarbon <= 3.777 &
MolWeight <= 4.83 &
SurfaceArea1 > 0.978 &
NumCarbon <= 2.508 &
```

---

[1] Also, note that the first three splits here involve the same predictors as the regression tree shown in Fig. 8.4 (and two of the three split values are identical).

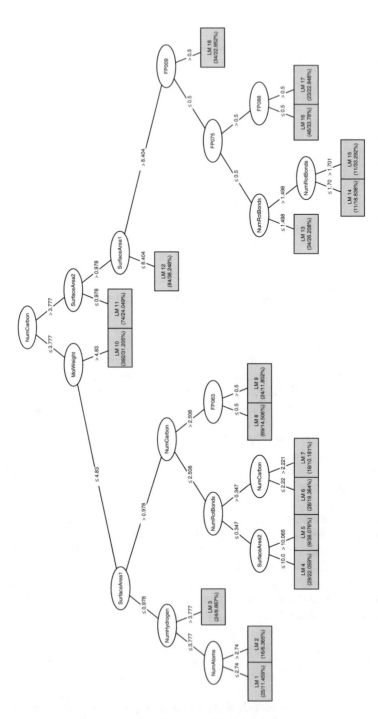

Fig. 8.10: The final model tree for the solubility data. The numbers at the bottom of each terminal node represent the number of samples and percent coverage of the node

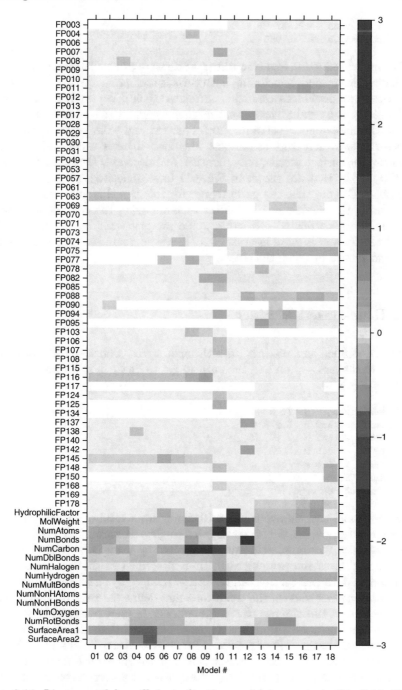

Fig. 8.11: Linear model coefficients for the model tree seen in Fig. 8.10. The coefficients have been normalized to be on the same scale. *White blocks* indicate that the predictor was not involved in the linear model

```
NumRotBonds  <=  0.347  &
SurfaceArea2  >    10.065
```

After model reduction and smoothing, there were 57 coefficients in the corresponding linear model, including both surface area predictors. In the training set, these two predictors are highly correlated (0.96). We would expect severe collinearity as a result. The two scaled coefficients for these predictors are almost complete opposites: 0.9 for `SurfaceArea1` and -0.8 for `SurfaceArea2`. Since the two predictors are almost identical, there is a contradiction: increasing the surface area equally increases and decreases the solubility. Many of the models that are shown in Fig. 8.11 have opposite signs for these two variables. Despite this, the performance for this model is fairly competitive; smoothing the models has the effect of minimizing the collinearity issues. Removing the correlated predictors would produce a model that has less inconsistencies and is more interpretable. However, there is a measurable drop in performance by using the strategy.

8.3 Rule-Based Models

A rule is defined as a distinct path through a tree. Consider the model tree shown in the last section and the path to get to linear model 15 in the lower right of Fig. 8.10:

```
NumCarbon  >    3.777  &
SurfaceArea2  >   0.978  &
SurfaceArea1  >   8.404  &
FP009  <=  0.5  &
FP075  <=  0.5  &
NumRotBonds  >   1.498  &
NumRotBonds  >   1.701
```

For the model tree shown in Fig. 8.10, there are a total of 18 rules. For the tree, a new sample can only travel down a single path through the tree defined by these rules. The number of samples affected by a rule is called its *coverage*.

In addition to the pruning algorithms described in the last section, the complexity of the model tree can be further reduced by either removing entire rules or removing some of the conditions that define the rule. In the previous rule, note that the number of rotatable bonds is used twice. This occurred because another path through the tree determined that modeling the data subset where the number of rotatable bonds is between 1.498 and 1.701 was important. However, when viewed in isolation, the rule above is unnecessarily complex because of this redundancy. Also, it may be advantageous to remove other conditions in the rule because they do not contribute much to the model.

Quinlan (1993b) describes methodologies for simplifying the rules generated from classification trees. Similar techniques can be applied to model trees to create a more simplistic set of rules from an initial model tree. This specific approach is described later in this chapter in the context of Cubist models (Sect. 8.7).

Another approach to creating rules from model trees is outlined in Holmes et al. (1993) that uses the "separate and conquer" strategy. This procedure derives rules from many different model trees instead of from a single tree. First, an initial model tree is created (they recommend using unsmoothed model trees). However, only the rule with the largest coverage is saved from this model. The samples covered by the rule are removed from the training set and another model tree is created with the remaining data. Again, only the rule with the maximum coverage is retained. This process repeats until all the training set data have been covered by at least one rule. A new sample is predicted by determining which rule(s) it falls under then applies the linear model associated with the largest coverage.

For the solubility data, a rule-based model was evaluated. Similar to the model tree tuning process, four models were fit using all combinations for pruning and smoothing. The same resampling data sets were used in the model tree analysis, so direct comparisons can be made. Figure 8.12 shows the results of this process. The right panel is the same as Fig. 8.9 while the left panel shows the results when the model trees are converted to rules. For these data, when smoothing and pruning are used, the model tree and rule-based version had equivalent error rates. As with the model trees, pruning had a large effect on the model and smoothing had a larger impact on the unpruned models.

The best fitting model tree was associated with a cross-validated RMSE of 0.737. The best rule-based model resulted in an RMSE value of 0.741. Based on this alone, the model tree would be used for prediction. However, for illustration, the rule-based model will be examined in more detail.

In all, nine rules were used to model these data, although the final rule has no associated conditions. The conditions for the rules are

```
Rule 1: NumCarbon <= 3.777 & MolWeight > 4.83
Rule 2: NumCarbon > 2.999
Rule 3: SurfaceArea1 > 0.978 & NumCarbon > 2.508 & NumRotBonds > 0.896
Rule 4: SurfaceArea1 > 0.978 & MolWeight <= 4.612 & FP063 <= 0.5
Rule 5: SurfaceArea1 > 0.978 & MolWeight <= 4.612
Rule 6: SurfaceArea1 <= 4.159 & NumHydrogen <= 3.414
Rule 7: SurfaceArea1 > 2.241 & FP046 <= 0.5 & NumBonds > 2.74
Rule 8: NumHydrogen <= 3.414
```

Looking back at the full model tree in Fig. 8.10, the rule corresponding to Model 10 has the largest coverage using the conditions NumCarbon $\geq$ 3.77 and MolWeight > 4.83. This rule was preserved as the first rule in the new model. The next model tree was created using the remaining samples. Here, the rule with the largest coverage has a condition similar to the previous rule: NumCarbon > 2.99. In this case, a sample with NumCarbon > 2.99 would be

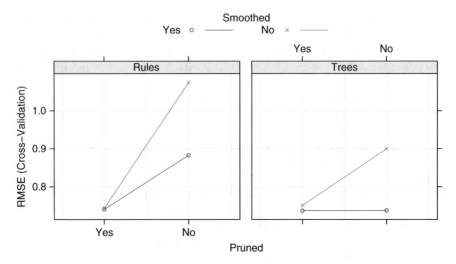

Fig. 8.12: Cross-validated RMSE profiles for the model trees before and after the conversion to rules

covered by at least two rules. The other rules used many of the same predictors: `SurfaceArea1` (five times), `MolWeight` (three times), and `NumCarbon` (also three times). Figure 8.13 shows the coefficients of the linear models for each rule (similar to Fig. 8.11 for the full model tree). Here, the linear models are more sparse; the number of terms in the linear models decreases as more rules are created. This makes sense because there are fewer data points to construct deep trees.

8.4 Bagged Trees

In the 1990s, ensemble techniques (methods that combine many models' predictions) began to appear. Bagging, short for *bootstrap agg*regation, was originally proposed by Leo Breiman and was one of the earliest developed ensemble techniques (Breiman 1996a). Bagging is a general approach that uses bootstrapping (Sect. 4.4) in conjunction with any regression (or classification; see Sect. 14.3) model to construct an ensemble. The method is fairly simple in structure and consists of the steps in Algorithm 8.1. Each model in the ensemble is then used to generate a prediction for a new sample and these m predictions are averaged to give the bagged model's prediction.

Bagging models provide several advantages over models that are not bagged. First, bagging effectively reduces the variance of a prediction through its aggregation process (see Sect. 5.2 for a discussion of the bias-variance trade-off). For models that produce an unstable prediction, like regression trees, aggregating over many versions of the training data actually reduces

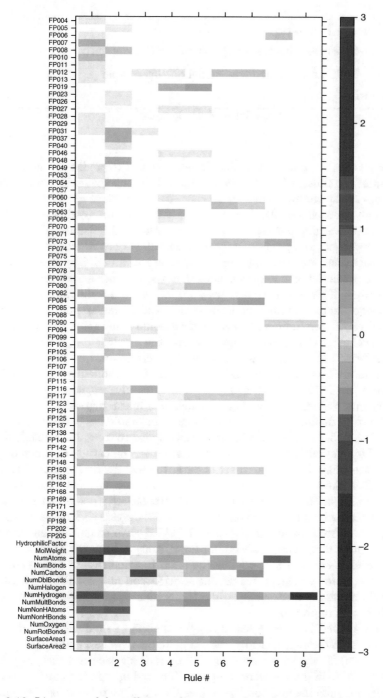

Fig. 8.13: Linear model coefficients for the rule-based version of M5. The coefficients have been normalized to be on the same scale as Fig. 8.11. *White
blocks* indicate that the predictor was not involved in linear regression equation for that rule

1	**for** $i = 1$ *to* m **do**
2	Generate a bootstrap sample of the original data
3	Train an unpruned tree model on this sample
4	**end**

Algorithm 8.1: Bagging

the variance in the prediction and, hence, makes the prediction more stable. Consider the illustration of trees in Fig. 8.14. In this example, six bootstrap samples of the solubility data were generated and a tree of maximum depth was built for each sample. These trees vary in structure (compare Fig. 8.14b, d, which have different structures on the right- and left-hand sides of each tree), and hence the prediction for samples will vary from tree to tree. When the predictions for a sample are averaged across all of the single trees, the average prediction has lower variance than the variance across the individual predictions. This means that if we were to generate a different sequence of bootstrap samples, build a model on each of the bootstrap samples, and average the predictions across models, then we would likely get a very similar predicted value for the selected sample as with the previous bagging model. This characteristic also improves the predictive performance of a bagged model over a model that is not bagged. If the goal of the modeling effort is to find the best prediction, then bagging has a distinct advantage.

Bagging stable, lower variance models like linear regression and MARS, on the other hand, offers less improvement in predictive performance. Consider Fig. 8.15, in which bagging has been applied to trees, linear models, and MARS for the solubility data and also for data from a study of concrete mixtures (see Chap. 10). For each set of data, the test set performance based on *RMSE* is plotted by number of bagging iterations. For the solubility data, the decrease in RMSE across iterations is similar for trees, linear regression, and MARS, which is not a typical result. This suggests that either the model predictions from linear regression and MARS have some inherent instability for these data which can be improved using a bagged ensemble or that trees are less effective at modeling the data. Bagging results for the concrete data are more typical, in which linear regression and MARS are least improved through the ensemble, while the predictions for regression trees are dramatically improved.

As a further demonstration of bagging's ability to reduce the variance of a model's prediction, consider the simulated *sin* wave in Fig. 5.2. For this illustration, 20 *sin* waves were simulated, and, for each data set, regression trees and MARS models were computed. The red lines in the panels show the true trend while the multiple black lines show the predictions for each model. Note that the CART panel has more noise around the true *sin* curve than the MARS model, which only shows variation at the change points of the pattern. This illustrates the high variance in the regression tree due to model

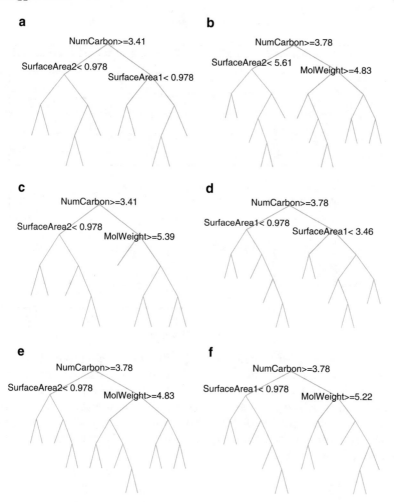

Fig. 8.14: Example of trees of maximum depth from bagging for the solubility data. Notice that the trees vary in structure, and hence the predictions will vary from tree to tree. The prediction variance for the ensemble of trees will be less than the variance of predictions from individual trees. (a) Sample 1. (b) Sample 2. (c) Sample 3. (d) Sample 4. (e) Sample 5. (f) Sample 6

instability. The bottom panels of the figure show the results for 20 bagged regression trees and MARS models (each with 50 model iterations). The variation around the true curve is greatly reduced for regression trees, and, for MARS, the variation is only reduced around the curvilinear portions on the pattern. Using a simulated test set for each model, the average reduction in RMSE by bagging the tree was 8.6 % while the more stable MARS model had a corresponding reduction of 2 % (Fig. 8.16).

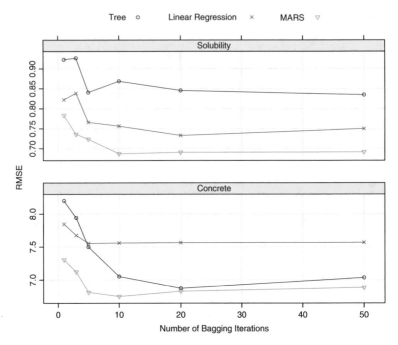

Fig. 8.15: Test set RMSE performance profiles for bagging trees, linear models, and MARS for the solubility data (*top plot*) and concrete data (*bottom plot*; see Chap. 10 for data details) by number of bootstrap samples. Bagging provides approximately the same magnitude of improvement in RMSE for all three methods for the solubility data, which is atypical. A more typical pattern of improvement from bagging is shown for the concrete data. In this case, trees benefit the most

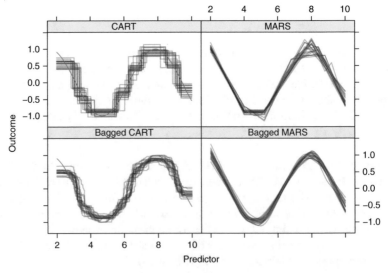

Fig. 8.16: The effect of bagging regression trees and MARS models

Another advantage of bagging models is that they can provide their own internal estimate of predictive performance that correlates well with either cross-validation estimates or test set estimates. Here's why: when constructing a bootstrap sample for each model in the ensemble, certain samples are left out. These samples are called *out-of-bag*, and they can be used to assess the predictive performance of that specific model since they were not used to build the model. Hence, every model in the ensemble generates a measure of predictive performance courtesy of the out-of-bag samples. The average of the out-of-bag performance metrics can then be used to gauge the predictive performance of the entire ensemble, and this value usually correlates well with the assessment of predictive performance we can get with either cross-validation or from a test set. This error estimate is usually referred to as the *out-of-bag* estimate.

In its basic form, the user has one choice to make for bagging: the number of bootstrap samples to aggregate, m. Often we see an exponential decrease in predictive improvement as the number of iterations increases; the most improvement in prediction performance is obtained with a small number of trees ($m < 10$). To illustrate this point, consider Fig. 8.17 which displays predictive performance ($RMSE$) for varying numbers of bootstrapped samples for CART trees. Notice predictive performance improves through ten trees and then tails off with very limited improvement beyond that point. In our experience, small improvements can still be made using bagging ensembles up to size 50. If performance is not at an acceptable level after 50 bagging iterations, then we suggest trying other more powerfully predictive ensemble methods such as random forests and boosting which will be described the following sections.

For the solubility data, CART trees without bagging produce an optimal cross-validated RMSE of 0.97 with a standard error of 0.021. Upon bagging, the performance improves and bottoms at an RMSE of 0.9, with a standard error of 0.019. Conditional inference trees, like CART trees, can also be bagged. As a comparison, conditional inference trees without bagging have an optimal RMSE and standard error of 0.93 and 0.034, respectively. Bagged conditional inference trees reduce the optimal RMSE to 0.8 with a standard error of 0.018. For both types of models, bagging improves performance and reduces variance of the estimate. In this specific example, bagging conditional inference trees appears to have a slight edge over CART trees in predictive performance as measured by RMSE. The test set R^2 values parallel the cross-validated RMSE performance with conditional inference trees doing slightly better (0.87) than CART trees (0.85).

Although bagging usually improves predictive performance for unstable models, there are a few caveats. First, computational costs and memory requirements increase as the number of bootstrap samples increases. This disadvantage can be mostly mitigated if the modeler has access to parallel computing because the bagging process can be easily parallelized. Recall that each bootstrap sample and corresponding model is independent of any other

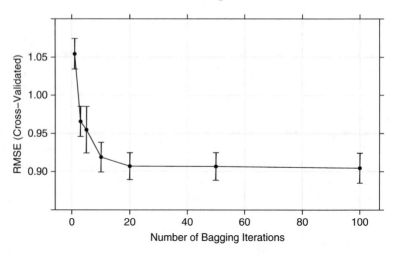

Fig. 8.17: Cross-validated performance profile for bagging CART trees for the solubility data by number of bootstrap samples. Vertical lines indicate ± one-standard error of $RMSE$. Most improvement in predictive performance is obtained aggregating across ten bootstrap replications

sample and model. This means that each model can be built separately and all models can be brought together in the end to generate the prediction.

Another disadvantage to this approach is that a bagged model is much less interpretable than a model that is not bagged. Convenient rules that we can get from a single regression tree like those displayed in Fig. 8.4 cannot be attained. However, measures of variable importance can be constructed by combining measures of importance from the individual models across the ensemble. More about variable importance will be discussed in the next section when we examine random forests.

8.5 Random Forests

As illustrated with the solubility data, bagging trees (or any high variance, low bias technique) improves predictive performance over a single tree by reducing variance of the prediction. Generating bootstrap samples introduces a random component into the tree building process, which induces a distribution of trees, and therefore also a distribution of predicted values for each sample. The trees in bagging, however, are not completely independent of each other since all of the original predictors are considered at every split of every tree. One can imagine that if we start with a sufficiently large number of original samples and a relationship between predictors and response that can be adequately modeled by a tree, then trees from different bootstrap samples may have similar structures to each other (especially at the top of the trees) due to the underlying relationship. This characteristic is known as tree correlation and prevents bagging from optimally reducing variance of the predicted values. Figure 8.14 provides a direct illustration of this phenomenon. Despite taking bootstrap samples, each tree starts splitting on the number of carbon atoms at a scaled value of approximately 3.5. The second-level splits vary a bit more but are restricted to both of the surface area predictors and molecular weight. While each tree is ultimately unique—no two trees are exactly the same—they all begin with a similar structure and are consequently related to each other. Therefore, the variance reduction provided by bagging could be improved. For a mathematical explanation of the tree correlation phenomenon, see Hastie et al. (2008). Reducing correlation among trees, known as de-correlating trees, is then the next logical step to improving the performance of bagging.

From a statistical perspective, reducing correlation among predictors can be done by adding randomness to the tree construction process. After Breiman unveiled bagging, several authors tweaked the algorithm by adding randomness into the learning process. Because trees were a popular learner for bagging, Dietterich (2000) developed the idea of random split selection, where trees are built using a random subset of the top k predictors at each split in the tree. Another approach was to build entire trees based on random subsets of descriptors (Ho 1998; Amit and Geman 1997). Breiman (2000) also tried adding noise to the response in order to perturb tree structure. After carefully evaluating these generalizations to the original bagging algorithm, Breiman (2001) constructed a unified algorithm called *random forests*. A general random forests algorithm for a tree-based model can be implemented as shown in Algorithm 8.2.

Each model in the ensemble is then used to generate a prediction for a new sample and these m predictions are averaged to give the forest's prediction. Since the algorithm randomly selects predictors at each split, tree correlation will necessarily be lessened. As an example, the first splits for the first six trees in the random forest for the solubility data are NumNonHBonds, NumCarbon, NumNonHAtoms, NumCarbon, NumCarbon, and NumCarbon, which are different from the trees illustrated in Fig. 8.14.

Random forests' tuning parameter is the number of randomly selected predictors, k, to choose from at each split, and is commonly referred to as m_{try}. In the regression context, Breiman (2001) recommends setting m_{try} to be one-third of the number of predictors. For the purpose of tuning the m_{try} parameter, since random forests is computationally intensive, we suggest starting with five values of k that are somewhat evenly spaced across the range from 2 to P. The practitioner must also specify the number of trees for the forest. Breiman (2001) proved that random forests is protected from over-fitting; therefore, the model will not be adversely affected if a large number of trees are built for the forest. Practically speaking, the larger the forest, the

---

1 Select the number of models to build, m

2 **for** $i = 1$ *to* m **do**

3 | Generate a bootstrap sample of the original data

4 | Train a tree model on this sample

5 | **for** *each split* **do**

6 | | Randomly select k $(< P)$ of the original predictors

7 | | Select the best predictor among the k predictors and partition the data

8 | **end**

9 | Use typical tree model stopping criteria to determine when a tree is complete (but do not prune)

10 end

Algorithm 8.2: Basic Random Forests

more computational burden we will incur to train and build the model. As a starting point, we suggest using at least 1,000 trees. If the cross-validation performance profiles are still improving at 1,000 trees, then incorporate more trees until performance levels off.

Breiman showed that the linear combination of many independent learners reduces the variance of the overall ensemble relative to any individual learner in the ensemble. A random forest model achieves this variance reduction by selecting strong, complex learners that exhibit low bias. This ensemble of many independent, strong learners yields an improvement in error rates. Because each learner is selected independently of all previous learners, random forests is robust to a noisy response. We elaborate more on this point in Sect. 20.2 and provide an illustration of the effect of noise on random forests as well as many other models. At the same time, the independence of learners can underfit data when the response is not noisy (Fig. 5.1).

Compared to bagging, random forests is more computationally efficient on a tree-by-tree basis since the tree building process only needs to evaluate a fraction of the original predictors at each split, although more trees are usually required by random forests. Combining this attribute with the ability to parallel process tree building makes random forests more computationally efficient than boosting (Sect. 8.6).

Like bagging, CART or conditional inference trees can be used as the base learner in random forests. Both of these base learners were used, as well as 10-fold cross-validation and out-of-bag validation, to train models on the solubility data. The m_{try} parameter was evaluated at ten values from 10 to 228. The RMSE profiles for these combinations are presented in Fig. 8.18. Contrary to bagging, CART trees have better performance than conditional inference trees at all values of the tuning parameter. Each of the profiles

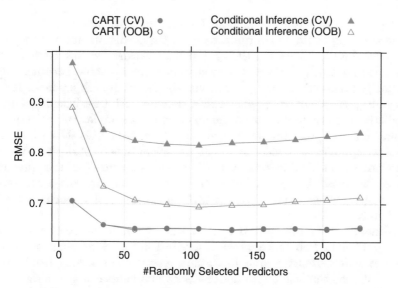

Fig. 8.18: Cross-validated RMSE profile for the CART and conditional inference approaches to random forests

shows a flat plateau between $m_{try} = 58$ and $m_{try} = 155$. The CART-based
random forest model was numerically optimal at $m_{try} = 131$ regardless of the
method of estimating the RMSE. Our experience is that the random forest
tuning parameter does not have a drastic effect on performance. In these
data, the only real difference in the RMSE comes when the smallest value
is used (10 in this case). It is often the case that such a small value is not
associated with optimal performance. However, we have seen rare examples
where small tuning parameter values generate the best results. To get a quick
assessment of how well the random forest model performs, the default tuning
parameter value for regression ($m_{try} = P/3$) tends to work well. If there is
a desire to maximize performance, tuning this value may result in a slight
improvement.

   In Fig. 8.18, also notice that random forest models built with CART trees
had extremely similar RMSE results with the out-of-bag error estimate and
cross-validation (when compared across tuning parameters). It is unclear
whether the pattern seen in these data generalizes, especially under different circumstances such as small sample sizes. Using the out-of-bag error rate
would drastically decrease the computational time to tune random forest
models. For forests created using conditional inference trees, the out-of-bag
error was much more optimistic than the cross-validated RMSE. Again, the
reasoning behind this pattern is unclear.

The ensemble nature of random forests makes it impossible to gain an understanding of the relationship between the predictors and the response. However, because trees are the typical base learner for this method, it is possible to quantify the impact of predictors in the ensemble. Breiman (2000) originally proposed randomly permuting the values of each predictor for the out-of-bag sample of one predictor at a time for each tree. The difference in predictive performance between the non-permuted sample and the permuted sample for each predictor is recorded and aggregated across the entire forest. Another approach is to measure the improvement in node purity based on the performance metric for each predictor at each occurrence of that predictor across the forest. These individual improvement values for each predictor are then aggregated across the forest to determine the overall importance for the predictor.

Although this strategy to determine the relative influence of a predictor is very different from the approach described in Sect. 8 for single regression trees, it suffers from the same limitations related to bias. Also, Strobl et al. (2007) showed that the correlations between predictors can have a significant impact on the importance values. For example, uninformative predictors with high correlations to informative predictors had abnormally large importance values. In some cases, their importance was greater than or equal to weakly important variables. They also demonstrated that the m_{try} tuning parameter has a serious effect on the importance values.

Another impact of between-predictor correlations is to dilute the importances of key predictors. For example, suppose a critical predictor had an importance of X. If another predictor is just as critical but is almost perfectly correlated as the first, the importance of these two predictors will be roughly $X/2$. If three such predictors were in the model, the values would further decrease to $X/3$ and so on. This can have profound implications for some problems. For example, RNA expression profiling data tend to measure the same gene at many locations, and, as a result, the within-gene variables tend to have very high correlations. If this gene were important for predicting some outcome, adding all the variables to a random forest model would make the gene appear to be less important than it actually is.

Strobl et al. (2007) developed an alternative approach for calculating importance in random forest models that takes between-predictor correlations into account. Their methodology reduces the effect of between-predictor redundancy. It does not adjust for the aforementioned dilution effect.

Random forest variable importance values for the top 25 predictors of the solubility data are presented in Fig. 8.19. For this model, MolWeight, NumCarbon, SurfaceArea2, and SurfaceArea1 percolate to the top of the importance metric, and importance values begin to taper with fingerprints. Importance values for fingerprints 116 and 75 are top fingerprint performers for importance, which may indicate that the structures represented by these fingerprints have an impact on a compound's solubility.

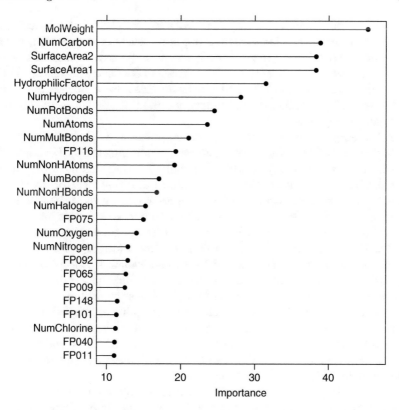

Fig. 8.19: Variable importance scores for the top 25 predictors used in the random forest CART tree model for solubility

Contrasting random forest importance results to a single CART tree (Fig. 8.6) we see that 2 of the top 4 predictors are the same (SurfaceArea2 and NumCarbon) and 14 of the top 16 are the same. However, the importance orderings are much different. For example NumNonHBonds is the top predictor for a CART tree but ends up ranked 14th for random forests; random forests identify MolWeight as the top predictor, whereas a CART tree ranks it 5th. These differences should not be disconcerting; rather they emphasize that a single tree's greediness prioritizes predictors differently than a random forest.

8.6 Boosting

Boosting models were originally developed for classification problems and were later extended to the regression setting. Readers unfamiliar with boosting may benefit by first reading about boosting for classification (Sect. 14.5) and then returning to this section. For completeness of this section, we will give a history of boosting to provide a bridge from boosting's original development in classification to its use in the regression context. This history begins with the AdaBoost algorithm and evolves to Friedman's stochastic gradient boosting machine, which is now widely accepted as the boosting algorithm of choice among practitioners.

In the early 1990s boosting algorithms appeared (Schapire 1990; Freund 1995; Schapire 1999), which were influenced by learning theory (Valiant 1984; Kearns and Valiant 1989), in which a number of weak classifiers (a classifier that predicts marginally better than random) are combined (or boosted) to produce an ensemble classifier with a superior generalized misclassification error rate. Researchers struggled for a time to find an effective implementation of boosting theory, until Freund and Schapire collaborated to produce the AdaBoost algorithm (Schapire 1999). AdaBoost (see Algorithm 14.2) provided a practical implementation of Kerns and Valiant's concept of boosting a weak learner into a strong learner (Kearns and Valiant 1989).

Boosting, especially in the form of the AdaBoost algorithm, was shown to be a powerful prediction tool, usually outperforming any individual model. Its success drew attention from the modeling community and its use became widespread with applications in gene expression (Dudoit et al. 2002; Ben-Dor et al. 2000), chemometrics (Varmuza et al. 2003), and music genre identification (Bergstra et al. 2006), to name a few.

The AdaBoost algorithm clearly worked, and after its successful arrival, several researchers (Friedman et al. 2000) connected the AdaBoost algorithm to statistical concepts of loss functions, additive modeling, and logistic regression and showed that boosting can be interpreted as a forward stagewise additive model that minimizes exponential loss. This fundamental understanding of boosting led to a new view of boosting that facilitated several algorithmic generalizations to classification problems (Sect. 14.5). Moreover, this new perspective also enabled the method to be extended to regression problems.

Friedman's ability to see boosting's statistical framework yielded a simple, elegant, and highly adaptable algorithm for different kinds of problems (Friedman 2001). He called this method "gradient boosting machines" which encompassed both classification and regression. The basic principles of gradient boosting are as follows: given a loss function (e.g., squared error for regression) and a weak learner (e.g., regression trees), the algorithm seeks to find an additive model that minimizes the loss function. The algorithm is typically initialized with the best guess of the response (e.g., the mean of the response in regression). The gradient (e.g., residual) is calculated, and a model is then fit to the residuals to minimize the loss function. The current model is added to the previous model, and the procedure continues for a user-specified number of iterations.

As described throughout this text, any modeling technique with tuning parameters can produce a range of predictive ability—from weak to strong. Because boosting requires a weak learner, almost any technique with tuning parameters can be made into a weak learner. Trees, as it turns out, make an excellent base learner for boosting for several reasons. First, they have the flexibility to be weak learners by simply restricting their depth. Second, separate trees can be easily added together, much like individual predictors can be added together in a regression model, to generate a prediction. And third, trees can be generated very quickly. Hence, results from individual trees can be directly aggregated, thus making them inherently suitable for an additive modeling process.

When regression tree are used as the base learner, simple gradient boosting for regression has two tuning parameters: tree depth and number of iterations. Tree depth in this context is also known as *interaction depth*, since each subsequential split can be thought of as a higher-level interaction term with all of the other previous split predictors. If squared error is used as the loss function, then a simple boosting algorithm using these tuning parameters can be found in Algorithm 8.3.

---

1 Select tree depth, D, and number of iterations, K

2 Compute the average response, $\bar{y}$, and use this as the initial predicted value for each sample

3 for $k = 1$ *to* K **do**

4   Compute the residual, the difference between the observed value and the *current* predicted value, for each sample

5   Fit a regression tree of depth, D, using the residuals as the response

6   Predict each sample using the regression tree fit in the previous step

7   Update the predicted value of each sample by adding the previous iteration's predicted value to the predicted value generated in the previous step

8 end

Algorithm 8.3: Simple Gradient Boosting for Regression

Clearly, the version of boosting presented in Algorithm 8.3 has similarities to random forests: the final prediction is based on an ensemble of models, and trees are used as the base learner. However, the way the ensembles are constructed differs substantially between each method. In random forests, all trees are created independently, each tree is created to have maximum depth, and each tree contributes equally to the final model. The trees in boosting, however, are dependent on past trees, have minimum depth, and contribute unequally to the final model. Despite these differences, both random forests and boosting offer competitive predictive performance. Computation time for boosting is often greater than for random forests, since random forests can be easily parallel processed given that the trees are created independently.

Friedman recognized that his gradient boosting machine could be susceptible to over-fitting, since the learner employed—even in its weakly defined learning capacity—is tasked with optimally fitting the gradient. This means that boosting will select the optimal learner at each stage of the algorithm. Despite using weak learners, boosting still employs the greedy strategy of choosing the optimal weak learner at each stage. Although this strategy generates an optimal solution at the current stage, it has the drawbacks of not finding the optimal global model as well as over-fitting the training data. A remedy for greediness is to constrain the learning process by employing regularization, or shrinkage, in the same manner as illustrated in Sect. 6.4. In Algorithm 8.3, a regularization strategy can be injected into the final line of the loop. Instead of adding the predicted value for a sample to previous iteration's predicted value, only a fraction of the current predicted value is added to the previous iteration's predicted value. This fraction is commonly referred to as the *learning rate* and is parameterized by the symbol, λ. This parameter can take values between 0 and 1 and becomes another tuning parameter for the model. Ridgeway (2007) suggests that small values of the learning parameter (< 0.01) work best, but he also notes that the value of the parameter is inversely proportional to the computation time required to find an optimal model, because more iterations are necessary. Having more iterations also implies that more memory is required for storing the model.

After Friedman published his gradient boosting machine, he considered some of the properties of Breiman's bagging technique. Specifically, the random sampling nature of bagging offered a reduction in prediction variance for bagging. Friedman updated the boosting machine algorithm with a random sampling scheme and termed the new procedure *stochastic gradient boosting*. To do this, Friedman inserted the following step before line within the loop: randomly select a fraction of the training data. The residuals and models in the remaining steps of the current iteration are based only on the sample of data. The fraction of training data used, known as the bagging fraction, then becomes another tuning parameter for the model. It turns out that this simple modification improved the prediction accuracy of boosting while also reducing the required computational resources. Friedman suggests using a bagging fraction of around 0.5; this value, however, can be tuned like any other parameter.

Figure 8.20 presents the cross-validated RMSE results for boosted trees across tuning parameters of tree depth (1–7), number of trees (100–1,000), and shrinkage (0.01 or 0.1); the bagging fraction in this illustration was fixed at 0.5. When examining this figure, the larger value of shrinkage (right-hand

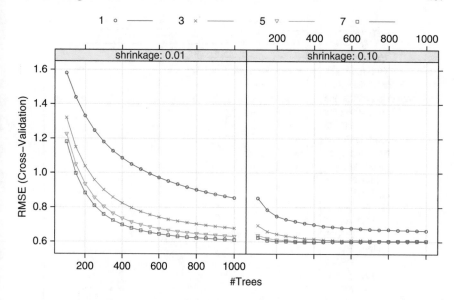

Fig. 8.20: Cross-validated RMSE profiles for the boosted tree model

plot) has an impact on reducing RMSE for all choices of tree depth and number of trees. Also, RMSE decreases as tree depth increases when shrinkage is 0.01. The same pattern holds true for RMSE when shrinkage is 0.1 and the number of trees is less than 300.

Using the one-standard-error rule, the optimal boosted tree has depth 3 with 400 trees and shrinkage of 0.1. These settings produce a cross-validated RMSE of 0.616.

Variable importance for boosting is a function of the reduction in squared error. Specifically, the improvement in squared error due to each predictor is summed within each tree in the ensemble (i.e., each predictor gets an improvement value for each tree). The improvement values for each predictor are then averaged across the entire ensemble to yield an overall importance value (Friedman 2002; Ridgeway 2007). The top 25 predictors for the model are presented in Fig. 8.21. NumCarbon and MolWeight stand out in this example as most important followed by SurfaceArea1 and SurfaceArea2; importance values tail off after about 7 predictors. Comparing these results to random forests we see that both methods identify the same top 4 predictors, albeit in different order. The importance profile for boosting has a much steeper importance slope than the one for random forests. This is due to the fact that the trees from boosting are dependent on each other and hence will have correlated structures as the method follows by the gradient. Therefore many of the same predictors will be selected across the trees, increasing their contribution to the importance metric. Differences between variable importance

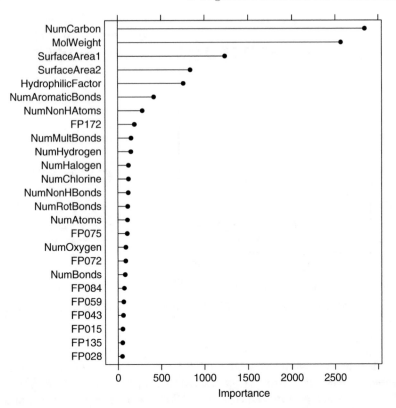

Fig. 8.21: Variable importance scores for the top 25 predictors used in the stochastic gradient boosting model for solubility

ordering and magnitude between random forests and boosting should not be disconcerting. Instead, one should consider these as two different perspectives of the data and use each view to provide some understanding of the gross relationships between predictors and the response.

8.7 Cubist

Cubist is a rule-based model that is an amalgamation of several methodologies published some time ago (Quinlan 1987, 1992, 1993a) but has evolved over this period. Previously, Cubist was only available in a commercial capacity, but in 2011 the source code was released under an open-source license. At this time, the full details of the current version of the model became public. Our description of the model stems from the open-source version of the model.[2] Some specific differences between Cubist and the previously described approaches for model trees and their rule-based variants are:

- The specific techniques used for linear model smoothing, creating rules, and pruning are different
- An optional boosting—like procedure called *committees*
- The predictions generated by the model rules can be adjusted using nearby points from the training set data

The model tree construction process is almost identical to the process described in Sect. 8.2, although the smoothing process between linear models is more complex than the approach described in Quinlan (1992). In Cubist, the models are still combined using a linear combination of two models:

$$\hat{y}_{\mathrm{par}} = a \times \hat{y}_{(k)} + (1 - a) \times \hat{y}_{(p)},$$

where $\hat{y}_{(k)}$ is the prediction from the current model and $\hat{y}_{(p)}$ is from parent model above it in the tree. Compared to model trees, Cubist calculates the mixing proportions using a different equation. Let $e_{(k)}$ be the collection of residuals of the child model (i.e., $y - \hat{y}_{(k)}$) and $e_{(p)}$ be similar values for the parent model. The smoothing procedure first determines the covariance between the two sets of model residuals (denoted as $\mathrm{Cov}[e_{(p)}, e_{(k)}]$). This is an overall measure of the linear relation between the two sets of residuals. If the covariance is large, this implies that the residuals generally have the same sign and relative magnitude, while a value near 0 would indicate no (linear) relationship between the errors of the two models. Cubist also calculates the variance of the difference between the residuals, e.g., $\mathrm{Var}[e_{(p)} - e_{(k)}]$. The smoothing coefficient used by Cubist is then

$$a = \frac{\mathrm{Var}[e_{(p)}] - \mathrm{Cov}[e_{(k)}, e_{(p)}]}{\mathrm{Var}[e_{(p)} - e_{(k)}]}.$$

The first part of the numerator is proportional to the parent model's RMSE. If variance of the parent model's errors is larger than the covariance, the smoothing procedure tends to weight the child more than the parent. Conversely, if the variance of the parent model is low, that model is given more weight.

In the end, the model with the smallest RMSE has a higher weight in the smoothed model. When the models have the same RMSE, they are equally weighted in the smooth procedure (regardless of the covariance).

Unlike the previously discussed "separate and conquer" methodology, the final model tree is used to construct the initial set of rules. Cubist collects the sequence of linear models at each node into a single, smoothed representation of the models so that there is one liner model associated with each rule. The

---

[2] We are indebted to the work of Chris Keefer, who extensively studied the Cubist source code.

adjusted error rate (Eq. 8.3) is the criterion for pruning and/or combining rules. Starting with splits made near the terminal nodes, each condition of the rules is tested using the adjusted error rate for the training set. If the deletion of a condition in the rule does not increase the error rate, it is dropped. This can lead to entire rules being removed from the overall model. Once the rule conditions have been finalized, a new sample is predicted using the average of the linear models from the appropriate rules (as opposed to the rule with the largest coverage).

Model committees can be created by generating a sequence of rule-based models. Like boosting, each model is affected by the result of the previous models. Recall that boosting uses new weights for each data point based on previous fits and then fits a new model utilizing these weights. Committees function differently. The training set outcome is adjusted based on the prior model fit and then builds a new set of rules using this pseudo-response. Specifically, the mth committee model uses an adjusted response:

$$y^*_{(m)} = y - (\hat{y}_{(m-1)} - y).$$

Basically, if a data point is underpredicted, the sample value is increased in the hope that the model will produce a larger prediction in the next iteration. Similarly, over-predicted points are adjusted so that the next model will lower its prediction. Once the full set of committee models are created, new samples are predicted using each model and the final rule-based prediction is the simple average of the individual model predictions (recall that boosting uses stage weights for the average).

Once the rule-based model is finalized (either using a single model or a committee), Cubist has the ability to adjust the model prediction with samples from the training set (Quinlan 1993a). When predicting a new sample, the K most similar neighbors are determined from the training set. Suppose that the model predicts the new sample to be $\hat{y}$ and then the final prediction would be

$$\frac{1}{K} \sum_{\ell=1}^{K} w_\ell \left[t_\ell + \left(\hat{y} - \hat{t}_\ell \right) \right],$$

where t_ℓ is the observed outcome for a training set neighbor, $\hat{t}_\ell$ is the model prediction of that neighbor, and w_ℓ is a weight calculated using the distance of the training set neighbors to the new sample. As the difference between the predictions of the new sample and its closest neighbor increases, the adjustment becomes larger.

There are several details that must be specified to enact this process. First, a distance metric to define the neighbors is needed. The implementation of Cubist uses Manhattan (a.k.a. city block) distances to determine the nearest neighbors. Also, neighbors are only included if they are "close enough" to the prediction sample. To filter the neighbors, the average pairwise distance of data points in the training set is used as a threshold. If the distance from

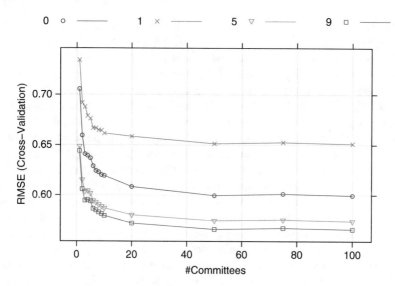

Fig. 8.22: Cross-validated RMSE profiles for the number of committees and neighbors used in Cubist

the potential neighbor to the prediction samples is greater than this average distance, the neighbor is excluded. The weights w_ℓ also use the distance to the neighbors. The raw weights are computed as

$$w_\ell = \frac{1}{D_\ell + 0.5},$$

where D_ℓ is the distance of the neighbor to the prediction sample. These weights are normalized to sum to one. Weighting has the effect of emphasizing neighbors that are more similar to the prediction sample. Quinlan (1993a) provides more information and further details can be found in the Cubist source code at www.RuleQuest.com.

To tune this model, different numbers of committees and neighbors were assessed. Figure 8.22 shows the cross-validation profiles. Independent of the number of neighbors used, there is a trend where the error is significantly reduced as the number of committees is increased and then stabilizes around 50 committees. The use of the training set to adjust the model predictions is interesting: a purely rule-based model does better than an adjustment with a single neighbor, but the error is reduced the most when nine neighbors are used. In the end, the model with the lowest error (0.57 log units) was associated with 100 committees and an adjustment using nine neighbors, although fewer committees could also be used without much loss of performance. For the final Cubist model, the average number of rules per committee was 5.1 but ranged from 1 to 15.

We can compare the Cubist model with a single committee member and no neighbor adjustment to the previous rule-based model. The M5 rule-based model had an estimated cross-validation error of 0.74 whereas the corresponding Cubist model had error rate of 0.71. Based on the variation in the results, this difference is slightly statistically significant (p-value: 0.0485). This might indicate that the methodological differences between the two methods for constructing rule-based models are not large, at least for these data.

There is no established technique for measuring predictor importance for Cubist models. Each linear model has a corresponding slope for each predictor, but, as previously shown, these values can be gigantic when there is significant collinearity in the data. A metric that relied solely on these values would also ignore which predictors were used in the splits. However, one can enumerate how many times a predictor variable was used in either a linear model or a split and use these tabulations to get a rough idea the impact each predictor has on the model. However, this approach ignores the neighbor-based correction that is sometimes used by Cubist. The modeler can choose how to weight the counts for the splits and the linear models in the overall usage calculation.

For the solubility data, predictor importance values were calculated for the model with 100 committees and correct the prediction using the 9-nearest neighbors. Figure 8.23 shows a visualization of the values, where the x-axis is the total usage of the predictor (i.e., the number of times it was used in a split or a linear model). Like many of the other models discussed for these data, the continuous predictors appear to have a greater impact on the model than the fingerprint descriptors. Unlike the boosted tree model, there is a more gradual decrease in importance for these data; there is not a small subset of predictors that are dominating the model fit.

8.8 Computing

The R packages used in this section are caret, Cubist, gbm, ipred, party, partykit, randomForest, rpart, RWeka.

Single Trees

Two widely used implementations for single regression trees in R are rpart and party. The rpart package makes splits based on the CART methodology using the rpart function, whereas the party makes splits based on the conditional inference framework using the ctree function. Both rpart and ctree functions use the formula method:

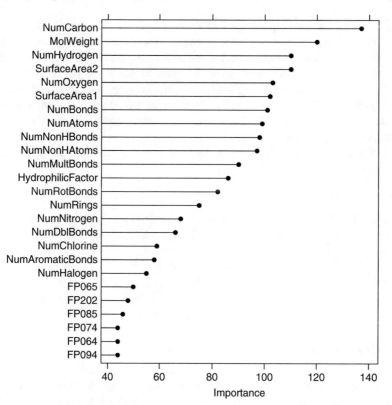

Fig. 8.23: Variable importance scores for the top 25 predictors used in the Cubist model for solubility

```
> library(rpart)
> rpartTree <- rpart(y ~ ., data = trainData)
> # or,
> ctreeTree <- ctree(y ~ ., data = trainData)
```

The rpart function has several control parameters that can be accessed through the rpart.control argument. Two that are commonly used in training and that can be accessed through the train function are the complexity parameter (cp) and maximum node depth (maxdepth). To tune an CART tree over the complexity parameter, the method option in the train function should be set to method = "rpart". To tune over maximum depth, the method option should be set to method="rpart2":

```
> set.seed(100)
> rpartTune <- train(solTrainXtrans, solTrainY,
+                    method = "rpart2",
+                    tuneLength = 10,
+                    trControl = trainControl(method = "cv"))
```

Likewise, the **party** package has several control parameters that can be accessed through the `ctree_control` argument. Two of these parameters are commonly used in training: `mincriterion` and `maxdepth`. `mincriterion` defines the statistical criterion that must be met in order to continue splitting; `maxdepth` is the maximum depth of the tree. To tune a conditional inference tree over `mincriterion`, the method option in the `train` function should be set to `method = "ctree"`. To tune over maximum depth, the method option should be set to `method="ctree2"`.

The `plot` method in the **party** package can produce the tree diagrams shown in Fig. 8.4 via

```
> plot(treeObject)
```

To produce such plots for **rpart** trees, the **partykit** can be used to first convert the `rpart` object to a `party` object and then use the `plot` function:

```
> library(partykit)
> rpartTree2 <- as.party(rpartTree)
> plot(rpartTree2)
```

Model Trees

The main implementation for model trees can be found in the **Weka** software suite, but the model can be accessed in R using the **RWeka** package. There are two different interfaces: `M5P` fits the model tree, while `M5Rules` uses the rule-based version. In either case, the functions work with formula methods:

```
> library(RWeka)
> m5tree <- M5P(y ~ ., data = trainData)
> # or, for rules:
> m5rules <- M5Rules(y ~ ., data = trainData)
```

In our example, the minimum number of training set points required to create additional splits was raised from the default of 4–10. To do this, the control argument is used:

```
> m5tree <- M5P(y ~ ., data = trainData,
+              control = Weka_control(M = 10))
```

The control argument also has options for toggling the use of smoothing and pruning. If the full model tree is used, a visualization similar to Fig. 8.10 can be created by the `plot` function on the output from `M5P`.

To tune these models, the `train` function in the **caret** package has two options: using `method = "M5"` evaluates model trees and the rule-based versions of the model, as well as the use of smoothing and pruning. Figure 8.12 shows the results of evaluating these models from the code:

```
> set.seed(100)
> m5Tune <- train(solTrainXtrans, solTrainY,
+                 method = "M5",
+                 trControl = trainControl(method = "cv"),
+                 ## Use an option for M5() to specify the minimum
+                 ## number of samples needed to further splits the
+                 ## data to be 10
+                 control = Weka_control(M = 10))
```

followed by plot(m5Tune). train with method = "M5Rules" evaluates only the
rule-based version of the model.

Bagged Trees

The ipred package contains two functions for bagged trees: bagging uses the
formula interface and ipredbagg has the non-formula interface:

```
> library(ipred)
> baggedTree <- ipredbagg(solTrainY, solTrainXtrans)
> ## or
> baggedTree <- bagging(y ~ ., data = trainData)
```

The function uses the rpart function and details about the type of tree can
be specified by passing rpart.control to the control argument for bagging and
ipredbagg. By default, the largest possible tree is created.

Several other packages have functions for bagging. The aforementioned
RWeka package has a function called Bagging and the caret package has a
general framework for bagging many model types, including trees, called bag.
Conditional inference trees can also be bagged using the cforest function in
the party package if the argument mtry is equal to the number of predictors:

```
> library(party)
> ## The mtry parameter should be the number of predictors (the
> ## number of columns minus 1 for the outcome).
> bagCtrl <- cforest_control(mtry = ncol(trainData) - 1)
> baggedTree <- cforest(y ~ ., data = trainData, controls = bagCtrl)
```

Random Forest

The primary implementation for random forest comes from the package with
the same name:

```
> library(randomForest)
> rfModel <- randomForest(solTrainXtrans, solTrainY)
> ## or
> rfModel <- randomForest(y ~ ., data = trainData)
```

The two main arguments are mtry for the number of predictors that are randomly sampled as candidates for each split and ntrees for the number of bootstrap samples. The default for mtry in regression is the number of predictors divided by 3. The number of trees should be large enough to provide a stable, reproducible results. Although the default is 500, at least 1,000 bootstrap samples should be used (and perhaps more depending on the number of predictors and the values of mtry). Another important option is importance; by default, variable importance scores are not computed as they are time consuming; importance = TRUE will generate these values:

```
> library(randomForest)
> rfModel <- randomForest(solTrainXtrans, solTrainY,
+                         importance = TRUE,
+                         ntrees = 1000)
```

For forests built using conditional inference trees, the cforest function in the **party** package is available. It has similar options, but the controls argument (note the plural) allows the user to pick the type of splitting algorithm to use (e.g., biased or unbiased).

Neither of these functions can be used with missing data.

The train function contains wrappers for tuning either of these models by specifying either method = "rf" or method = "cforest". Optimizing the mtry parameter may result in a slight increase in performance. Also, train can use standard resampling methods for estimating performance (as opposed to the out-of-bag estimate).

For **randomForest** models, the variable importance scores can be accessed using a function in that package called importance. For cforest objects, the analogous function in the **party** package is varimp.

Each package tends to have its own function for calculating importance scores, similar to the situation for class probabilities shown in Table B.1 of the first Appendix. **caret** has a unifying function called varImp that is a wrapper for variable importance functions for the following tree-model objects: rpart, classbagg (produced by the **ipred** package's bagging functions) randomForest, cforest, gbm, and cubist.

Boosted Trees

The most widely used package for boosting regression trees via stochastic gradient boosting machines is **gbm**. Like the random forests interface, models can be built in two distinct ways:

```
> library(gbm)
> gbmModel <- gbm.fit(solTrainXtrans, solTrainY, distribution = "gaussian")
> ## or
> gbmModel <- gbm(y ~ ., data = trainData, distribution = "gaussian")
```

The distribution argument defines the type of loss function that will be optimized during boosting. For a continuous response, distribution should be set to "gaussian." The number of trees (n.trees), depth of trees (interaction.depth), shrinkage (shrinkage), and proportion of observations to be sampled (bag.fraction) can all be directly set in the call to gbm.

Like other parameters, the train function can be used to tune over these parameters. To tune over interaction depth, number of trees, and shrinkage, for example, we first define a tuning grid. Then we train over this grid as follows:

```
> gbmGrid <- expand.grid(.interaction.depth = seq(1, 7, by = 2),
+                        .n.trees = seq(100, 1000, by = 50),
+                        .shrinkage = c(0.01, 0.1))
> set.seed(100)
> gbmTune <- train(solTrainXtrans, solTrainY,
+                  method = "gbm",
+                  tuneGrid = gbmGrid,
+                  ## The gbm() function produces copious amounts
+                  ## of  output, so pass in the verbose option
+                  ## to avoid printing a lot to the screen.
+                  verbose = FALSE)
```

Cubist

As previously mentioned, the implementation for this model created by Rule-Quest was recently made public using an open-source license. An R package called Cubist was created using the open-source code. The function does not have a formula method since it is desirable to have the Cubist code manage the creation and usage of dummy variables. To create a simple rule-based model with a single committee and no instance-based adjustment, we can use the simple code:

```
> library(Cubist)
> cubistMod <- cubist(solTrainXtrans, solTrainY)
```

An argument, committees, fits multiple models. The familiar predict method would be used for new samples:

```
> predict(cubistMod, solTestXtrans)
```

The choice of instance-based corrections does not need to be made until samples are predicted. The predict function has an argument, neighbors, that can take on a single integer value (between 0 and 9) to adjust the rule-based predictions from the training set.

Once the model is trained, the summary function generates the exact rules that were used, as well as the final smoothed linear model for each rule. Also,

as with most other models, the `train` function in the **caret** package can tune
the model over values of `committees` and `neighbors` through resampling:

```
> cubistTuned <- train(solTrainXtrans, solTrainY, method = "cubist")
```

Exercises

8.1. Recreate the simulated data from Exercise 7.2:

```
> library(mlbench)
> set.seed(200)
> simulated <- mlbench.friedman1(200, sd = 1)
> simulated <- cbind(simulated$x, simulated$y)
> simulated <- as.data.frame(simulated)
> colnames(simulated)[ncol(simulated)] <- "y"
```

(a) Fit a random forest model to all of the predictors, then estimate the
variable importance scores:

```
> library(randomForest)
> library(caret)
> model1 <- randomForest(y ~ ., data = simulated,
+                        importance = TRUE,
+                        ntree = 1000)
> rfImp1 <- varImp(model1, scale = FALSE)
```

Did the random forest model significantly use the uninformative predictors (V6 – V10)?

(b) Now add an additional predictor that is highly correlated with one of the
informative predictors. For example:

```
> simulated$duplicate1 <- simulated$V1 + rnorm(200) * .1
> cor(simulated$duplicate1, simulated$V1)
```

Fit another random forest model to these data. Did the importance score
for V1 change? What happens when you add another predictor that is
also highly correlated with V1?

(c) Use the `cforest` function in the **party** package to fit a random forest model
using conditional inference trees. The **party** package function `varimp` can
calculate predictor importance. The `conditional` argument of that function toggles between the traditional importance measure and the modified
version described in Strobl et al. (2007). Do these importances show the
same pattern as the traditional random forest model?

(d) Repeat this process with different tree models, such as boosted trees and
Cubist. Does the same pattern occur?

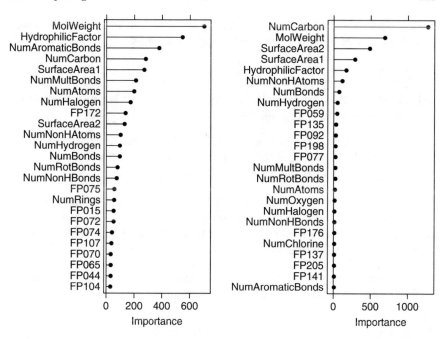

Fig. 8.24: A comparison of variable importance magnitudes for differing values of the bagging fraction and shrinkage parameters. Both tuning parameters are set to 0.1 in the *left* figure. Both are set to 0.9 in the *right* figure

8.2. Use a simulation to show tree bias with different granularities.

8.3. In stochastic gradient boosting the bagging fraction and learning rate will govern the construction of the trees as they are guided by the gradient. Although the optimal values of these parameters should be obtained through the tuning process, it is helpful to understand how the magnitudes of these parameters affect magnitudes of variable importance. Figure 8.24 provides the variable importance plots for boosting using two extreme values for the bagging fraction (0.1 and 0.9) and the learning rate (0.1 and 0.9) for the solubility data. The left-hand plot has both parameters set to 0.1, and the right-hand plot has both set to 0.9:

(a) Why does the model on the right focus its importance on just the first few of predictors, whereas the model on the left spreads importance across more predictors?

(b) Which model do you think would be more predictive of other samples?

(c) How would increasing interaction depth affect the slope of predictor importance for either model in Fig. 8.24?

8.4. Use a single predictor in the solubility data, such as the molecular weight or the number of carbon atoms and fit several models:

(a) A simple regression tree
(b) A random forest model
(c) Different Cubist models with a single rule or multiple committees (each with and without using neighbor adjustments)

Plot the predictor data versus the solubility results for the test set. Overlay the model predictions for the test set. How do the model differ? Does changing the tuning parameter(s) significantly affect the model fit?

8.5. Fit different tree- and rule-based models for the Tecator data discussed in Exercise 6.1. How do they compare to linear models? Do the between-predictor correlations seem to affect your models? If so, how would you transform or re-encode the predictor data to mitigate this issue?

8.6. Return to the permeability problem described in Exercises 6.2 and 7.4. Train several tree-based models and evaluate the resampling and test set performance:

(a) Which tree-based model gives the optimal resampling and test set performance?
(b) Do any of these models outperform the covariance or non-covariance based regression models you have previously developed for these data? What criteria did you use to compare models' performance?
(c) Of all the models you have developed thus far, which, if any, would you recommend to replace the permeability laboratory experiment?

8.7. Refer to Exercises 6.3 and 7.5 which describe a chemical manufacturing process. Use the same data imputation, data splitting, and pre-processing steps as before and train several tree-based models:

(a) Which tree-based regression model gives the optimal resampling and test set performance?
(b) Which predictors are most important in the optimal tree-based regression model? Do either the biological or process variables dominate the list? How do the top 10 important predictors compare to the top 10 predictors from the optimal linear and nonlinear models?
(c) Plot the optimal single tree with the distribution of yield in the terminal nodes. Does this view of the data provide additional knowledge about the biological or process predictors and their relationship with yield?

Chapter 9
A Summary of Solubility Models

Across the last few chapters, a variety of models have been fit to the solubility data set. How do the models compare for these data and which one should be selected for the final model? Figs. 9.1 and 9.2 show scatter plots of the performance metrics calculated using cross-validation and the test set data.

With the exception of poorly performing models, there is a fairly high correlation between the results derived from resampling and the test set (0.9 for the RMSE and 0.88 for R^2). For the most part, the models tend to rank order similarly. K-nearest neighbors were the weakest performer, followed by the two single tree-based methods. While bagging these trees did help, it did not make the models very competitive. Additionally, conditional random forest models had mediocre results.

There was a "pack" of models that showed better results, including model trees, linear regression, penalized linear models, MARS, and neural networks. These models are more simplistic but would not be considered interpretable given the number of predictors involved in the linear models and the complexity of the model trees and MARS. For the most part, they would be easy to implement. Recall that this type of model might be used by a pharmaceutical company to screen *millions* of potential compounds, so ease of implementation should not be taken lightly.

The group of high-performance models include support vector machines (SVMs), boosted trees, random forests, and Cubist. Each is essentially a black box with a highly complex prediction equation. The performance of these models is head and shoulders above the rest so there is probably some value in finding computationally efficient implementations that can be used to predict large numbers of new samples.

Are there any real differences between these models? Using the resampling results, a set of confidence intervals were constructed to characterize the differences in RMSE in the models using the techniques shown in Sect. 4.8. Figure 9.3 shows the intervals. There are very few statistically significant

M. Kuhn and K. Johnson, *Applied Predictive Modeling*,
DOI 10.1007/978-1-4614-6849-3_9,
© Springer Science+Business Media New York 2013

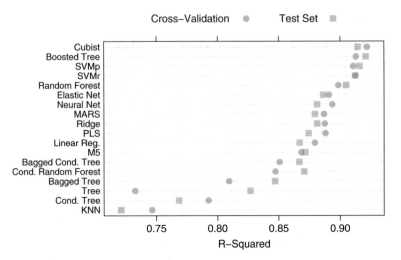

Fig. 9.1: A plot of the R^2 solubility models estimated by 10-fold cross-validation and the test set

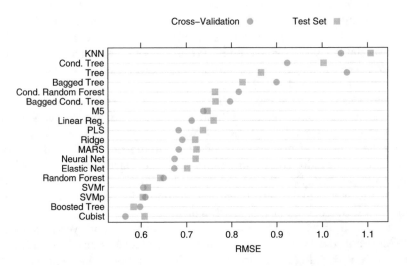

Fig. 9.2: A plot of the RMSE solubility models estimated by 10-fold cross-validation and the test set

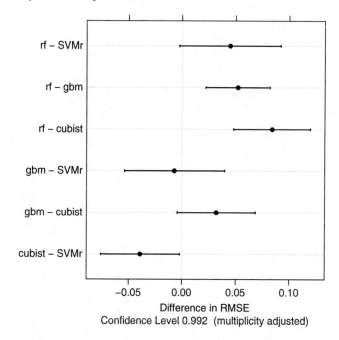

Fig. 9.3: Confidence intervals for the differences in RMSE for the high-performance models

differences. Additionally, most of the estimated mean differences are less than 0.05 log units, which are not scientifically meaningful. Given this, any of these models would be a reasonable choice.

Chapter 10
Case Study: Compressive Strength of Concrete Mixtures

Thus far, the focus has been on observational data sets where the values of the predictors were not pre-specified. For example, the QSAR data used in the previous chapters involved a collection of diverse compounds that captured a sufficient amount of the "chemical space." This particular data set was not created by specifying exact values for the chemical properties (such as molecular weight). Instead compounds were sampled from an appropriate population for use in the model.

Designed experiments are created by planning the exact values of the predictors (referred to as the factors in this context) using some sort of strategic methodology. The configurations of predictor settings are created so that they have good mathematical and experimental properties. One such property is *balance*. A balanced design is one where no one experimental factor (i.e., the predictors) has more focus than the others. In most cases, this means that each predictor has the same number of possible levels and that the frequencies of the levels are equivalent for each factor. The properties used to choose the best experimental design are driven by the stage of experimentation.

Box et al. (1978) popularized the concept of *sequential experimentation* where a large number of possible experimental factors are screened with low resolution (i.e., "casting a wide net") to determine the *active* or important factors that relate to the outcome. Once the importance of the predictors are quantified, more focused experiments are created with the subset of important factors. In subsequent experiments, the nature of the relationship between the important factors can be further elucidated. The last step in the sequence of experiments is to fine-tune a small number of important factors. *Response surface experiments* (Myers and Montgomery 2009) use a smaller set of predictor values. Here, the primary goal is to optimize the experimental settings based on a nonlinear model of the experimental predictors.

M. Kuhn and K. Johnson, *Applied Predictive Modeling*,
DOI 10.1007/978-1-4614-6849-3_10,
© Springer Science+Business Media New York 2013

Designed experiments and predictive models have several differences[1]:

- A sequence of studies is preferred over a single, comprehensive data set that attempts to include all possible predictors (i.e., experimental factors) with many values per predictor. The iterative paradigm of planning, designing, and then analyzing an experiment is, on the surface, different than most predictive modeling problems.
- Until the final stages of sequential experimentation, the focus is on understanding which predictors affect the outcome and how. Once response surface experiments are utilized, the focus of the activities is solely about prediction.

This case study will focus on the prediction of optimal formulations of concrete mixture-based data from designed experiments.

Concrete is an integral part of most industrialized societies. It is used to some extent in nearly all structures and in many roads. One of the main properties of interest (beside cost) is the compressive strength of the hardened concrete. The composition of many concretes includes a number of dry ingredients which are mixed with water and then are allowed to dry and harden. Given its abundance and critical role in infrastructure, the composition is important and has been widely studied. In this chapter, models will be created to help find potential recipes to maximize compressive strength.

Yeh (2006) describes a standard type of experimental setup for this scenario called a *mixture design* (Cornell 2002; Myers and Montgomery 2009). Here, boundaries on the upper and lower limits on the mixture *proportion* for each ingredient are used to create multiple mixtures that methodically fill the space within the boundaries. For a specific type of mixture design, there is a corresponding linear regression model that is typically used to model the relationship between the ingredients and the outcome. These linear models can include interaction effects and higher-order terms for the ingredients. The ingredients used in Yeh (2006) were:

- Cement (kg/m^3)
- Fly ash (kg/m^3), small particles produced by burning coal
- Blast furnace slag (kg/m^3)
- Water (kg/m^3)

---

[1] There are cases where specialized types of experimental designs are utilized with predictive models. In the field of chemometrics, an orthogonal array-type design followed by the sequential elimination of level combination algorithm has been shown to improve QSAR models (Mandal et al. 2006, 2007). Also, the field of *active learning* sequentially added samples based on the training set using the predictive model results (Cohn et al. 1994; Saar-Tsechansky and Provost 2007a).

- Superplasticizer (kg/m^3), an additive that reduces particle aggregation
- Coarse aggregate (kg/m^3)
- Fine aggregate (kg/m^3)

Yeh (2006) also describes an additional non-mixture factor related to compressive strength: the age of the mixture (at testing). Since this is not an ingredient, it is usually referred to as a *process factor*. Specific experimental designs (and linear model forms) exist for experiments that combine mixture and process variables (see Cornell (2002) for more details).

Yeh (1998) takes a different approach to modeling concrete mixture experiments. Here, separate experiments from 17 sources with common experimental factors were combined into one "meta-experiment" and the author used neural networks to create predictive models across the whole mixture space. Age was also included in the model. The public version of the data set includes 1030 data points across the different experiments, although Yeh (1998) states that some mixtures were removed from his analysis due to nonstandard conditions. There is no information regarding exactly which mixtures were removed, so the analyses here will use all available data points. Table 10.1 shows a summary of the predictor data (in amounts) and the outcome.

Figure 10.1 shows scatter plots of each predictor versus the compressive strength. Age shows a strong nonlinear relationship with the predictor, and the cement amount has a linear relationship. Note that several of the ingredients have a large frequency of a single amount, such as zero for the superplasticizer and the amount of fly ash. In these cases, the compressive strength varies widely for those values of the predictors. This might indicate that some of the partitioning methods, such as trees or MARS, may be able to isolate these mixtures within the model and more effectively predict the compressive strength. For example, there are 53 mixtures with no superplasticizer or fly ash but with exactly $228\,kg/m^3$ of water. This may represent an important sub-population of mixtures that may benefit from a model that is specific to these types of mixtures. A tree- or rule-based model has the ability to model such a sub-group while classical regression models would not.

Although the available data do not denote which formulations came from each source, there are 19 distinct mixtures with replicate data points. The majority of these mixtures had only two or three duplicate conditions, although some conditions have as many as four replicates. When modeling these data, the replicate results should not be treated as though they are independent observations. For example, having replicate mixtures in both the training and test sets can result in overly optimistic assessments of how well the model works. A common approach here is to average the outcomes within each unique mixture. Consequentially, the number of mixtures available for modeling drops from 1030 to 992.

Table 10.1: Data for the concrete mixtures

9 Variables   1030 Observations

Cement

n	missing	unique	Mean	0.05	0.10	0.25	0.50	0.75	0.90	0.95
1,030	0	278	281.2	143.7	153.5	192.4	272.9	350.0	425.0	480.0

```
lowest : 102.0 108.3 116.0 122.6 132.0
highest: 522.0 525.0 528.0 531.3 540.0
```

BlastFurnaceSlag

n	missing	unique	Mean	0.05	0.10	0.25	0.50	0.75	0.90	0.95
1,030	0	185	73.9	0.0	0.0	0.0	22.0	142.9	192.0	236.0

```
lowest :   0.0  11.0  13.6  15.0  17.2
highest: 290.2 305.3 316.1 342.1 359.4
```

FlyAsh

n	missing	unique	Mean	0.05	0.10	0.25	0.50	0.75	0.90	0.95
1,030	0	156	54.19	0.0	0.0	0.0	0.0	118.3	141.1	167.0

```
lowest :   0.0  24.5  59.0  60.0  71.0
highest: 194.0 194.9 195.0 200.0 200.1
```

Water

n	missing	unique	Mean	0.05	0.10	0.25	0.50	0.75	0.90	0.95
1030	0	195	181.6	146.1	154.6	164.9	185.0	192.0	203.5	228.0

```
lowest : 121.8 126.6 127.0 127.3 137.8
highest: 228.0 236.7 237.0 246.9 247.0
```

Superplasticizer

n	missing	unique	Mean	0.05	0.10	0.25	0.50	0.75	0.90	0.95
1,030	0	111	6.205	0.00	0.00	0.00	6.40	10.20	12.21	16.05

```
lowest :  0.0  1.7  1.9  2.0  2.2,
highest: 22.0 22.1 23.4 28.2 32.2
```

CoarseAggregate

n	missing	unique	Mean	0.05	0.10	0.25	0.50	0.75	0.90	0.95
1,030	0	284	972.9	842.0	852.1	932.0	968.0	1029.4	1076.5	1104.0

```
lowest :  801.0  801.1  801.4  811.0  814.0
highest: 1124.4 1125.0 1130.0 1134.3 1145.0
```

FineAggregate

n	missing	unique	Mean	0.05	0.10	0.25	.50	0.75	.90	0.95
1030	0	302	773.6	613.0	664.1	730.9	779.5	824.0	880.8	898.1

```
lowest : 594.0 605.0 611.8 612.0 613.0
highest: 925.7 942.0 943.1 945.0 992.6
```

Age

n	missing	unique	Mean	0.05	0.10	0.25	0.50	0.75	0.90	0.95
1,030	0	14	45.66	3	3	7	28	56	100	180

	1	3	7	14	28	56	90	91	100	120	180	270	360	365
Frequency	2	134	126	62	425	91	54	22	52	3	26	13	6	14
%	0	13	12	6	41	9	5	2	5	0	3	1	1	1

CompressiveStrength

n	missing	unique	Mean	0.05	0.10	0.25	0.50	0.75	0.90	0.95
1,030	0	845	35.82	10.96	14.20	23.71	34.45	46.14	58.82	66.80

```
lowest :  2.33  3.32  4.57  4.78  4.83
highest: 79.40 79.99 80.20 81.75 82.60
```

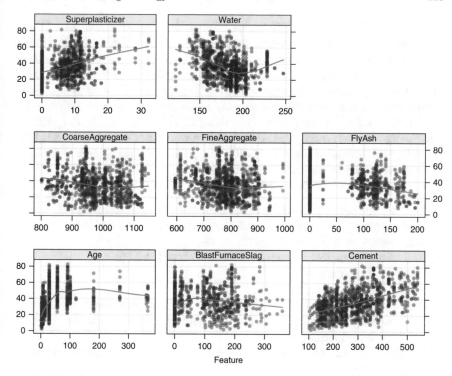

Fig. 10.1: Scatter plots of the concrete predictors versus the compressive strength

10.1 Model Building Strategy

The neural network models used in Yeh (1998) were single-layer networks with eight hidden units. Multiple data splitting approaches were used by the original author. Four models were fit with different training sets such that all the data from a single source were held out each time. These models resulted in test set R^2 values ranging from 0.814 to 0.895. They also used a random sample of 25 % of the data for holdout test sets. This was repeated four times to produce test set R^2 values between 0.908 and 0.922.

Although an apples-to-apples comparison cannot be made with the analyses of Yeh (1998), a similar data splitting approach will be taken for this case study. A random holdout set of 25 % ($n = 247$) will be used as a test set and five repeats of 10-fold cross-validation will be used to tune the various models.

In this case study, a series of models will be created and evaluated. Once a final model is selected, the model will be used to predict mixtures with optimal compressive strength within practical limitations.

How should the predictors be used to model the outcome? Yeh (1998) discusses traditional approaches, such as relying on the water-to-cement ratio, but suggests that the existing experimental data are not consistent with historical strategies. In this chapter, the predictors will enter the models as the proportion of the total amount. Because of this, there is a built-in dependency in the predictor values (any predictor can be automatically determined by knowing the values of the other seven). Despite this, the pairwise correlations are not large, and, therefore, we would not expect methods that are designed to deal with collinearity (e.g., PLS, ridge regression) to have performance that is superior to other models.

A suite of models were tested:

- Linear regression, partial least squares, and the elastic net. Each model used an expanded set of predictors that included all two-factor interactions (e.g., age × water) and quadratic terms.
- Radial basis function support vector machines (SVMs).
- Neural network models.
- MARS models.
- Regression trees (both CART and conditional inference trees), model trees (with and without rules), and Cubist (with and without committees and neighbor-based adjustments).
- Bagged and boosted regression trees, along with random forest models.

The details of how the models were tuned are given in the Computing section at the end of the chapter.

10.2 Model Performance

The same cross-validation folds were used for each model. Figure 10.2 shows *parallel-coordinate plots* for the resampling results across the models. Each line corresponds to a common cross-validation holdout. From this, the top performing models were tree ensembles (random forest and boosting), rule ensembles (Cubist), and neural networks. Linear models and simple trees did not perform well. Bagged trees, SVMs, and MARS showed modest results but are clearly worse than the top cluster of models. The averaged R^2 statistics ranged from 0.76 to 0.92 across the models. The top three models (as ranked by resampling) were applied to the test set. The RMSE values are roughly consistent with the cross-validation rankings: 3.9 (boosted tree), 4.2 (neural networks), and 4.5 (cubist).

Figure 10.3 shows plots of the raw data, predictions, and residuals for the three models. The plots for each model are fairly similar; each shows good concordance between the observed and predicted values with a slight "fanning out" at the high end of compressive strength. The majority of the residuals

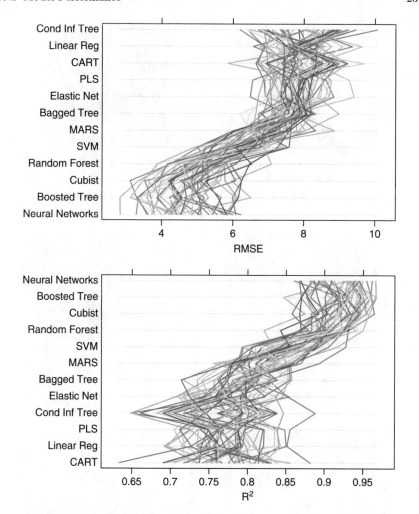

Fig. 10.2: Parallel coordinate plots for the cross-validated RMSE and R^2 across different models. Each line represents the results for a common cross-validation holdout set

are within ± 2.8 MPa with the largest errors slightly more than 15 MPa. There is no clear winner or loser in the models based on these plots.

The neural network model used 27 hidden units with a weight decay value of 0.1. The performance profile for this model (not shown, but can be reproduced using syntax provided in the Computing section below) showed that weight decay had very little impact on the effectiveness of the model. The final Cubist model used 100 committees and adjusted the predictions with 3-nearest neighbors. Similar to the Cubist profiles shown for the

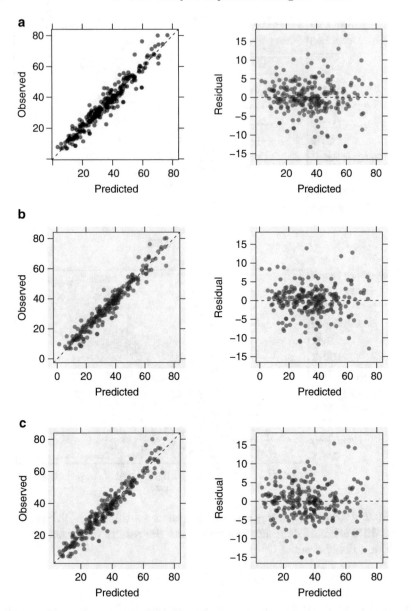

Fig. 10.3: Diagnostic plots of the test set results for three models. (**a**) Neural network (**b**) Boosted trees (**c**) Cubist

computational chemistry data (see the figure on page 211), performance suffered when the number of neighbors was either too low or too high. The boosted tree preferred a fast learning rate and deep trees.

10.3 Optimizing Compressive Strength

The neural network and Cubist models were used to determine possible mixtures with improved compressive strength. To do this, a numerical search routine can be used to find formulations with high compressive strength (as predicted by the model). Once a candidate set of mixtures is found, additional experiments would then be executed for the mixtures to verify that the strength has indeed improved. For illustrative purposes, the age of the formulation was fixed to a value of 28 days (there are a large number of data points in the training set with this value) and only the mixture ingredients will be optimized.

How, exactly, should the search be conducted? There are numerous numerical optimization routines that can search seven-dimensional space. Many rely on determining the gradient (i.e., first derivative) of the prediction equation. Several of the models have smooth prediction equations (e.g., neural networks and SVMs). However, others have many discontinuities (such as tree- and rule-based models and multivariate adaptive regression splines) that are not conducive to gradient-based search methods.

An alternative is to use a class of optimizers called *direct methods* that would not use derivatives to find the settings with optimal compressive strength and evaluate the prediction equation many more times than derivative-based optimizers. Two such search procedures are the Nelder–Mead simplex method (Nelder and Mead 1965; Olsson and Nelson 1975) and simulated annealing (Bohachevsky et al. 1986). Of these, the simplex search procedure had the best results for these data.[2] The Nelder–Mead method has the potential to get "stuck" in a sub-optimal region of the search space, which would generate poor mixtures. To counter-act this issue, it is common to repeat the search using different starting points and choosing the searches that are associated with the best results. To do this, 15–28-day-old mixtures were selected from the training set. The first of the 15 was selected at random and the remaining starting points were selected using the maximum dissimilarity sampling procedure discussed in Sect. 4.3.

Before beginning the search, constraints were used to avoid searching parts of the formulation space that were impractical or impossible. For example, the amount of water ranged from 5.1 % to 11.2 %. The search procedure was set to only consider mixtures with at least 5 % water.

---

[2] The reader can also try simulated annealing using the code at the end of the chapter.

Table 10.2: The top three optimal mixtures predicted from two models where the age was fixed at a value of 28. In the training set, matching on age, the strongest mixtures had compressive strengths of 81.75, 79.99, and 78.8

Model	Cement	Slag	Ash	Plast.	C. Agg.	F. Agg.	Water	Prediction
Cubist								
New mix 1	12.7	14.9	6.8	0.5	34.0	25.7	5.4	89.1
New mix 2	21.7	3.4	5.7	0.3	33.7	29.9	5.3	88.4
New mix 3	14.6	13.7	0.4	2.0	35.8	27.5	6.0	88.2
Neural network								
New mix 4	34.4	7.9	0.2	0.3	31.1	21.1	5.1	88.7
New mix 5	21.2	11.6	0.1	1.1	32.4	27.8	5.8	85.7
New mix 6	40.8	4.9	6.7	0.7	20.3	20.5	6.1	83.9

In the training set, there were 416 formulations that were tested at 28 days. Of these, the top three mixtures had compressive strengths of 81.75, 79.99, and 78.8. Table 10.2 shows the top three predicted mixtures for a smooth and non-smooth model (neural networks and Cubist, respectively). The models are able to find formulations that are predicted to have better strength than those seen in the data.

The Cubist mixtures were predicted to have similar compressive strengths. Their formulations were differentiated by the cement, slag, ash, and plasticizer components. The neural network mixtures were in a nearby region of mixture space and had predicted values that were lower than the Cubist model predictions but larger than the best-observed mixtures. In each of the six cases, the mixtures have very low proportions of water. Principal component analysis was used to represent the training set mixture (in seven-dimensional space) using two components. A PCA plot of the 28-day data is shown in Fig. 10.4. The principal component values for the 15 mixtures used as starting points for the search procedure are shown (as × symbols) as are the other 401 time-matched data points in the training set (shown as small grey dots). The top three predictions from the two models are also shown. Many of the predicted mixtures are near the outskirts of the mixture space and are likely to suffer some model inaccuracy due to extrapolation. Given this, it is extremely important to validate these new formulations scientifically and experimentally.

More complex approaches to finding optimal mixtures can also be used. For example, it may be important to incorporate the cost of the mixture (or other factors) into the search. Such a *multivariate* or *multiparameter* optimization can be executed a number of ways. One simple approach is *desirability functions* (Derringer and Suich 1980; Costa et al. 2011). Here, the impor-

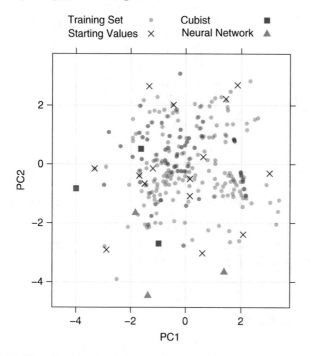

Fig. 10.4: A PCA plot of the training set data where the mixtures were aged 28 days. The search algorithm was executed across 15 different training set mixtures (shown as × in the plot). The top three optimal mixtures predicted from two models are also shown

tant characteristics of a mixture (e.g., strength and cost) are mapped to a common desirability scale between 0 and 1, where one is most desirable and zero is completely undesirable. For example, mixtures above a certain cost may be unacceptable. Mixtures associated with costs at or above this value would have zero desirability (literally). As the cost decreases the relationship between cost and desirability might be specified to be linearly decreasing. Figure 10.5 shows two hypothetical examples of desirability function for cost and strength. Here, formulations with costs greater than 20 and strength less than 70 are considered completely unacceptable. Once desirability functions are created by the user for every characteristic to be optimized, the overall desirability is combined, usually using a geometric mean. Note that, since the geometric mean multiplies values, if any one desirability function has a score of 0, all other characteristics would be considered irrelevant (since the overall value is also 0). The overall desirability would be optimized by a search procedure to find a solution that takes all the characteristics into account. Wager et al. (2010) and Cruz-Monteagudo et al. (2011) show examples of this approach.

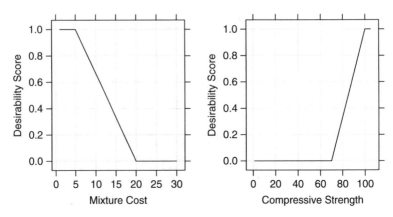

Fig. 10.5: Examples of individual desirability functions for mixture cost and compression strength. The geometric mean of these scores can be optimized for the purpose of finding strong, low-cost mixtures

10.4 Computing

This section uses functions from the caret, desirability, Hmisc, and plyr packages.

The concrete data can be found in the UCI Machine Learning repository. The AppliedPredictiveModeling package contains the original data (in amounts) and an alternate version that has the mixture proportions:

```
> library(AppliedPredictiveModeling)
> data(concrete)
> str(concrete)

  'data.frame':   1030 obs. of  9 variables:
   $ Cement            : num  540 540 332 332 199 ...
   $ BlastFurnaceSlag  : num  0 0 142 142 132 ...
   $ FlyAsh            : num  0 0 0 0 0 0 0 0 0 0 ...
   $ Water             : num  162 162 228 228 192 228 228 228 228 228 ...
   $ Superplasticizer  : num  2.5 2.5 0 0 0 0 0 0 0 0 ...
   $ CoarseAggregate   : num  1040 1055 932 932 978 ...
   $ FineAggregate     : num  676 676 594 594 826 ...
   $ Age               : int  28 28 270 365 360 90 365 28 28 28 ...
   $ CompressiveStrength: num  80 61.9 40.3 41 44.3 ...
> str(mixtures)

  'data.frame':   1030 obs. of  9 variables:
   $ Cement            : num  0.2231 0.2217 0.1492 0.1492 0.0853 ...
   $ BlastFurnaceSlag  : num  0 0 0.0639 0.0639 0.0569 ...
   $ FlyAsh            : num  0 0 0 0 0 0 0 0 0 0 ...
   $ Water             : num  0.0669 0.0665 0.1023 0.1023 0.0825 ...
   $ Superplasticizer  : num  0.00103 0.00103 0 0 0 ...
   $ CoarseAggregate   : num  0.43 0.433 0.418 0.418 0.42 ...
```

```
  $ FineAggregate       : num   0.279 0.278 0.266 0.266 0.355 ...
  $ Age                 : int   28 28 270 365 360 90 365 28 28 28 ...
  $ CompressiveStrength: num   80 61.9 40.3 41 44.3 ...
```

Table 10.1 was created using the describe function in the Hmisc package, and Fig. 10.1 was create using the featurePlot function in caret:

```
> featurePlot(x = concrete[, -9],
+             y = concrete$CompressiveStrength,
+             ## Add some space between the panels
+             between = list(x = 1, y = 1),
+             ## Add a background grid ('g') and a smoother ('smooth')
+             type = c("g", "p", "smooth"))
```

The code for averaging the replicated mixtures and splitting the data into training and test sets is

```
> averaged <- ddply(mixtures,
+                    .(Cement, BlastFurnaceSlag, FlyAsh, Water,
+                      Superplasticizer, CoarseAggregate,
+                      FineAggregate, Age),
+                    function(x) c(CompressiveStrength =
+                                  mean(x$CompressiveStrength)))
> set.seed(975)
> forTraining <- createDataPartition(averaged$CompressiveStrength,
+                                     p = 3/4)[[1]]
> trainingSet <- averaged[ forTraining,]
> testSet   <- averaged[-forTraining,]
```

To fit the linear models with the expanded set of predictors, such as inter-actions, a specific model formula was created. The dot in the formula below is shorthand for all predictors and (.)^2 expands into a model with all the linear terms and all two-factor interactions. The quadratic terms are created manually and are encapsulated inside the I() function. This "as-is" function tells R that the squaring of the predictors should be done arithmetically (and not symbolically).

The formula is first created as a character string using the paste command, then is converted to a bona fide R formula.

```
> modFormula <- paste("CompressiveStrength ~ (.)^2 + I(Cement^2) + ",
+                      "I(BlastFurnaceSlag^2) + I(FlyAsh^2) + I(Water^2) +",
+                      " I(Superplasticizer^2) + I(CoarseAggregate^2) + ",
+                      "I(FineAggregate^2) + I(Age^2)")
> modFormula <- as.formula(modFormula)
```

Each model used repeated 10-fold cross-validation and is specified with the trainControl function:

```
> controlObject <- trainControl(method = "repeatedcv",
+                                repeats = 5,
+                                number = 10)
```

To create the exact same folds, the random number generator is reset to a common seed prior to running `train`. For example, to fit the linear regression model:

```
> set.seed(669)
> linearReg <- train(modFormula,
+                     data = trainingSet,
+                     method = "lm",
+                     trControl = controlObject)
> linearReg
  745 samples
   44 predictors

  No pre-processing
  Resampling: Cross-Validation (10-fold, repeated 5 times)

  Summary of sample sizes: 671, 671, 672, 670, 669, 669, ...

  Resampling results

    RMSE  Rsquared  RMSE SD  Rsquared SD
    7.85  0.771     0.647    0.0398
```

The output shows that 44 predictors were used, indicating the expanded model formula was used.

The other two linear models were created with:

```
> set.seed(669)
> plsModel <- train(modForm, data = trainingSet,
+                    method = "pls",
+                    preProc = c("center", "scale"),
+                    tuneLength = 15,
+                    trControl = controlObject)
> enetGrid <- expand.grid(.lambda = c(0, .001, .01, .1),
+                          .fraction = seq(0.05, 1, length = 20))
> set.seed(669)
> enetModel <- train(modForm, data = trainingSet,
+                     method = "enet",
+                     preProc = c("center", "scale"),
+                     tuneGrid = enetGrid,
+                     trControl = controlObject)
```

MARS, neural networks, and SVMs were created as follows:

```
> set.seed(669)
> earthModel <- train(CompressiveStrength ~ ., data = trainingSet,
+                      method = "earth",
+                      tuneGrid = expand.grid(.degree = 1,
+                                             .nprune = 2:25),
+                      trControl = controlObject)
> set.seed(669)
> svmRModel <- train(CompressiveStrength ~ ., data = trainingSet,
+                     method = "svmRadial",
+                     tuneLength = 15,
+                     preProc = c("center", "scale"),
```

```
+                    trControl = controlObject)
> nnetGrid <- expand.grid(.decay = c(0.001, .01, .1),
+                          .size = seq(1, 27, by = 2),
+                          .bag = FALSE)
> set.seed(669)
> nnetModel <- train(CompressiveStrength ~ .,
+                    data = trainingSet,
+                    method = "avNNet",
+                    tuneGrid = nnetGrid,
+                    preProc = c("center", "scale"),
+                    linout = TRUE,
+                    trace = FALSE,
+                    maxit = 1000,
+                    trControl = controlObject)
```

The regression and model trees were similarly created:

```
> set.seed(669)
> rpartModel <- train(CompressiveStrength ~ .,
+                     data = trainingSet,
+                     method = "rpart",
+                     tuneLength = 30,
+                     trControl = controlObject)


> set.seed(669)
> ctreeModel <- train(CompressiveStrength ~ .,
+                     data = trainingSet,
+                     method = "ctree",
+                     tuneLength = 10,
+                     trControl = controlObject)


> set.seed(669)
> mtModel <- train(CompressiveStrength ~ .,
+                  data = trainingSet,
+                  method = "M5",
+                  trControl = controlObject)
```

The following code creates the remaining model objects:

```
> set.seed(669)
> treebagModel <- train(CompressiveStrength ~ .,
+                       data = trainingSet,
+                       method = "treebag",
+                       trControl = controlObject)
> set.seed(669)
> rfModel <- train(CompressiveStrength ~ .,
+                  data = trainingSet,
+                  method = "rf",
+                  tuneLength = 10,
+                  ntrees = 1000,
+                  importance = TRUE,
+                  trControl = controlObject)
> gbmGrid <- expand.grid(.interaction.depth = seq(1, 7, by = 2),
+                        .n.trees = seq(100, 1000, by = 50),
```

```
+                        .shrinkage = c(0.01, 0.1))
> set.seed(669)
> gbmModel <- train(CompressiveStrength ~ .,
+                   data = trainingSet,
+                   method = "gbm",
+                   tuneGrid = gbmGrid,
+                   verbose = FALSE,
+                   trControl = controlObject)
> cubistGrid <- expand.grid(.committees = c(1, 5, 10, 50, 75, 100),
+                           .neighbors = c(0, 1, 3, 5, 7, 9))
> set.seed(669)
> cbModel <- train(CompressiveStrength ~ .,
+                  data = trainingSet,
+                  method = "cubist",
+                  tuneGrid = cubistGrid,
+                  trControl = controlObject)
```

The resampling results for these models were collected into a single object using caret's resamples function. This object can then be used for visualizations or to make formal comparisons between the models.

```
> allResamples <- resamples(list("Linear Reg" = lmModel,
+                                "PLS" = plsModel,
+                                "Elastic Net" = enetModel,
+                                MARS = earthModel,
+                                SVM = svmRModel,
+                                "Neural Networks" = nnetModel,
+                                CART = rpartModel,
+                                "Cond Inf Tree" = ctreeModel,
+                                "Bagged Tree" = treebagModel,
+                                "Boosted Tree" = gbmModel,
+                                "Random Forest" = rfModel,
+                                Cubist = cbModel))
```

Figure 10.2 was created from this object as

```
> ## Plot the RMSE values
> parallelPlot(allResamples)
> ## Using R-squared:
> parallelplot(allResamples, metric = "Rsquared")
```

Other visualizations of the resampling results can also be created (see ?xyplot.resamples for other options).

The test set predictions are achieved using a simple application of the predict function:

```
> nnetPredictions <- predict(nnetModel, testData)
> gbmPredictions <- predict(gbmModel, testData)
> cbPredictions <- predict(cbModel, testData)
```

To predict optimal mixtures, we first use the 28-day data to generate a set of random starting points from the training set.

Since distances between the formulations will be used as a measure of dissimilarity, the data are pre-processed to have the same mean and variance for each predictor. After this, a single random mixture is selected to initialize the maximum dissimilarity sampling process:

```
> age28Data <- subset(trainingData, Age == 28)
> ## Remove the age and compressive strength columns and
> ## then center and scale the predictor columns
> pp1 <- preProcess(age28Data[, -(8:9)], c("center", "scale"))
> scaledTrain <- predict(pp1, age28Data[, 1:7])
> set.seed(91)
> startMixture <- sample(1:nrow(age28Data), 1)
> starters <- scaledTrain[startMixture, 1:7]
```

After this, the maximum dissimilarity sampling method from Sect. 4.3 selects 14 more mixtures to complete a diverse set of starting points for the search algorithms:

```
> pool <- scaledTrain
> index <- maxDissim(starters, pool, 14)
> startPoints <- c(startMixture, index)
> starters <- age28Data[startPoints,1:7]
```

Since all seven mixture proportions should add to one, the search procedures will conduct the search without one ingredient (water), and the water proportion will be determined by the sum of the other six ingredient proportions. Without this step, the search procedures would pick candidate mixture values that would not add to one.

```
> ## Remove water
> startingValues <- starters[, -4]
```

To maximize the compressive strength, the R function optim searches the mixture space for optimal formulations. A custom R function is needed to translate a candidate mixture to a prediction. This function can find settings to *minimize* a function, so it will return the negative of the compressive strength. The function below checks to make sure that (a) the proportions are between 0 and 1 and (b) the proportion of water does not fall below 5 %. If these conditions are violated, the function returns a large positive number which the search procedure will avoid (as optim is for minimization).

```
> ## The inputs to the function are a vector of six mixture proportions
> ## (in argument 'x') and the model used for prediction ('mod')
> modelPrediction <- function(x, mod)
+ {
+   ## Check to make sure the mixture proportions are
+   ## in the correct range
+   if(x[1] < 0 | x[1] > 1) return(10^38)
+   if(x[2] < 0 | x[2] > 1) return(10^38)
+   if(x[3] < 0 | x[3] > 1) return(10^38)
+   if(x[4] < 0 | x[4] > 1) return(10^38)
+   if(x[5] < 0 | x[5] > 1) return(10^38)
+   if(x[6] < 0 | x[6] > 1) return(10^38)
+
+   ## Determine the water proportion
```

```
+    x <- c(x, 1 - sum(x))
+
+    ## Check the water range
+    if(x[7] < 0.05) return(10^38)
+
+    ## Convert the vector to a data frame, assign names
+    ## and fix age at 28 days
+    tmp <- as.data.frame(t(x))
+    names(tmp) <- c('Cement','BlastFurnaceSlag','FlyAsh',
+                    'Superplasticizer','CoarseAggregate',
+                    'FineAggregate', 'Water')
+    tmp$Age <- 28
+    ## Get the model prediction, square them to get back to the
+    ## original units, then return the negative of the result
+    -predict(mod, tmp)
+    }
```

First, the Cubist model is used:

```
> cbResults <- startingValues
> cbResults$Water <- NA
> cbResults$Prediction <- NA
> ## Loop over each starting point and conduct the search
> for(i in 1:nrow(cbResults))
+    {
+      results <- optim(unlist(cbResults[i,1:6]),
+                       modelPrediction,
+                       method = "Nelder-Mead",
+                       ## Use method = 'SANN' for simulated annealing
+                       control=list(maxit=5000),
+                       ## The next option is passed to the
+                       ## modelPrediction() function
+                       mod = cbModel)
+      ## Save the predicted compressive strength
+      cbResults$Prediction[i] <- -results$value
+      ## Also save the final mixture values
+      cbResults[i,1:6] <- results$par
+    }
> ## Calculate the water proportion
> cbResults$Water <- 1 - apply(cbResults[,1:6], 1, sum)
> ## Keep the top three mixtures
> cbResults <- cbResults[order(-cbResults$Prediction),][1:3,]
> cbResults$Model <- "Cubist"
```

We then employ the same process for the neural network model:

```
> nnetResults <- startingValues
> nnetResults$Water <- NA
> nnetResults$Prediction <- NA
> for(i in 1:nrow(nnetResults))
+    {
+      results <- optim(unlist(nnetResults[i, 1:6,]),
+                       modelPrediction,
+                       method = "Nelder-Mead",
+                       control=list(maxit=5000),
```

```
+                      mod = nnetModel)
+      nnetResults$Prediction[i] <- -results$value
+      nnetResults[i,1:6] <- results$par
+    }
> nnetResults$Water <- 1 - apply(nnetResults[,1:6], 1, sum)
> nnetResults <- nnetResults[order(-nnetResults$Prediction),][1:3,]
> nnetResults$Model <- "NNet"
```

To create Fig. 10.4, PCA was conducted on the 28-day-old mixtures and the six predicted mixtures were projected. The components are combined and plotted:

```
> ## Run PCA on the data at 28\,days
> pp2 <- preProcess(age28Data[, 1:7], "pca")
> ## Get the components for these mixtures
> pca1 <- predict(pp2, age28Data[, 1:7])
> pca1$Data <- "Training Set"
> ## Label which data points were used to start the searches
> pca1$Data[startPoints] <- "Starting Values"

> ## Project the new mixtures in the same way (making sure to
> ## re-order the columns to match the order of the age28Data object).
> pca3 <- predict(pp2, cbResults[, names(age28Data[, 1:7])])
> pca3$Data <- "Cubist"
> pca4 <- predict(pp2, nnetResults[, names(age28Data[, 1:7])])
> pca4$Data <- "Neural Network"
> ## Combine the data, determine the axis ranges and plot
> pcaData <- rbind(pca1, pca3, pca4)
> pcaData$Data <- factor(pcaData$Data,
+                         levels = c("Training Set","Starting Values",
+                                    "Cubist","Neural Network"))

> lim <- extendrange(pcaData[, 1:2])
> xyplot(PC2 ~ PC1, data = pcaData, groups = Data,
+        auto.key = list(columns = 2),
+        xlim = lim, ylim = lim,
+        type = c("g", "p"))
```

Desirability functions can be calculated with the **desirability** package. The functions dMin and dMax can be used to create desirability function curve definitions for minimization and maximization, respectively.

Part III
Classification Models

Chapter 11
Measuring Performance in Classification Models

In the previous part of this book we focused on building and evaluating models for a continuous response. We now turn our focus to building and evaluating models for a categorical response. Although many of the regression modeling techniques can also be used for classification, the way we evaluate model performance is necessarily very different since metrics like RMSE and R^2 are not appropriate in the context of classification. We begin this part of the book by discussing metrics for evaluating classification model performance. In the first section of this chapter we take an in-depth look at the different aspects of classification model predictions and how these relate to the question of interest. The two subsequent sections explore strategies for evaluating classification models using statistics and visualizations.

11.1 Class Predictions

Classification models usually generate two types of predictions. Like regression models, classification models produce a continuous valued prediction, which is usually in the form of a probability (i.e., the predicted values of class membership for any individual sample are between 0 and 1 and sum to 1). In addition to a continuous prediction, classification models generate a predicted class, which comes in the form of a discrete category. For most practical applications, a discrete category prediction is required in order to make a decision. Automated spam filtering, for example, requires a definitive judgement for each e-mail.

Although classification models produce both of these types of predictions, often the focus is on the discrete prediction rather than the continuous prediction. However, the probability estimates for each class can be very useful for gauging the model's confidence about the predicted classification. Returning to the spam e-mail filter example, an e-mail message with a predicted probability of being spam of 0.51 would be classified the same as a message with

M. Kuhn and K. Johnson, *Applied Predictive Modeling*,
DOI 10.1007/978-1-4614-6849-3_11,
© Springer Science+Business Media New York 2013

a predicted probability of being spam of 0.99. While both messages would be treated the same by the filter, we would have more confidence that the second message was, in fact, truly spam. As a second example, consider building a model to classify molecules by their *in-vivo* safety status (i.e., non-toxic, weakly toxic, and strongly toxic; e.g., Piersma et al. 2004). A molecule with predicted probabilities in each respective toxicity category of 0.34, 0.33, and 0.33, would be classified the same as a molecule with respective predicted probabilities of 0.98, 0.01, and 0.01. However in this case, we are much more confident that the second molecule is non-toxic as compared to the first.

In some applications, the desired outcome is the predicted class probabilities which are then used as inputs for other calculations. Consider an insurance company that wants to uncover and prosecute fraudulent claims. Using historical claims data, a classification model could be built to predict the probability of claim fraud. This probability would then be combined with the company's investigation costs and potential monetary loss to determine if pursuing the investigation is in the best financial interest of the insurance company. As another example of classification probabilities as inputs to a subsequent model, consider the customer lifetime value (CLV) calculation which is defined as the amount of profit associated with a customer over a period of time (Gupta et al. 2006). To estimate the CLV, several quantities are required, including the amount paid by a consumer over a given time frame, the cost of servicing the consumer, and the probability that the consumer will make a purchase in the time frame.

As mentioned above, most classification models generate predicted class probabilities. However, when some models are used for classification, like neural networks and partial least squares, they produce continuous predictions that do not follow the definition of a probability-the predicted values are not necessarily between 0 and 1 and do not sum to 1. For example, a partial least squares classification model (described in more detail in Sect. 12.4) would create 0/1 dummy variables for each class and simultaneously model these values as a function of the predictors. When samples are predicted, the model predictions are not guaranteed to be within 0 and 1. For classification models like these, a transformation must be used to coerce the predictions into "probability-like" values so that they can be interpreted and used for classification. One such method is the *softmax transformation* (Bridle 1990) which is defined as

$$\hat{p}_\ell^* = \frac{e^{\hat{y}_\ell}}{\sum_{l=1}^{C} e^{\hat{y}_l}}$$

where $\hat{y}_\ell$ is the numeric model prediction for the ℓth class and $\hat{p}_\ell^*$ is the transformed value between 0 and 1. Suppose that an outcome has three classes and that a PLS model predicts values of $\hat{y}_1 = 0.25$, $\hat{y}_2 = 0.76$, and $\hat{y}_3 =$-0.1. The softmax function would transform these values to $\hat{p}_1^* = 0.30$, $\hat{p}_2^* = 0.49$, and $\hat{p}_3^* = 0.21$. To be clear, no probability statement is being created by this transformation; it merely ensures that the predictions have the same mathematical qualities as probabilities.

Well-Calibrated Probabilities

Whether a classification model is used to predict spam e-mail, a molecule's toxicity status, or as inputs to insurance fraud or customer lifetime value calculations, we desire that the estimated class probabilities are reflective of the true underlying probability of the sample. That is, the predicted class probability (or probability-like value) needs to be well-calibrated. To be well-calibrated, the probabilities must effectively reflect the true likelihood of the event of interest. Returning to the spam filter illustration, if a model produces a probability or probability-like value of 20% for the likelihood of a particular e-mail to be spam, then this value would be well-calibrated if similar types of messages would truly be from that class on average in 1 of 5 samples.

One way to assess the quality of the class probabilities is using a *calibration plot*. For a given set of data, this plot shows some measure of the observed probability of an event versus the predicted class probability. One approach for creating this visualization is to score a collection of samples with known outcomes (preferably a test set) using a classification model. The next step is to bin the data into groups based on their class probabilities. For example, a set of bins might be [0, 10%], (10%, 20%], ..., (90%, 100%]. For each bin, determine the observed event rate. Suppose that 50 samples fell into the bin for class probabilities less than 10% and there was a single event. The midpoint of the bin is 5% and the observed event rate would be 2%. The calibration plot would display the midpoint of the bin on the x-axis and the observed event rate on the y-axis. If the points fall along a 45° line, the model has produced well-calibrated probabilities.

As an illustration, a data set was simulated in a way that the true event probabilities are known. For two classes (classes 1 and 2) and two predictors (A and B), the true probability (p) of the event is generated from the equation:

$$\log\left(\frac{p}{1-p}\right) = -1 - 2A - .2A^2 + 2B^2$$

Figure 11.1 shows a simulated test set along with the a contour line for a $p = 0.50$ event probability. Two models were fit to the training set: quadratic discriminant analysis (QDA, Sect. 13.1) and a random forest model (Sect. 14.4). A test set of $n = 1000$ samples was used to score the model and create the calibration plot also shown in Fig. 11.1. Both classification models have similar accuracy for the test set (about 87.1% for either model). The calibration plot shows that the QDA class probabilities tend to perform poorly compared to the random forest model. For example, in the bin with class probabilities ranging from 20 to 30%, the observed percentage of events for QDA was 4.6%, far lower than the percentage in the random forest model (35.4%).

The class probabilities can be calibrated to more closely reflect the likelihood of the event (or, at least the likelihood seen in the actual data).

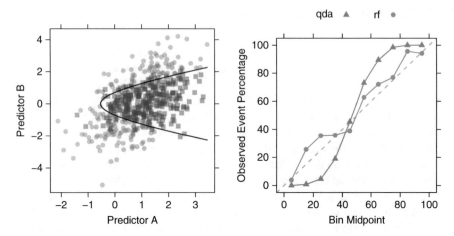

Fig. 11.1: *Left*: A simulated two-class data set with two predictors. The *solid black line* denotes the 50 % probability contour. *Right*: A calibration plot of the test set probabilities for random forest and quadratic discriminant analysis models

For example, Fig. 11.1 shows a sigmoidal pattern such that the QDA model under-predicts the event probability when the true likelihood is moderately high or low. An additional model could be created to adjust for this pattern. One equation that is consistent with this sigmoidal pattern is the logistic regression model (described in Sect. 12.2). The class predictions and true outcome values from the training set can be used to post-process the probably estimates with the following formula (Platt 2000):

$$\hat{p}^* = \frac{1}{1 + \exp\left(-\beta_0 - \beta_1 \hat{p}\right)} \tag{11.1}$$

where the β parameters are estimated by predicting the true classes as a function of the uncalibrated class probabilities ($\hat{p}$). For the QDA model, this process resulted in estimates $\hat{\beta}_0 = -5.7$ and $\hat{\beta}_1 = 11.7$. Figure 11.2 shows the results for the test set samples using this correction method. The results show improved calibration with the test set data. Alternatively, an application of Bayes' Rule (described model is Sect. 13.6) can be similarly applied to recalibrate the predictions. The Bayesian approach also improves the predictions (Fig. 11.2). Note that, after calibration, the samples must be reclassified to ensure consistency between the new probabilities and the predicted classes.

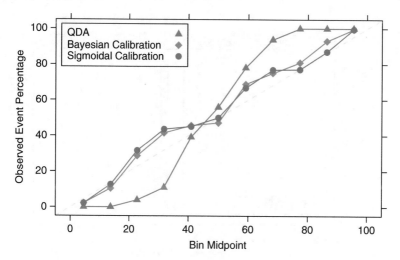

Fig. 11.2: The original QDA class probabilities and recalibrated versions using two different methodologies

Presenting Class Probabilities

Visualizations of the class probabilities are an effective method of communicating model results. For two classes, histograms of the predicted classes for each of the true outcomes illustrate the strengths and weaknesses of a model. In Chap. 4 we introduced the credit scoring example. Two classification models were created to predict the quality of a customer's credit: a support vector machine (SVM) and logistic regression. Since the performance of the two models were roughly equivalent, the logistic regression model was favored due to its simplicity. The top panel of Fig. 11.3 shows histograms of the test set probabilities for the logistic regression model (the panels indicate the true credit status). The probability of bad credit for the customers with good credit shows a skewed distribution where most customers' probabilities are quite low. In contrast, the probabilities for the customers with bad credit are flat (or uniformly distributed), reflecting the model's inability to distinguish bad credit cases.

This figure also presents a calibration plot for these data. The accuracy of the probability of bad credit degrades as it becomes larger to the point where no samples with bad credit were predicted with a probability above 82.7 %. This pattern is indicative of a model that has both poor calibration and poor performance.

When there are three or more classes, a *heat map* of the class probabilities can help gauge the confidence in the predictions. Figure 11.4 shows the test set results with eight classes (denotes A through I) and 48 samples. The

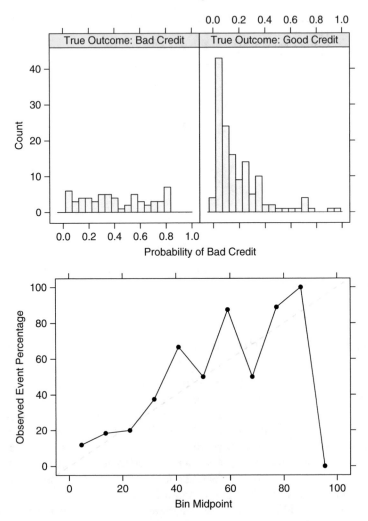

Fig. 11.3: *Top*: Histograms for a set of probabilities associated with bad credit. The two panels split the customers by their true class. *Bottom*: A calibration plot for these probabilities

true classes are shown in the rows (along with the sample identifiers) and the columns reflect the class probabilities. In some cases, such as Sample 20, there was a clear signal associated with the predicted class (the class C probability was 78.5 %), while in other cases, the situation is murky. Consider Sample 7. The four largest probabilities (and associated classes) were 19.6 % (B), 19.3 % (C), 17.7 % (A), and 15 % (E). While the model places the highest individual probability for this sample in the correct class, it is uncertain that it could also be of class C, A, or E.

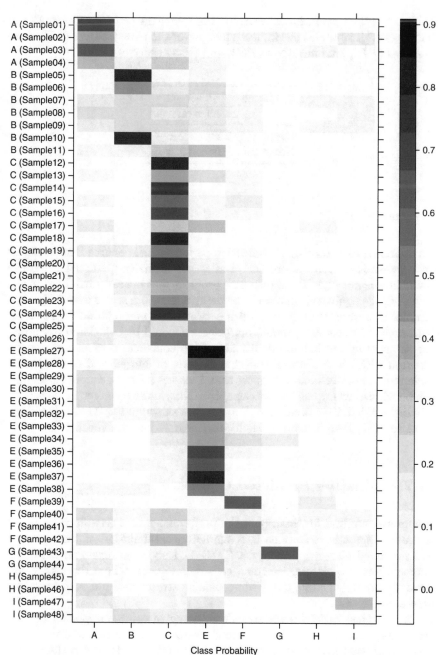

Fig. 11.4: A heat map of a test set with eight classes. The true classes are shown in the row labels while columns quantify the probabilities for each category (labeled as A through I)

Table 11.1: The confusion matrix for the two-class problem ("events" and "nonevents." The table cells indicate number of the true positives (TP), false positives (FP), true negatives (TN), and false negatives (FN)

Predicted	Observed	
	Event	Nonevent
Event	TP	FP
Nonevent	FN	TN

Equivocal Zones

An approach to improving classification performance is to create an *equivocal* or *indeterminate zone* where the class is not formally predicted when the confidence is not high. For a two-class problem that is nearly balanced in the response, the equivocal zone could be defined as $0.50 \pm z$. If z were 0.10, then samples with prediction probabilities between 0.40 and 0.60 would be called "equivocal." In this case, model performance would be calculated excluding the samples in the indeterminate zone. The equivocal rate should also be reported with the performance so that the rate of unpredicted results is well understood. For data sets with more than 2 classes $(C > 2)$, similar thresholds can be applied where the largest class probability must be larger than $(1/C) + z$ to make a definitive prediction. For the data shown in Fig. 11.4, if $(1/C) + z$ is set to 30%, then 5 samples would be designated as equivocal.

11.2 Evaluating Predicted Classes

A common method for describing the performance of a classification model is the *confusion matrix*. This is a simple cross-tabulation of the observed and predicted classes for the data. Table 11.1 shows an example when the outcome has two classes. Diagonal cells denote cases where the classes are correctly predicted while the off-diagonals illustrate the number of errors for each possible case.

The simplest metric is the overall accuracy rate (or, for pessimists, the error rate). This reflects the agreement between the observed and predicted classes and has the most straightforward interpretation. However, there are a few disadvantages to using this statistic. First, overall accuracy counts make no distinction about the *type* of errors being made. In spam filtering, the cost of erroneous deleting an important email is likely to be higher than incorrectly allowing a spam email past a filter. In situations where the costs are different, accuracy may not measure the important model characteristics. Provost et al. (1998) provide a comprehensive discussion of this issue, which is examined further below.

Second, one must consider the natural frequencies of each class. For example, in the USA, pregnant women routinely have blood drawn for alpha-fetoprotein testing, which attempts to detect genetic problems such as Down syndrome. Suppose the rate of this disorder[1] in fetuses is approximately 1 in 800 or about one-tenth of one percent. A predictive model can achieve almost perfect accuracy by predicting all samples to be negative for Down syndrome.

What benchmark accuracy rate should be used to determine whether a model is performing adequately? The no-information rate is the accuracy rate that can be achieved without a model. There are various ways to define this rate. For a data set with C classes, the simplest definition, based on pure randomness, is $1/C$. However, this does not take into account the relative frequencies of the classes in the training set. For the Down syndrome example, if 1,000 random samples are collected from the population who would receive the test, the expected number of positive samples would be small (perhaps 1 or 2). A model that simply predicted all samples to be negative for Down syndrome would easily surpass the no-information rate based on random guessing (50 %). An alternate definition of the no-information rate is the percentage of the largest class in the training set. Models with accuracy greater than this rate might be considered reasonable. The effect of severe class imbalances and some possible remedies are discussed in Chap. 16.

Rather than calculate the overall accuracy and compare it to the no-information rate, other metrics can be used that take into account the class distributions of the training set samples. The *Kappa statistic* (also known as Cohen's Kappa) was originally designed to assess the agreement between two raters (Cohen 1960). Kappa takes into account the accuracy that would be generated simply by chance. The form of the statistic is

$$Kappa = \frac{O - E}{1 - E}$$

where O is the observed accuracy and E is the expected accuracy based on the marginal totals of the confusion matrix. The statistic can take on values between -1 and 1; a value of 0 means there is no agreement between the observed and predicted classes, while a value of 1 indicates perfect concordance of the model prediction and the observed classes. Negative values indicate that the prediction is in the *opposite* direction of the truth, but large negative values seldom occur, if ever, when working with predictive models.[2]

---

[1] In medical terminology, this rate is referred to as the prevalence of a disease while in Bayesian statistics it would be the prior distribution of the event.

[2] This is true since predictive models seek to find a concordant relationship with the truth. A large negative Kappa would imply that there is relationship between the predictors and the response and the predictive model would seek to find the relationship in the correct direction.

When the class distributions are equivalent, overall accuracy and Kappa are proportional. Depending on the context, Kappa values within 0.30 to 0.50 indicate reasonable agreement. Suppose the accuracy for a model is high (90 %) but the expected accuracy is also high (85 %), the Kappa statistic would show moderate agreement (Kappa = 1/3) between the observed and predicted classes.

The Kappa statistic can also be extended to evaluate concordance in problems with more than two classes. When there is a natural ordering to the classes (e.g., "low," "medium," and "high"), an alternate form of the statistic called *weighted Kappa* can be used to enact more substantial penalties on errors that are further away from the true result. For example, a "low" sample erroneously predicted as "high" would reduce the Kappa statistic more than an error were "low" was predicted to be "medium." See (Agresti 2002) for more details.

Two-Class Problems

Consider the case where there are two classes. Table 11.1 shows the confusion matrix for generic classes "event" and "nonevent." The top row of the table corresponds to samples predicted to be events. Some are predicted correctly (the true positives, or TP) while others are inaccurately classified (false positives or FP). Similarly, the second row contains the predicted negatives with true negatives (TN) and false negatives (FN).

For two classes, there are additional statistics that may be relevant when one class is interpreted as the event of interest (such as Down syndrome in the previous example). The *sensitivity* of the model is the rate that the event of interest is predicted correctly for all samples having the event, or

$$Sensitivity = \frac{\# \text{ samples with the event } and \text{ predicted to have the event}}{\# \text{ samples having the event}}$$

The sensitivity is sometimes considered the *true positive rate* since it measures the accuracy in the event population. Conversely, the *specificity* is defined as the rate that nonevent samples are predicted as nonevents, or

$$Specificity = \frac{\# \text{ samples without the event } and \text{ predicted as nonevents}}{\# \text{ samples without the event}}$$

The *false-positive rate* is defined as one minus the specificity. Assuming a fixed level of accuracy for the model, there is typically a trade-off to be made between the sensitivity and specificity. Intuitively, increasing the sensitivity of a model is likely to incur a loss of specificity, since more samples are being predicted as events. Potential trade-offs between sensitivity and specificity may be appropriate when there are different penalties associated with each

Table 11.2: Test set confusion matrix for the logistic regression model training with the credit scoring data from Sect. 4.5

Predicted	Observed	
	Bad	Good
Bad	24	10
Good	36	130

type of error. In spam filtering, there is usually a focus on specificity; most people are willing to accept seeing some spam if emails from family members or coworkers are not deleted. The *receiver operating characteristic (ROC) curve* is one technique for evaluating this trade-off and is discussed in the next section.

In Chap. 4 we introduced the credit scoring example. Two classification models were created to predict the quality of a customer's credit: a SVM and logistic regression. Since the performance of the two models were roughly equivalent, the logistic regression model was favored due to its simplicity. Using the previously chosen test set of 200 customers, Table 11.2 shows the confusion matrix associated with the logistic regression model. The overall accuracy was 77 %, which is slightly better than the no-information rate of 70 %. The test set had a Kappa value of 0.375, which suggests moderate agreement. If we choose the event of interest to be a customer with bad credit, the sensitivity from this model would be estimated to be 40 % and the specificity to be 92.9 %. Clearly, the model has trouble predicting when customers have bad credit. This is likely due to the imbalance of the classes and a lack of a strong predictor for bad credit.

Often, there is interest in having a single measure that reflects the false-positive and false-negative rates. Youden's J Index (Youden 1950), which is

$$J = Sensitivity + Specificity - 1$$

measures the proportions of correctly predicted samples for both the event and nonevent groups. In some contexts, this may be an appropriate method for summarizing the magnitude of both types of errors. The most common method for combining sensitivity and specificity into a single value uses the receiver operating characteristic (ROC) curve, discussed below.

One often overlooked aspect of sensitivity and specificity is that they are *conditional* measures. Sensitivity is the accuracy rate for only the event population (and specificity for the nonevents). Using the sensitivity and specificity, the obstetrician can make statements such as "assuming that the fetus does not have Down syndrome, the test has an accuracy of 95 %." However, these statements might not be helpful to a patient since, for new samples, all that is known is the prediction. The person using the model prediction is typically interested in *unconditional* queries such as "what are the chances that the fetus has the genetic disorder?" This depends on three values: the sensitivity and specificity of the diagnostic test and the prevalence of the event in the population. Intuitively, if the event is rare, this should be reflected in the answer. Taking the prevalence into account, the analog to sensitivity is the *positive predicted value*, and the analog to specificity is the *negative predicted value*. These values make unconditional evaluations of the data.[3] The positive predicted value answers the question "what is the probability that this sample is an event?" The formulas are

$$PPV = \frac{Sensitivity \times Prevalence}{(Sensitivity \times Prevalence) + ((1 - Specificity) \times (1 - Prevalence))}$$

$$NPV = \frac{Specificity \times (1 - Prevalence)}{(Prevalence \times (1 - Sensitivity)) + (Specificity \times (1 - Prevalence))}$$

Clearly, the predictive values are nontrivial combinations of performance and the rate of events. The top panel in Fig. 11.5 shows the effect of prevalence on the predictive values when the model has a specificity of 95 % and a sensitivity of either 90 % or 99 %. Large negative predictive values can be achieved when the prevalence is low. However, as the event rate becomes high, the negative predictive value becomes very small. The opposite is true for the positive predictive values. This figure also shows that a sizable difference in sensitivity (90 % versus 99 %) has little effect on the positive predictive values.

The lower panel of Fig. 11.5 shows the positive predictive value as a function of sensitivity and specificity when the event rate is balanced (50 %). In this case, the positive predicted value would be

$$PPV = \frac{Sensitivity}{Sensitivity(1 - Specificity)} = \frac{TP}{TP + FP}$$

This figure also shows that the value of the sensitivity has a smaller effect than specificity. For example, if specificity is high, say $\geq 90\%$, a large positive predicted value can be achieved across a wide range of sensitivities.

Predictive values are not often used to characterize the model. There are several reasons why, most of which are related to prevalence. First, prevalence is hard to quantify. Our experience is that very few people, even experts, are willing to propose an estimate of this quantity based on prior knowledge. Also, the prevalence is dynamic. For example, the rate of spam emails increases when new schemes are invented but later fall off to baseline levels. For medical diagnoses, the prevalence of diseases can vary greatly depend-

---

[3] In relation to Bayesian statistics, the sensitivity and specificity are the conditional probabilities, the prevalence is the prior, and the positive/negative predicted values are the posterior probabilities.

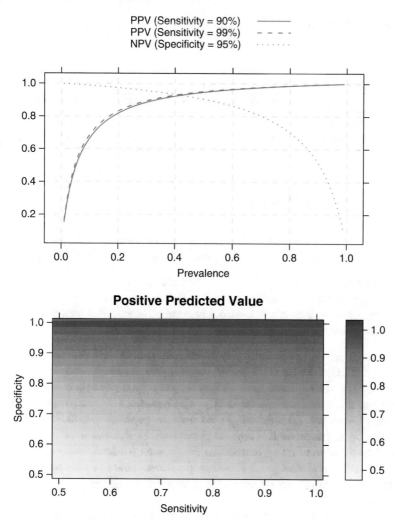

Fig. 11.5: *Top*: The effect of prevalence on the positive and negative predictive values. The PPV was computed using a specificity of 95 % and two values of sensitivity. The NPV was computed with 90 % sensitivity and 95 % specificity. *Bottom*: For a fixed prevalence of 50 %, positive predictive values are shown as a function of sensitivity and specificity

ing on the geographic location (e.g., urban versus rural). For example, in a multicenter clinical trial of a diagnostic test for *Neisseria gonorrhoeae*, the prevalence within the patient population varied from 0 % to 42.9 % across nine clinical sites (Becton Dickinson and Company 1991).

Table 11.3: The confusion matrix and profit costs/benefits for the direct mailing example of Larose (2006)

Predicted	Observed		Observed	
	Response	Nonresponse	Response	Nonresponse
Response	TP	FP	$26.40	−$2.00
Nonresponse	FN	TN	−$28.40	−

Non-Accuracy-Based Criteria

For many commercial applications of predictive models, accuracy is not the primary goal for the model. Often, the purpose of the model might be to:

- Predict investment opportunities that maximize return
- Improve customer satisfaction by market segmentation
- Lower inventory costs by improving product demand forecasts or
- Reduce costs associated with fraudulent transactions

While accuracy is important, it only describes how well the model predicts the data. If the model is *fit for purpose*, other more direct metrics of performance should be considered. These metrics quantify the consequences of correct and incorrect predictions (i.e., the benefits and costs). For example, in fraud detection, a model might be used to quantify the likelihood that a transaction is fraudulent. Suppose that fraud is the event of interest. Any model predictions of fraud (correct or not) have an associated cost for a more in-depth review of the case. For true positives, there is also a quantifiable benefit to catching bad transactions. Likewise, a false negative results in a loss of income.

Consider the direct marketing application in Larose (2006, Chap. 7) where a clothing company is interested in offering promotions by mail to its customers. Using existing customer data on shopping habits, they wish to predict who would respond (i.e., the two classes and "responders" and "nonresponders"). The 2×2 table of possible outcomes is shown in Table 11.3 where the type of decisions is presented on the left and the revenue or cost per decision is on the right. For example, if the model were to accurately predict a responder, the average profit when the customer responds to the promotion is estimated to be $28.40. There is a small $2.00 cost for mailing the promotion, so the net profit of a correct decision is $26.40. If we inaccurately predict that a customer will respond (a false positive), the only loss is the cost of the promotion ($2.00).

Table 11.4: Left: A hypothetical test confusion matrix for a predictive model with a sensitivity of 75 % and a specificity of 94.4 %. Right: The confusion matrix when a mass mailing is used for all customers

Predicted	Observed		Observed	
	Response	Nonresponse	Response	Nonresponse
Response	1,500	1,000	2,000	18,000
Nonresponse	500	17,000	0	0

If the model accurately predicts a nonresponse, there is no gain or loss since they would not have made a purchase and the mailer was not sent.[4] However, incorrectly predicting that a true responder would not respond means that a potential $28.40 was lost, so this is the cost of a false-negative. The total profit for a particular model is then

$$profit = \$26.40TP - \$2.00FP - \$28.40FN \qquad (11.2)$$

However, the prevalence of the classes should be taken into account. The response rate in direct marketing is often very low (Ling and Li 1998) so the expected profit for a given marketing application may be driven by the false-negative costs since this value is likely to be larger than the other two in Eq. 11.2.

Table 11.4 shows hypothetical confusion matrices for 20,000 customers with a 10 % response rate. The table on the left is the result of a predicted model with a sensitivity of 75 % and a specificity of 94.4 %. The total profit would be $23,400 or $1.17 per customer. Suppose another model had the same sensitivity but 100 % specificity. In this case, the total profit would increase to $25,400, a marginal gain given a significant increase in model performance (mostly due to the low cost of mailing the promotion).

The right side of Table 11.4 shows the results when a mass mailing for all the customers is used. This approach has perfect sensitivity and the worst possible specificity. Here, due to the low costs, the profit is $16,800 or $0.84 per customer. This should be considered the baseline performance for any predictive model to beat. The models could alternatively be characterized using the profit *gain* or *lift*, estimated as the model profit above and beyond the profit from a mass mailing.

With two classes, a general outline for incorporating unequal costs with performance measures is given by Drummond and Holte (2000). They define the probability-cost function (PCF) as

---

[4] This depends on a few assumptions which may or may not be true. Section 20.1 discusses this aspect of the example in more detail in the context of *net lift modeling*.

$$PCF = \frac{P \times C(+|-)}{P \times C(-|+) + (1 - P) \times C(+|-)}$$

where P is the (prior) probability of the event, $C(-|+)$ is the cost associated with incorrectly predicting an event $(+)$ as a nonevent, and $C(+|-)$ is the cost of incorrectly predicting a nonevent. The PCF is the proportion of the total costs associated with a false-positive sample. They suggest using the normalized expected cost (NEC) function to characterize the model

$$NEC = PCF \times (1 - TP) + (1 - PCF) \times FP$$

for a specific set of costs. Essentially, the NEC takes into account the prevalence of the event, model performance, and the costs and scales the total cost to be between 0 and 1. Note that this approach only assigns costs to the two types of errors and might not be appropriate for problems where there are other cost or benefits (such as the direct marketing costs shown in Table 11.3).

11.3 Evaluating Class Probabilities

Class probabilities potentially offer more information about model predictions than the simple class value. This section discussed several approaches to using the probabilities to compare models.

Receiver Operating Characteristic (ROC) Curves

ROC curves (Altman and Bland 1994; Brown and Davis 2006; Fawcett 2006) were designed as a general method that, given a collection of continuous data points, determine effective threshold such that values above the threshold are indicative of a specific event. This tool will be examined in this context in Chap. 19, but here, we describe how the ROC curve can be used for determining alternate cutoffs for class probabilities.

For the credit model test set previously discussed, the sensitivity was poor for the logistic regression model (40 %), while the specificity was fairly high (92.9 %). These values were calculated from classes that were determined with the default 50 % probability threshold. Can we improve the sensitivity by lowering the threshold[5] to capture more true positives? Lowering the threshold for classifying bad credit to 30 % results in a model with improved sensi-

---

[5] In this analysis, we have used the test set to investigate the effects of alternative thresholds. Generally, a new threshold should be derived from a separate data set than those used to train the model or evaluate performance.

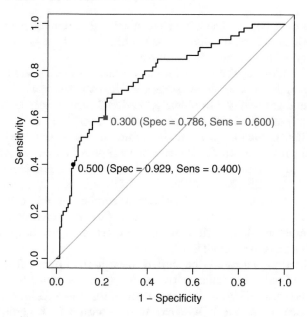

Fig. 11.6: A receiver operator characteristic (ROC) curve for the logistic regression model results for the credit model. The dot indicates the value corresponding to a cutoff of 50 % while the green square corresponds to a cutoff of 30 % (i.e., probabilities greater than 0.30 are called events)

tivity (60 %) but decrease specificity (79.3 %). Referring to Fig. 11.3, we see that decreasing the threshold begins to capture more of the customers with bad credit but also begins to encroach on the bulk of the customers with good credit.

The ROC curve is created by evaluating the class probabilities for the model across a continuum of thresholds. For each candidate threshold, the resulting true-positive rate (i.e., the sensitivity) and the false-positive rate (one minus the specificity) are plotted against each other. Figure 11.6 shows the results of this process for the credit data. The solid black point is the default 50 % threshold while the green square corresponds to the performance characteristics for a threshold of 30 %. In this figure, the numbers in parentheses are (*specificity*, *sensitivity*). Note that the trajectory of the curve between (0, 0) and the 50 % threshold is steep, indicating that the sensitivity is increasing at a greater rate than the decrease in specificity. However, when the sensitivity is greater than 70 %, there is a more significant decrease in specificity than the gain in sensitivity.

This plot is a helpful tool for choosing a threshold that appropriately maximizes the trade-off between sensitivity and specificity. However, altering the threshold only has the effect of making samples more positive (or negative as the case may be). In the confusion matrix, it cannot move samples out of *both* off-diagonal table cells. There is almost always a decrease in either sensitivity or specificity as 1 is increased.

The ROC curve can also be used for a quantitative assessment of the model. A perfect model that completely separates the two classes would have 100 % sensitivity and specificity. Graphically, the ROC curve would be a single step between (0, 0) and (0, 1) and remain constant from (0, 1) to (1, 1). The area under the ROC curve for such a model would be one. A completely ineffective model would result in an ROC curve that closely follows the 45° diagonal line and would have an area under the ROC curve of approximately 0.50. To visually compare different models, their ROC curves can be superimposed on the same graph. Comparing ROC curves can be useful in contrasting two or more models with different predictor sets (for the same model), different tuning parameters (i.e., within model comparisons), or complete different classifiers (i.e., between models).

The optimal model should be shifted towards the upper left corner of the plot. Alternatively, the model with the largest area under the ROC curve would be the most effective. For the credit data, the logistic model had an estimated area under the ROC curve of 0.78 with a 95 % confidence interval of (0.7, 0.85) determined using the bootstrap confidence interval method (Hall et al. 2004). There is a considerable amount of research on methods to formally compare multiple ROC curves. See Hanley and McNeil (1982), DeLong et al. (1988), Venkatraman (2000), and Pepe et al. (2009) for more information.

One advantage of using ROC curves to characterize models is that, since it is a function of sensitivity and specificity, the curve is insensitive to disparities in the class proportions (Provost et al. 1998; Fawcett 2006). A disadvantage of using the area under the curve to evaluate models is that it obscures information. For example, when comparing models, it is common that no individual ROC curve is uniformly better than another (i.e., the curves cross). By summarizing these curves, there is a loss of information, especially if one particular area of the curve is of interest. For example, one model may produce a steep ROC curve slope on the left but have a lower AUC than another model. If the lower end of the ROC curve was of primary interest, then AUC would not identify the best model. The partial area under the ROC curve (McClish 1989) is an alternative that focuses on specific parts of the curve.

The ROC curve is only defined for two-class problems but has been extended to handle three or more classes. Hand and Till (2001), Lachiche and Flach (2003), and Li and Fine (2008) use different approaches extending the definition of the ROC curve with more than two classes.

Lift Charts

Lift charts (Ling and Li 1998) are a visualization tool for assessing the ability of a model to detect events in a data set with two classes. Suppose a group of samples with M events is *scored* using the event class probability. When ordered by the class probability, one would hope that the events are ranked higher than the nonevents. Lift charts do just this: rank the samples by their scores and determine the cumulative event rate as more samples are evaluated. In the optimal case, the M highest-ranked samples would contain all M events. When the model is non-informative, the highest-ranked $X\%$ of the data would contain, on average, X events. The *lift* is the number of samples detected by a model above a completely random selection of samples.

To construct the *lift chart* we would take the following steps:

1. Predict a set of samples that were not used in the model building process but have known outcomes.
2. Determine the *baseline* event rate, i.e., the percent of true events in the entire data set.
3. Order the data by the classification probability of the event of interest.
4. For each unique class probability value, calculate the percent of true events in all samples below the probability value.
5. Divide the percent of true events for each probability threshold by the baseline event rate.

The lift chart plots the cumulative gain/lift against the cumulative percentage of samples that have been screened. Figure 11.7 shows the best and worse case lift curves for a data set with a 50% event rate. The non-informative model has a curve that is close to the 45° reference line, meaning that the model has no benefit for ranking samples. The other curve is indicative of a model that can perfectly separate two classes. At the 50% point on the x-axis, all of the events have been captured by the model.

Like ROC curves, the lift curves for different models can be compared to find the most appropriate model and the area under the curve can be used as a quantitative measure of performance. Also like ROC curves, some parts of the lift curve are of more interest than others. For example, the section of the curve associated with the highest-ranked samples should have an enriched true-positive rate and is likely to be the most important part of the curve.

Consider the direct marketing application. Using this curve, a quasi-threshold can be determined for a model. Again, suppose there is a 10% response rate and that most of the responders are found in the top 7% of model predictions. Sending the promotions to this subset of customers effectively imposes a new threshold for customer response since samples below the threshold will not be acted on.

In this application, recall that a predictive model would have to generate more profit than the baseline profit associated with sending the promotion

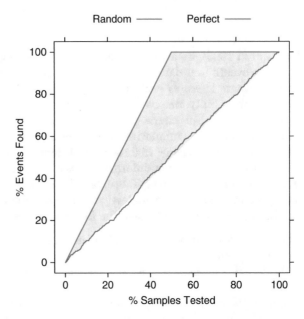

Fig. 11.7: An example lift plot with two models: one that perfectly separates two classes and another that is completely non-informative

to all customers. Using the lift plot, the expected profit can be calculated for each point on the curve to determine if the lift is sufficient to beat the baseline profit.

11.4 Computing

The R packages AppliedPredictiveModeling, caret, klaR, MASS, pROC, and randomForest will be utilized in this section.

For illustration, the simulated data set shown in Fig. 11.1 will be used in this section. To create these data, the quadBoundaryFunc function in the AppliedPredictiveModeling package is used to generate the predictors and outcomes:

```
> library(AppliedPredictiveModeling)
> set.seed(975)
> simulatedTrain <- quadBoundaryFunc(500)
> simulatedTest <- quadBoundaryFunc(1000)
> head(simulatedTrain)
           X1          X2      prob  class
  1  2.4685709  2.28742015 0.9647251 Class1
  2 -0.1889407 -1.63949455 0.9913938 Class1
```

```
3 -1.9101460 -2.89194964 1.0000000 Class1
4  0.3481279  0.06707434 0.1529697 Class1
5  0.1401153  0.86900555 0.5563062 Class1
6  0.7717148 -0.91504835 0.2713248 Class2
```

The random forest and quadratic discriminant models will be fit to the data:

```
> library(randomForest)
> rfModel <- randomForest(class ~ X1 + X2,
+                         data = simulatedTrain,
+                         ntree = 2000)
> library(MASS) ## for the qda() function
> qdaModel <- qda(class ~ X1 + X2, data = simulatedTrain)
```

The output of the predict function for qda objects includes both the predicted classes (in a slot called class) and the associated probabilities are in a matrix called posterior. For the QDA model, predictions will be created for the training and test sets. Later in this section, the training set probabilities will be used in an additional model to calibrate the class probabilities. The calibration will then be applied to the test set probabilities:

```
> qdaTrainPred <- predict(qdaModel, simulatedTrain)
> names(qdaTrainPred)

[1] "class"     "posterior"
> head(qdaTrainPred$class)

[1] Class1 Class1 Class1 Class2 Class1 Class2
Levels: Class1 Class2
> head(qdaTrainPred$posterior)

      Class1      Class2
1 0.7313136 0.268686374
2 0.8083861 0.191613899
3 0.9985019 0.001498068
4 0.3549247 0.645075330
5 0.5264952 0.473504846
6 0.3604055 0.639594534
> qdaTestPred <- predict(qdaModel, simulatedTest)
> simulatedTrain$QDAprob <- qdaTrainPred$posterior[,"Class1"]
> simulatedTest$QDAprob <- qdaTestPred$posterior[,"Class1"]
```

The random forest model requires two calls to the predict function to get the predicted classes and the class probabilities:

```
> rfTestPred <- predict(rfModel, simulatedTest, type = "prob")
> head(rfTestPred)

   Class1 Class2
1 0.4300 0.5700
2 0.5185 0.4815
3 0.9970 0.0030
4 0.9395 0.0605
5 0.0205 0.9795
6 0.2840 0.7160
> simulatedTest$RFprob <- rfTestPred[,"Class1"]
> simulatedTest$RFclass <- predict(rfModel, simulatedTest)
```

Sensitivity and Specificity

caret has functions for computing sensitivity and specificity. These functions require the user to indicate the role of each of the classes:

```
> # Class 1 will be used as the event of interest
> sensitivity(data = simulatedTest$RFclass,
+              reference = simulatedTest$class,
+              positive = "Class1")
  [1] 0.8278867
> specificity(data = simulatedTest$RFclass,
+              reference = simulatedTest$class,
+              negative = "Class2")
  [1] 0.8946396
```

Predictive values can also be computed either by using the prevalence found in the data set (46 %) or by using prior judgement:

```
> posPredValue(data = simulatedTest$RFclass,
+              reference = simulatedTest$class,
+              positive = "Class1")
  [1] 0.8695652
> negPredValue(data = simulatedTest$RFclass,
+              reference = simulatedTest$class,
+              positive = "Class2")
  [1] 0.8596803
> # Change the prevalence manually
> posPredValue(data = simulatedTest$RFclass,
+              reference = simulatedTest$class,
+              positive = "Class1",
+              prevalence = .9)
  [1] 0.9860567
```

Confusion Matrix

There are several functions in R to create the confusion matrix. The confusionMatrix function in the **caret** package produces the table and associated statistics:

```
> confusionMatrix(data = simulatedTest$RFclass,
+                 reference = simulatedTest$class,
+                 positive = "Class1")

  Confusion Matrix and Statistics

            Reference
  Prediction Class1 Class2
      Class1    380     57
      Class2     79    484
```

```
            Accuracy : 0.864
              95% CI : (0.8412, 0.8846)
  No Information Rate : 0.541
  P-Value [Acc > NIR] : < 2e-16

               Kappa : 0.7252
Mcnemar's Test P-Value : 0.07174

         Sensitivity : 0.8279
         Specificity : 0.8946
      Pos Pred Value : 0.8696
      Neg Pred Value : 0.8597
          Prevalence : 0.4590
      Detection Rate : 0.3800
Detection Prevalence : 0.4370

     'Positive' Class : Class1
```

There is also an option in this function to manually set the prevalence. If there were more than two classes, the sensitivity, specificity, and similar statistics are calculated on a "one-versus-all" basis (e.g., the first class versus a pool of classes two and three).

Receiver Operating Characteristic Curves

The pROC package (Robin et al. 2011) can create the curve and derive various statistics.[6] First, an R object must be created that contains the relevant information using the pROC function roc. The resulting object is then used to generate the ROC curve or calculate the area under the curve. For example,

```
> library(pROC)
> rocCurve <-  roc(response = simulatedTest$class,
+                  predictor = simulatedTest$RFprob,
+                  ## This function assumes that the second
+                  ## class is the event of interest, so we
+                  ## reverse the labels.
+                  levels = rev(levels(simulatedTest$class)))
```

From this object, we can produce statistics (such as the area under the ROC curve and its confidence interval):

```
> auc(rocCurve)
  Area under the curve: 0.9328
> ci.roc(rocCurve)
  95% CI: 0.9176-0.948 (DeLong)
```

---

[6] R has a number of packages that can compute the ROC curve, including ROCR, caTools, PresenceAbsence, and others.

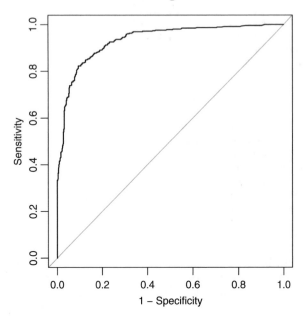

Fig. 11.8: An example of an ROC curve produced using the `roc` and `plot.roc` functions in the pROC package

We can also use the `plot` function to produce the ROC curve itself:

```
> plot(rocCurve, legacy.axes = TRUE)
> ## By default, the x-axis goes backwards, used
> ## the option legacy.axes = TRUE to get 1-spec
> ## on the x-axis moving from 0 to 1
>
> ## Also, another curve can be added using
> ## add = TRUE the next time plot.auc is used.
```

Figure 11.8 shows the results of this function call.

Lift Charts

The lift curve can be created using the `lift` function in the caret package. It takes a formula as the input where the true class is on the left-hand side of the formula, and one or more columns for model class probabilities are on the right. For example, to produce a lift plot for the random forest and QDA test set probabilities,

```
> labs <- c(RFprob = "Random Forest",
+           QDAprob = "Quadratic Discriminant Analysis")
> liftCurve <- lift(class ~ RFprob + QDAprob, data = simulatedTest,
+                   labels = labs)
> liftCurve

  Call:
  lift.formula(x = class ~ RFprob + QDAprob, data = simulatedTest, labels
   = labs)


  Models: Random Forest, Quadratic Discriminant Analysis
  Event: Class1 (45.9%)
```

To plot two lift curves, the `xyplot` function is used to create a lattice plot:

```
> ## Add lattice options to produce a legend on top
> xyplot(liftCurve,
+        auto.key = list(columns = 2,
+                        lines = TRUE,
+                        points = FALSE))
```

See Fig. 11.9.

Calibrating Probabilities

Calibration plots as described above are available in the `calibration.plot` function in the PresenceAbsence package and in the caret function `calibration` (details below). The syntax for the `calibration` function is similar to the `lift` function:

```
> calCurve <- calibration(class ~ RFprob + QDAprob, data = simulatedTest)
> calCurve
  Call:
  calibration.formula(x = class ~ RFprob + QDAprob, data = simulatedTest)

  Models: RFprob, QDAprob
  Event:  Class1
  Cuts:   11
> xyplot(calCurve, auto.key = list(columns = 2))
```

Figure 11.9 also shows this plot. An entirely different approach to calibration plots that model the observed event rate as a function of the class probabilities can be found in the `calibrate.plot` function of the gbm package.

To recalibrate the QDA probabilities, a post-processing model is created that models the true outcome as a function of the class probability. To fit a sigmoidal function, a logistic regression model is used (see Sect. 12.2 for more details) via the `glm` function in base R. This function is an interface to a broad set of methods called generalized linear models (Dobson 2002), which includes logistic regression. To fit the model, the function requires the

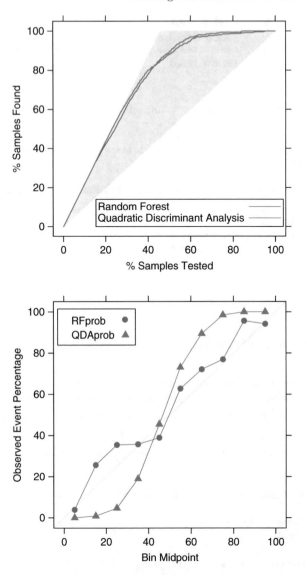

Fig. 11.9: Examples of lift and calibration curves for the random forest and QDA models

family argument to specify the type of outcome data being modeled. Since our outcome is a discrete category, the binomial distribution is selected:

```
> ## The glm() function models the probability of the second factor
> ## level, so the function relevel() is used to temporarily reverse the
> ## factors levels.
```

```
> sigmoidalCal <- glm(relevel(class, ref = "Class2") ~ QDAprob,
+                      data = simulatedTrain,
+                      family = binomial)
> coef(summary(sigmoidalCal))
                Estimate Std. Error   z value      Pr(>|z|)
  (Intercept) -5.701055  0.5005652 -11.38924 4.731132e-30
  QDAprob      11.717292  1.0705197  10.94542 6.989017e-28
```

The corrected probabilities are created by taking the original model and applying Eq. 11.1 with the estimated slope and intercept. In R, the `predict` function can be used:

```
> sigmoidProbs <- predict(sigmoidalCal,
+                         newdata = simulatedTest[,"QDAprob", drop = FALSE],
+                         type = "response")
> simulatedTest$QDAsigmoid <- sigmoidProbs
```

The Bayesian approach for calibration is to treat the training set class probabilities to estimate the probabilities $Pr[X]$ and $Pr[X|Y = C_\ell]$ (see Eq. 13.5 on page 354). In R, the naïve Bayes model function `NaiveBayes` in the klaR package can be used for the computations:

```
> BayesCal <- NaiveBayes(class ~ QDAprob, data = simulatedTrain,
+                        usekernel = TRUE)
> ## Like qda(), the predict function for this model creates
> ## both the classes and the probabilities
> BayesProbs <- predict(BayesCal,
+                       newdata = simulatedTest[, "QDAprob", drop = FALSE])
> simulatedTest$QDABayes <- BayesProbs$posterior[, "Class1"]
> ## The probability values before and after calibration
> head(simulatedTest[, c(5:6, 8, 9)])
      QDAprob RFprob QDAsigmoid  QDABayes
 1 0.3830767 0.4300 0.22927068 0.2515696
 2 0.5440393 0.5185 0.66231139 0.6383383
 3 0.9846107 0.9970 0.99708776 0.9995061
 4 0.5463540 0.9395 0.66835048 0.6430232
 5 0.2426705 0.0205 0.05428903 0.0566883
 6 0.4823296 0.2840 0.48763794 0.5109129
```

The option `usekernel = TRUE` allows a flexible function to model the probability distribution of the class probabilities.

These new probabilities are evaluated using another plot:

```
> calCurve2 <- calibration(class ~ QDAprob + QDABayes + QDAsigmoid,
+                          data = simulatedTest)
> xyplot(calCurve2)
```

Chapter 12
Discriminant Analysis and Other Linear Classification Models

In general, discriminant or classification techniques seek to categorize samples into groups based on the predictor characteristics, and the route to achieving this minimization is different for each technique. Some techniques take a mathematical path [e.g., linear discriminant analysis (LDA)], and others take an algorithmic path (e.g., k-nearest neighbors).

Classical methods such as LDA and its closely related mathematical cousins (partial least squares discriminant analysis (PLSDA), logistic regression, etc.) will be discussed in this chapter and will focus on separating samples into groups based on characteristics of predictor variation.

12.1 Case Study: Predicting Successful Grant Applications

These data are from a 2011 Kaggle competition sponsored by the University of Melbourne where there was interest in predicting whether or not a grant application would be accepted. Since public funding of grants had decreased over time, triaging grant applications based on their likelihood of success could be important for estimating the amount of potential funding to the university. In addition to predicting grant success, the university sought to understand factors that were important in predicting success. As we have discussed throughout the regression chapters, there is often a trade-off between models that are developed for understanding and models that are developed for prediction. The same is true for classification models; this will be illustrated in this and the following chapters.

In the contest, data on 8,708 grants between the years 2005 and 2008 were available for model building and the test set contained applications from 2009 to 2010. The winning entry achieved an area under the ROC curve of 0.968

M. Kuhn and K. Johnson, *Applied Predictive Modeling*,
DOI 10.1007/978-1-4614-6849-3_12,
© Springer Science+Business Media New York 2013

on the test set. The first and second place winners discuss their approaches to the data and modeling on the Kaggle blog.[1]

The data can be found at the Kaggle web site,[2] but only the training set data contain the outcomes for the grants. Many pieces of information were collected across grants, including whether or not the grant application was successful. The original data contained many predictors such as:

- The role of each individual listed on the grant. Possible values include chief investigator (shortened to "CI" in the data), delegated researcher (DR), principal supervisor (PS), external advisor (EA), external chief investigator (ECI), student chief investigator (SCI), student researcher (SR), honorary visitor (HV), or unknown (UNK). The total number of individuals listed on the grant ranged from 1 to 14.
- Several characteristics of each individual on the grant, such as their date of birth, home language, highest degree, nationality, number of prior successful (and unsuccessful) grants, department, faculty status, level of seniority, length of employment at the university, and number of publications in four different grades of journals.
- One or more codes related to Australia's research fields, courses and disciplines (RFCD) classification. Using this, the grant can be classified into subgroups, such as Applied Economics, Microbiology, and Librarianship. There were 738 possible values of the RFCD codes in the data. If more than one code was specified for a grant, their relative percentages were recorded. The RFCD codes listed by the Australian Bureau of Statistics[3] range from 210,000 to 449,999. There were many grants with nonsensical codes (such as 0 or 999,999) that were grouped into an unknown category for these analyses.
- One or more codes corresponding to the socio-economic objective (SEO) classification. This classification describes the intended purpose of the grant, such as developing construction activities or health services. If more than one code was specified for a grant, their relative percentages were recorded. Like the RFCD codes, there were some values in the data that did not map to any of the codes listed by the Australian government and were grouped into an unknown category.
- The submission date of the grant
- The monetary value of the grant, binned into 17 groups
- A grant category code which describes the type sponsor as well as a code for the specific sponsor

One of the first steps in the model building process is to transform, or encode, the original data structure into a form that is most informative for the model (i.e., *feature engineering*). This encoding process is critical and must be done

---

[1] http://blog.kaggle.com/.

[2] http://www.kaggle.com/c/unimelb.

[3] The RFCD codes can be found at http://tinyurl.com/25zvts while the SEO codes can be found at http://tinyurl.com/8435ae4.

with foresight into the analyses that will be performed so that appropriate predictors can be elucidated from the original data. Failure to appropriately format the predictors can prevent developing effective predictive models.

The original form of the grant data is not conducive to modeling. For example, many fields are broken down for each individual involved in the grant. As such, there are 15 columns in the data for each individual. Since there could be as many as 14 individuals associated with a grant, there are a large number of columns for a grant, many of which have no data.

How to encode these data is a primary first question. For example, since there are often multiple individuals associated with the grant, how should this information be represented in the data? Similarly, when there are multiple RFCD codes and associated percentages, in what manner should these data enter the models? Additionally, these data contain many missing values which we must also handle before building a predictive model. We must think through all of these questions while keeping in mind the goal of predicting the success of a grant application.

Given this goal, we took the following steps. First, a group of predictors was created that describe how many investigators were on the grant broken up by role (e.g., chief investigator). Second, groups of role-specific count variables were also created for the home language, nationality, degree, birth year, department, and grant history. For example, one variable counts the number of chief investigators from Australia while another counts the total number of successful grants from all delegated researchers on the grant. For publication data, the total number of publications in the four tiers of journals was aggregated across all roles. The duration of employment was similarly aggregated across all roles.

Indicator variables for each sponsor code and grant category were also created. For the RFCD and SEO codes, the number of non-zero percentages for each grant was used. Finally, indicators were generated for the month and day or the week that the grant was submitted. In all, 1,784 possible predictors were created using this encoding scheme.

As a result, the vast majority of these predictors are discrete in nature (i.e., either 0/1 dummy variables or counts) with many 0 values. Since many of the predictors are categorical in nature, missing values were encoded as "unknown." For example, 912 grants had missing category codes. A binary predictor for missing grant categories was created to capture this information.

As described in Chap. 3, some predictive models have different constraints on the type of predictors that they can utilize. For example, in these data, a significant number of predictors had pair-wise absolute correlations that were larger than 0.99. Because of this, a high-correlation filter was used on the predictor set to remove these highly redundant predictors from the data. In the end, 56 predictors were eliminated from the data for this reason. The binary nature of many of predictors also resulted in many cases where the data were very sparse and unbalanced. For the RFCD codes, 95 % of the predictors had less than 50 non-zero indicators. This high degree of class imbalance

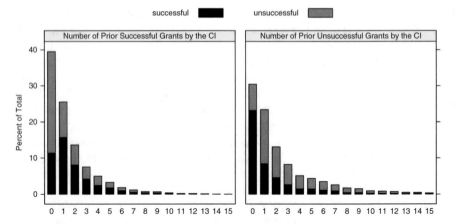

Fig. 12.1: The top two continuous predictors associated with grant success based on the pre-2008 data. Prior success in receiving a grant by the chief investigator as well as prior failure in receiving a grant are most highly associated with the success or failure of receiving a future grant. The x-axis is truncated to 15 grants so that the long tails of the distribution do not obfuscate the differences

indicates that many of the predictors could be classified as *near-zero variance predictors* described in Chap. 3, which can lead to computational issues in many of the models.

Since not all models are affected by this issue, two different sets of predictors were used, depending on the model. The "full set" of predictors included all the variables regardless of their distribution (1,070 predictors). The "reduced set" was developed for models that are sensitive to sparse and unbalanced predictors and contained 252 predictors. In subsequent chapters and sections, the text will describe which predictor set was used for each model.[4] As a reminder, the process of removing predictors without measuring their association with the outcome is *unsupervised feature selection*. Although a few models that use supervised feature selection are described in this chapter, a broader discussion of feature selection is tabled until Chap. 19.

A cursory, univariate review of the newly encoded data uncovers a few interesting relationships with the response. Two continuous predictors, the number of prior successful and unsuccessful grant applications by the chief investigator, were highly associated with grant application success. The distributions of these predictors by current grant application success are displayed in Fig. 12.1. Not surprisingly these histograms suggest that prior success or

---

[4] However, there are several tree-based methods described in Chap. 14 that are more effective if the categorical predictors are not converted to dummy variables. In these cases, the full set of categories are used.

Table 12.1: Statistics for the three categorical predictors with highest univariate association with the success funding of a grant

| | Grant success | | | | | |
	Yes	No	N	Percent	Odds	Odds ratio
Contract value band						
A	1,501	818	2,319	64.7	1.835	2.84
Other bands	2,302	3,569	5,871	39.2	0.645	
Sponsor						
Unknown	732	158	890	82.2	4.633	6.38
Known	3,071	4,229	7,300	42.1	0.726	
Month						
January	480	45	525	91.4	10.667	13.93
Other months	3,323	4,342	7,665	43.4	0.765	

failure shifts the respective distribution towards current success or failure. Given this knowledge, we would expect these predictors to play significant roles for most any classification model.

Three categorical predictors (Contract Value Band A, Sponsor Unknown, and January) had the highest univariate associations with grant application success. The associations for these three predictors were not strong but do reveal some useful patterns. Table 12.1 shows the data and suggests that grant submissions with a large monetary value, an unknown sponsor, or a submission in January are associated with greater funding success. Looking at the problem a different way, unsuccessful grant applications are likely to have a smaller monetary value, to have a known sponsor, and are submitted in a month other than January. The table has the success rates for each group and also the *odds*, which is ratio of the probability of a success grant over the probability of an unsuccessful grant. One common method for quantifying the predictive ability of a binary predictor (such as these) is the *odds ratio*. For example, when a grant is submitted in January the odds are much higher (10.7) than other months (0.8). The ratio of the odds for this predictor suggests that grants submitted in January are 13.9 times more likely to be successful than the other months. Given the high odds ratios, we would expect that these predictors will also have impact on the development of most classification models.

Finally, we must choose how to split the data which is not directly obvious. Before deciding on the splitting approach, it is important to note that the percentage of successful grants varied over the years: 45 % (2005), 51.7 % (2006), 47.2 % (2007), and 36.6 % (2008). Although 2008 had the lowest percentage in the data, there is not yet enough information to declare a downward trend. The data splitting scheme should take into account the *application domain* of the model: how will it be used and what should the criterion be to assess if it is fit for purpose? The purpose of the model exercise is to create a predictive model to quantify the likelihood of success for new grants, which is why the competition used the most recent data for testing purposes.

If the grant success rate were relatively constant over the years, a reasonable data splitting strategy would be relatively straightforward: take all the available data from 2005 to 2008, reserve some data for a test set, and use resampling with the remainder of the samples for tuning the various models. However, a random test sample across all of the years is likely to lead to a substantially less *relevant* test set; in effect, we would be building models that are focused on the *past* grant application environment.

An alternative strategy would be to create models using the data before 2008, but tune them based on how well they fit the 2008 data. Essentially, the 2008 data would serve as a single test set that is more relevant in time to the original test set of data from 2009 to 2010. However, this is a single "look" at the data that do not provide any real measure of uncertainty for model performance. More importantly, this strategy may lead to substantial over-fitting to this particular set of 2008 data and may not generalize well to subsequent years. For example, as with regression models, there are a number of classification models that automatically perform feature selection while building the model. One potential methodology error that may occur with a single test set that is evaluated many times is that a set of predictors may be selected that work only for these particular 2008 grant applications. We would have no way of knowing if this is the case until another set of recent grant applications are evaluated.

How do these two approaches compare for these data? Figure 12.2 shows the results for a support vector machine classification model discussed in detail in Sect. 13.4 but is similar to the support vector regression model described in Sect. 7.3. Using the radial basis function kernel previously discussed, the tuning parameters are the kernel parameter, σ, and the cost value, C, used to control for over-fitting. Several values of the radial basis function kernel parameter were evaluated as well as several values of the cost function.

Figure 12.2 shows both approaches to tuning the model. Two tuning parameter profiles for the support vector machine are shown:

- The first model is built on 8,189 grants that include all the pre-2008 data and 25 % of the 2008 data ($n = 290$). To choose the regularization and kernel parameter(s), 10-fold cross-validation is used. The performance profile across the cost parameter is shown as a blue line in Fig. 12.2 (this profile uses the optimal value of the kernel parameter). A set of 2008 grants ($n = 1,785$) is held back to validate the choice of the final tuning parameter (blue profile).
- The second model is exclusively built on pre-2008 data, and the value of the tuning parameter is chosen to maximize the area under the ROC curve for the 2008 grants. No additional samples are held back for verifying the parameter choice (red profile).

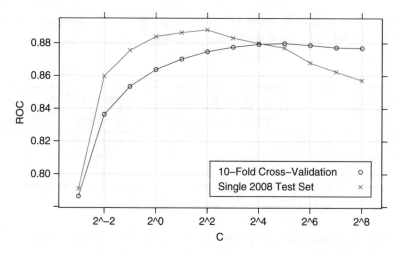

Fig. 12.2: Two models for grant success based on the pre-2008 data but with different data sets used to tune the model

The blue profile suggests that a value of 32 for the cost parameter will yield an area under the ROC curve of 0.88. The red profile shows the results of evaluating only the 2008 data (i.e., no resampling). Here, the tuning process suggests that a smaller cost value is needed (4) to achieve an optimal model with an area under the ROC curve of 0.89. Firstly, given the amount of data to evaluate the model, it is problematic that the curves suggest different tuning parameters. Secondly, when the cross-validated model is evaluated on the 2008 data, the area under the ROC curve is substantially smaller (0.83) than the cross-validation results indicate.

The compromise taken here is to build models on the pre-2008 data and tune them by evaluating a random sample of 2,075 grants from 2008. Once the optimal parameters are determined, final model is built using these parameters and the entire training set (i.e., the data prior to 2008 and the additional 2,075 grants). A small holdout set of 518 grants from 2008 will be used to ensure that no gross methodology errors occur from repeatedly evaluating the 2008 data during model tuning. In the text, this set of samples is called the *2008 holdout set*. This small set of year 2008 grants will be referred to as the *test set* and will not be evaluated until set of candidate models are identified (in Chap. 15). These strategies are summarized in Table 12.2.

To be clear, there is no single, clean approach to handling this issue for data that appear to be evolving over time. Therefore the practitioner must understand the modeling objectives and carefully craft a plan for training and testing models. In this case, the grant data have the luxury of a moderate amount of recent data; there are enough data to split out a small holdout set

Table 12.2: A schematic for the data splitting strategy for the grant application data used in this and subsequent chapters

	Model tuning		Final model	
	Training	Holdout	Training	Holdout
Pre-2008 ($n = 6,633$)	×		×	
2008 ($n = 1,557$)		×	×	
2008 ($n = 518$)				×

without significantly impairing the tuning process. The disadvantages of this approach are:

1. An assumption is being made that the model parameters derived from the tuning process will be appropriate for the final model, which uses pre-2008 data as well as the 2,075 grants from 2008.
2. Since the final model uses some 2008 grants, the performance on the test set is likely to be better than the results generated in the tuning process (where the model parameters were not exposed to year 2008 grants).

In Chap. 15, the test set results will be compared to those generated during model tuning.

12.2 Logistic Regression

Linear regression (Sect. 6.2) forms a model that is linear in the parameters, and these parameters are obtained by minimizing the sum of the squared residuals. It turns out that the model that minimizes the sum of the squared residuals also produces *maximum likelihood estimates* of the parameters when it is reasonable to assume that the model residuals follow a normal (i.e., Gaussian) distribution.

Maximum likelihood parameter estimation is a technique that can be used when we are willing to make assumptions about the probability distribution of the data. Based on the theoretical probability distribution and the observed data, the likelihood function is a probability statement that can be made about a particular set of parameter values. If two sets of parameters values are being identified, the set with the larger likelihood would be deemed more consistent with the observed data.

The probability distribution that is most often used when there are two classes is the binomial distribution.[5] This distribution has a single parameter, p, that is the probability of an event or a specific class. For the grant data, suppose p is the probability of a successful grant. In the pre-2008 grants, there were a total of 6,633 grants and, of these, 3,233 were successful. Here, the form of the binomial likelihood function would be

$$L(p) = \binom{6633}{3233} p^{3233} (1-p)^{6633-3233}, \qquad (12.1)$$

where the exponents for p and $1-p$ reflect the frequencies of the classes in the observed data. The first part of the equation is "n choose r" and accounts for the possible ways that there could be 3,233 successes and 3,400 failures in the data.

The maximum likelihood estimator would find a value of p that produces the largest value for $f(p)$. It turns out that the sample proportion, $3233/6633 = 0.487$, is the maximum likelihood estimate in this situation.

However, we know that the success rate is affected by multiple factors and we would like to build a model that uses those factors to produce a more refined probability estimate. In this case, we would *re-parameterize* the model so that p is a function of these factors. Like linear regression, the logistic regression model has an intercept in addition to slope parameters for each model term. However, since the probability of the event is required to be between 0 and 1, we cannot be guaranteed that a slope and intercept model would constrain values within this range. As discussed earlier in the chapter, if p is the probability of an event, the odds of the event are then $p/(1-p)$. Logistic regression models the log odds of the event as a linear function:

$$\log\left(\frac{p}{1-p}\right) = \beta_0 + \beta_1 x_1 + \cdots + \beta_P x_P. \qquad (12.2)$$

Here, P is the number of predictors. The right-hand side of the equation is usually referred to as the *linear predictor*. Since the log of the odds can range from $-\infty$ to ∞, there is no concern about the range of values that the linear predictors may produce. By moving some terms around, we get back to a function of the event probability:

$$p = \frac{1}{1 + \exp\left[-(\beta_0 + \beta_1 x_1 + \cdots + \beta_P x_P)\right]} \qquad (12.3)$$

This nonlinear function is a sigmoidal function of the model terms and constrains the probability estimates to between 0 and 1. Also, this model produces linear class boundaries, unless the predictors used in the model are

---

[5] Data with three or more classes are usually modeled using the *multinomial distribution*. See Agresti (2002) for more details.

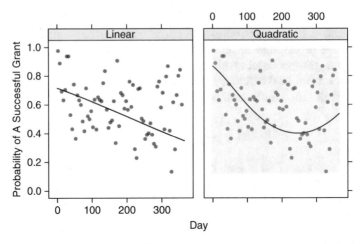

Fig. 12.3: Two logistic regression models that relate the probability of a successful grant to the numeric day of the year. In this plot, the day values were binned into 5-day periods. The model fits did not use the binned version of the predictor; the log odds were modeled as a function of the day of the year (e.g., 1, 2, ..., 365)

nonlinear versions of the data (e.g., the squared values of a predictor are used as one of the x_j model terms).

Now that we have a way to relate our model to the parameter of the binomial distribution, we can find candidate values of the parameters (β) and, with our observed data, compute a value of the likelihood function. Once we find β values that appear to maximize the likelihood for our data, these values would be used to predict sample outcomes.

Logistic regression and ordinary linear regression fall into a larger class of techniques called generalized linear models (GLMs) that encompass many different probability distributions. Dobson (2002) provides an excellent introduction to these models. They are linear in the sense that some function of the outcome is modeled using the linear predictors, such as the log odds in Eq. 12.2. They often produce nonlinear equations (such as the one for p in Eq. 12.3). Again, note that even though the equation for p is nonlinear, it produces linear classification boundaries.

For example, we could fit a simple logistic regression model to the grant data using a single predictor, such as the numeric day of the year. Figure 12.3 shows the observed probability of a successful grant when the data are binned into 5-day intervals. In this plot, there is a higher success rate associated with the beginning and end of the year. In fact, for the data prior to 2008, there were zero unsuccessful grants in the pool of 343 grants submitted on the first day of the year. During the middle of the year the acceptance rate is roughly decreasing but increases near the end of the year. A simple logistic regression model would try to estimate a slope corresponding to the day as well as an intercept term. Using the training data, the model fitting routine searches across different values of these two parameters to find a combination that, given the observed training data, maximizes the likelihood of the binomial distribution. In the end, the estimated intercept was 0.919 and the slope parameter was determined to be −0.0042. This means that there was a per day *decrease* in the log odds of 0.0042. The model fit is shown on the left panel of Fig. 12.3. This does not adequately represent the trend in the later part of the year. Another model can be created where a third parameter corresponds to a squared day term. For this model, the estimated intercept now becomes 1.88, the slope for the linear day term is −0.019, and the slope for the quadratic term was estimated to be −0.000038. The right-hand panel of Fig. 12.3 shows a clear improvement in the model but does not quite capture the increase in the success rate at the end of the year. As evidence of the need for an additional term, the area under the ROC curve for the linear model was 0.56, which improves to 0.66 once the additional model term is utilized.

An effective logistic regression model would require an inspection of how the success rate related to each of the continuous predictors and, based on this, may parameterize the model terms to account for nonlinear effects. One efficient method for doing this is discussed in Harrell (2001), where restricted cubic splines are used to create flexible, adaptive versions of the predictors that can capture many types of nonlinearities. The chapter's Computing section has more details on this methodology. Another approach is a generalized additive model (Hastie and Tibshirani 1990; Hastie et al. 2008), which also uses flexible regression methods (such as splines) to adaptively model the log odds. We refer the reader to the reference texts to learn more about these methods.

For the grant data, the full set of predictors was used in a logistic regression model. The other continuous predictors were evaluated for nonlinearities. However, many of the predictors have few data points on one or more extremes of the distributions, such as the two predictors shown in Fig. 12.1. This increases the difficulty in prescribing an exact functional form for the predictors. Using this predictor set, the logistic regression model was able to achieve an area under the ROC curve of 0.78, a sensitivity of 77 % and a specificity of 76.1 %, on the 2008 holdout set.

Many of the categorical predictors have sparse and unbalanced distributions. Because of this, we would expect that a model using the full set of predictors would perform worse than the set that has near-zero variance predictors removed. For the reduced set of 253 variables, the area under the ROC curve was 0.87, the sensitivity was 80.4 %, and the specificity was 82.2 % (Fig. 12.4). The confusion matrix is shown in Table 12.3. With this particular model, there was a substantial improvement gained by removing these predictors.

For logistic regression, formal statistical hypothesis tests can be conducted to assess whether the slope coefficients for each predictor are statistically significant. A Z statistic is commonly used for these models (Dobson 2002), and

Table 12.3: The 2008 holdout set confusion matrix for the logistic regression model

| | Observed class | |
	Successful	Unsuccessful
Successful	439	236
Unsuccessful	131	751

This model had an overall accuracy of 76.4 %, a sensitivity of 77 %, and a specificity of 76.1 %

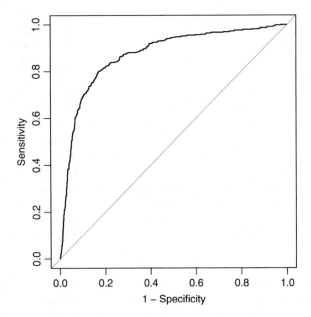

Fig. 12.4: The ROC curve for the grant data test set using a logistic regression model. The AUC is 0.87

is essentially a measure of the signal-to-noise ratio: the estimated slope is divided by its corresponding standard error. Using this statistic, the predictors can be ranked to understand which terms had the largest effect on the model. For these data, the five most important predictors were the number of unsuccessful grants by chief investigators, the number of successful grants by chief investigators, contract value band F, contract value band E, and numeric day of the year (squared).

The logistic regression model is very popular due to its simplicity and ability to make inferential statements about model terms. For example, a researcher may want to formally evaluate whether the day of the calendar year has a statistically significant relationship with the probability of grant acceptance. Harrell (2001) is an excellent resource for developing statistical models for the purpose of making inferential statements about model parameters.

This model can also be effective when the goal is solely prediction, but, as demonstrated above, it does require the user to identify effective representations of the predictor data that yield the best performance. As will be shown in the later sections, there are other classification models that empirically derive these relationships in the course of model training. If the model will only be utilized for prediction, these techniques may be more advantageous.

12.3 Linear Discriminant Analysis

The roots of LDA date back to Fisher (1936) and Welch (1939). Each of these researchers took a different perspective on the problem of obtaining optimal classification rules. Yet, as we will see, each came to find the same rule in the two-group classification setting. In this section we will provide highlights of both of these approaches to capture their necessary technical details while also discussing a few mathematical constructs required for connecting it with other methods discussed later in this chapter.

For the classification problem, Welch (1939) took the approach of minimizing the total probability of misclassification, which depends on class probabilities and multivariate distributions of the predictors. To see Welch's approach, we first need a basic understanding of Bayes' Rule[6] which is

$$Pr[Y = C_\ell | X] = \frac{Pr[Y = C_\ell]Pr[X | Y = C_\ell]}{\sum_{l=1}^{C} Pr[Y = C_l]Pr[X | Y = C_l]} \qquad (12.4)$$

$Pr[Y = C_\ell]$ is known as the *prior probability* of membership in class C_ℓ. In practice these values are either known, are determined by the proportions of samples in each class, or are unknown in which case all values of the priors are set to be equal. $Pr[X | Y = C_\ell]$ is the *conditional probability* of observing predictors X, given that the data stem from class C_ℓ. Here we assume that the data are generated from a probability distribution (e.g., multivariate normal distribution), which then defines this quantity's mathematical form. The result of this equation is $Pr[Y = C_\ell | X]$, which is commonly referred to as the *posterior probability* that the sample, X, is a member of class C_ℓ. For a more detailed description of this equation, we refer you to Sect. 13.6.

For a two-group classification problem, the rule that minimizes the total probability of misclassification would be to classify X into group 1 if $Pr[Y = C_1 | X] > Pr[Y = C_2 | X]$ and into group 2 if the inequality is reversed. Using Eq. 12.4, this rule directly translates to classifying X into group 1 if

$$Pr[Y = C_1]Pr[X | Y = C_1] > Pr[Y = C_2]Pr[X | Y = C_2]. \qquad (12.5)$$

---

[6] Bayes' Rule is examined in more detail in Sect. 13.6.

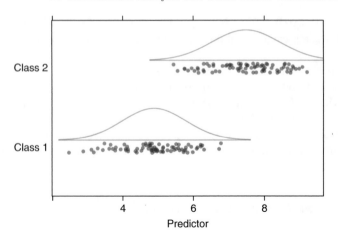

Fig. 12.5: A single predictor is used to classify samples into two groups. The *blue figures* above each group represent the probability density function for a normal distribution determined by the class-specific means and variances

We can easily extend this rule to the more-than-two group case. In this setting, we would classify X into group C_ℓ if $Pr[Y = C_\ell]Pr[X|Y = C_\ell]$ has the largest value across all of the C classes.

Figure 12.5 illustrates this with a single predictor and two classes (the individual data points have been "jittered" to reduce their overlap). The blue illustrations above each group of data points are the probability density function for the normal distribution for each of the classes (i.e., $Pr[X|Y = C_1]$ and $Pr[X|Y = C_2]$). Since there is a single predictor, a new sample is classified by finding its value on the x-axis, then determining the value for each of the probability density functions for each class (in addition to the overall probability, $Pr[X]$, found by pooling both groups). Suppose a new sample had a value of 4 for the predictor. The probability for Class 2 is virtually 0, so this sample would be predicted to belong to the first class.

Since a single predictor is used for this example, it belies the complexity of using Bayes' Rule in practice. For classification, the number of predictors is almost always greater than one and can be extremely large. In more realistic situations, how does one compute quantities such as $Pr[X|Y = C_\ell]$ in many dimensions?[7] What multivariate probability distributions can be used to this effect?

One special, often used scenario is to assume that the distribution of the predictors is multivariate normal. This distribution has two parameters: the multidimensional mean vector $\boldsymbol{\mu}_\ell$ and covariance matrix $\boldsymbol{\Sigma}_\ell$. Further, if we assume that the means of the groups are unique (i.e., a different $\boldsymbol{\mu}_\ell$ for each group), but the covariance matrices are identical across groups, we can solve

---

[7] This situation is addressed again for the naïve Bayes models in the next chapter.

Eq. 12.5 or the more general multi-class problem to find the linear discriminant function of the ℓth group:

$$X'\Sigma^{-1}\mu_\ell - 0.5\mu_\ell'\Sigma^{-1}\mu_\ell + \log\left(Pr[Y = C_\ell]\right). \tag{12.6}$$

In practice, the theoretical means, μ_ℓ, are estimated by using the class-specific means $(\bar{x}_\ell)$. The theoretical covariance matrix, Σ, is likewise estimated by the observed covariance matrix of the data, S, and X is replaced with an observed sample, u. In the simple example in Fig. 12.5, the sample mean and variance of the data were sufficient to produce the probability distributions shown in blue. For two classes, the class-specific means and variances would be computed along with the sample covariance between the two predictors (to fill out the sample covariance matrix).

Notice that Eq. 12.6 is a linear function in X and defines the separating class boundaries. Hence the method's name: LDA. A slight alteration in the assumptions—that the covariance matrices are not identical across the groups—leads to quadratic discriminant analysis, which will be described in Sect. 13.1.

Fisher formulated the classification problem in a different way. In this approach, he sought to find the linear combination of the predictors such that the between-group variance was maximized relative to the within-group variance. In other words, he wanted to find the combination of the predictors that gave maximum separation between the centers of the data while at the same time minimizing the variation within each group of data.

To illustrate this concept, Fig. 12.6 is an analog to Fig. 12.5. Here, the blue bars indicate the class-specific means. Since there is a single predictor, the between group variance is the square of the difference in these means. The within-group variance would be estimated by a variance that pools the variances of the predictor within each group (illustrated using the red bars in the figure). Taking a ratio of these two quantities is, in effect, a signal-to-noise ratio. Fisher's approach determines linear combinations of the predictors to maximize the signal-to-noise ratio. Similar to the previous discussion of Welch's approach, the situation becomes increasingly more complicated by adding additional predictors. The between- and within-group variances become complex calculations that involve the covariance structure of the predictors, etc.

Mathematically, let B represent the between-group covariance matrix and W represent the within-group covariance matrix. Then Fisher's problem can be formulated as finding the value of b such that

$$\frac{b'\mathbf{B}b}{b'\mathbf{W}b} \tag{12.7}$$

is maximized. The solution to this optimization problem is the eigenvector corresponding to the largest eigenvalue of $\mathbf{W}^{-1}\mathbf{B}$. This vector is a linear discriminant, and subsequent discriminants are found through the same op-

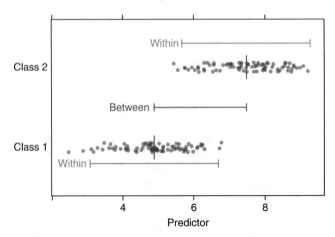

Fig. 12.6: The same data as shown in Fig. 12.5. Here, the between- and within-class variances are illustrated. The within-class ranges are based on the mean ± two standard deviations

timization subject to the constraint that the new directions are uncorrelated with the previous discriminants.

To make Fisher's approach more concrete, let's consider the two-group setting. Solving Eq. 12.7 for two groups gives the discriminant function of $S^{-1}(\bar{\mathbf{x}}_1 - \bar{\mathbf{x}}_2)$, where S^{-1} is the inverse of the covariance matrix of the data and is multiplied by the difference between the mean vectors of predictors for each group (i.e., $\bar{\mathbf{x}}_1$ contains the means of each predictor calculated from the class 1 data). In practice, a new sample, $\mathbf{u}$, is projected onto the discriminant function as $\mathbf{u}'S^{-1}(\bar{\mathbf{x}}_1 - \bar{\mathbf{x}}_2)$, which returns a discriminant score. A new sample is then classified into group 1 if the sample is closer to the group 1 mean than the group 2 mean in the projection:

$$\left| b'(\mathbf{u} - \bar{\mathbf{x}}_1) \right| - \left| b'(\mathbf{u} - \bar{\mathbf{x}}_2) \right| < 0. \tag{12.8}$$

As a more complex illustration, Fig. 12.7 shows a data set with two classes and two predictors, A and B. The line $A = B$ easily separates these two sets of points into distinct groups. However, this line is *not* the discriminant function. Rather, the discriminant function is instead orthogonal to the line that separates them in space (see Fig. 12.8). With two predictors, the discriminant function for an unknown sample u is

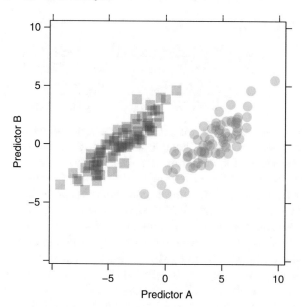

Fig. 12.7: A simple example of two groups of samples that are clearly separable

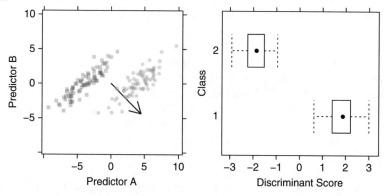

Fig. 12.8: The line at approximately $A = B$ is the vector that visually separates the two groups. Assessing class membership is determined by projecting a sample onto the discriminant vector (*red arrow*) and then calculating its distance from the mean for each group. The sample is then classified into the group which mean is closer. The *box plots* are the distribution of the samples for each class after LDA has been performed, illustrating the maximization of between-to-within group variation

$$D(u) = \mathbf{u}'S^{-1}(\bar{\mathbf{x}}_1 - \bar{\mathbf{x}}_2)$$
$$= u_A \left(\frac{(\bar{x}_{1A} - \bar{x}_{2A})s_B^2}{s_A^2 s_B^2 - s_{AB}^2} - \frac{(\bar{x}_{1B} - \bar{x}_{2B})s_{AB}}{s_A^2 s_B^2 - s_{AB}^2} \right)$$
$$+ u_B \left(\frac{(\bar{x}_{1B} - \bar{x}_{2B})s_A^2}{s_A^2 s_B^2 - s_{AB}^2} - \frac{(\bar{x}_{1A} - \bar{x}_{2A})s_{AB}}{s_A^2 s_B^2 - s_{AB}^2} \right).$$

Here, $\bar{x}_{1A}$ is the sample mean for predictor A calculated using the data from only the first class; $\bar{x}_{2A}$ is the sample mean for A for the second class (the notation is analogous for predictor B). Also, s_A^2 is the sample variance for predictor A (computed with data from both classes), s_B^2 is the sample variance for predictor B, and s_{AB} is the sample covariance between the two predictors.

For this function, note that all of the predictor variances and the between-predictor covariance are used in this equation. When the number of predictors is large, the prediction equation requires a very large number of parameters to be estimated. For $P = 2$ and two classes, this equation uses four means and three variance parameters. In general, the model would require $CP + P(P + 1)/2$ parameters with P predictors and C classes. In comparison to logistic regression, a similar model would only estimate three parameters. This difference between the models becomes more significant as the number of predictors grow. However, the value of the extra parameters in LDA models is that the between-predictor correlations are explicitly handled by the model. This should provide some advantage to LDA over logistic regression when there are substantial correlations, although both models will break down when the multicollinearity becomes extreme.

Fisher's formulation of the problem makes intuitive sense, is easy to solve mathematically, and, unlike Welch's approach, involves no assumptions about the underlying distributions of the data. The mathematical optimization constrains the maximum number of discriminant functions that can be extracted to be the lesser of the number of predictors or one less than the number of groups. For example, if we have ten predictors and three groups, we can at most extract two linear discriminant vectors. Similar to PCA, the eigenvalues in this problem represent the amount of variation explained by each component of $\mathbf{W}^{-1}\mathbf{B}$. Hence, LDA is a member of the latent variable routines like PCA and partial least squares (PLS). In practice, the number of discriminant vectors is a tuning parameter that we would estimate using the usual approach of cross-validation or resampling with the appropriate performance criteria.

Closely examining the linear discriminant function leads to two findings which are similar to what we observed with multiple linear regression (Sect. 6.2). First, the LDA solution depends on inverting a covariance matrix, and a unique solution exists only when this matrix is invertible. Just like in regression, this means that the data must contain more samples than predictors, and the predictors must be independent (see the computing section for an approach to determining if the covariance matrix is invertible). When there are more predictors than samples, or when the predictors are extremely correlated, then just like in regression, a popular approach is to first perform PCA to reduce dimension and generate new uncorrelated predictor combinations. While this approach has been shown to work, the dimension reduction is uninformed about the class structure of the data. To incorporate the class structure into the dimension reduction, we recommend using PLSDA or regularization methods (see following sections). Second, the linear discriminant function is a P-dimensional vector, the values of which are directly paired to the original predictors. The magnitudes of these values can be used to understand the contribution of each predictor to the classification of samples and provide some understanding and interpretation about the underlying system.

From the above discussion, practitioners should be particularly rigorous in pre-processing data before using LDA. We recommend that predictors be centered and scaled and that near-zero variance predictors be removed. If the covariance matrix is still not invertible, then we recommend using PLS or a regularization approach. Similarly, we recommend using PLS or regularization methods (described in sections in this chapter) if there are more predictors than samples. Along the same lines, the practitioner must be aware of the number of samples relative to the number of predictors when using cross-validation routines for methods that depend on inverting a covariance matrix. For example, if the number of samples is 5 % greater than the number of predictors for the training set, and we choose 10-fold cross-validation, then the covariance matrix will not be invertible for any of the folds since all of the folds will have fewer samples than predictors.

We will now illustrate how LDA performs on the grant data. Since LDA is sensitive to near zero variance predictors and collinear predictors,we have reduced the predictor set to 253 predictors (including the squared day term as in logistic regression). Using this subset of predictors, the area under the ROC curve for the 2008 holdout set is 0.89. Table 12.4 shows the confusion matrix for these data and Fig. 12.9 displays the corresponding ROC curve. The light grey line in this plot also shows the ROC curve for the previous logistic regression model.

As we mentioned above, examining the coefficients of the linear discriminant function can provide an understanding of the relative importance of predictors. The top 5 predictors based on absolute magnitude of discriminant function coefficient are numeric day of the year (squared) (2.2), numeric day of the year (-1.9), the number of unsuccessful grants by chief investigators (-0.62), the number of successful grants by chief investigators (0.58), and contract value band A (0.56). Note that this list contains several predictors that the univariate approach identified as being associated with the success of a grant submission. Here, the number of previous unsuccessful grant submissions by the chief investigator is inversely related to the number of previous successful grant submissions by the chief investigator and largest monetary categorization, which is intuitive.

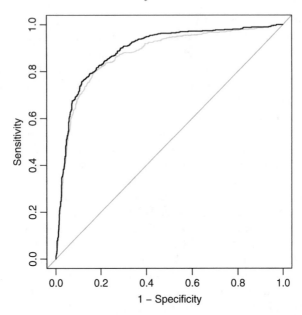

Fig. 12.9: The ROC curve for the 2008 holdout using LDA. The AUC is 0.89. The *lightly shaded line* is the ROC curve for the previous logistic regression model

Table 12.4: The 2008 holdout set confusion matrix for the LDA model

	Observed class	
	Successful	Unsuccessful
Successful	458	175
Unsuccessful	112	812

This model had an overall accuracy of 81.6 %, a sensitivity of 80.4 %, and a specificity of 82.3 %

We can then project the 2008 holdout grants onto this linear discriminant vector and examine the distribution of the discriminant scores (Fig. 12.10). While there is overlap of the distributions for successful and unsuccessful grant applications, LDA yields decent classification performance—especially given that LDA is summarizing the entirety of the underlying relationships in one dimension (Table 12.4).

When we have more samples than predictors, the covariance matrix is invertible, and the data can be decently separated by a linear hyperplane, then LDA will produce a predictively satisfying model that also provides some understanding of the underlying relationships between predictors and response.

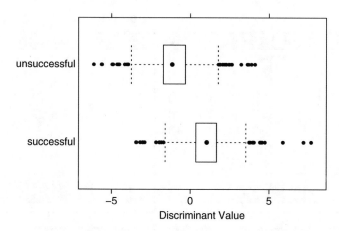

Fig. 12.10: Box plots of the discriminant scores for the 2008 holdout set

The user should be aware, however, that there is a data set scenario that meets these basic requirements but will yield class probability estimates that are overly optimistic. Specifically, the user should be very cautious with LDA predicted class probabilities when the number of samples begins to approach the number of predictors. We will use a simple simulation to illustrate this cautionary note. For 500 samples we have generated data sets containing 10, 100, 200, and 450 predictors all from a random normal population. The response for the samples was also randomly generated placing 250 samples in each category. Therefore, the predictors and response for each of these data sets have no relationship with each other. We will then build LDA models on each of these data sets and examine performance. As we would expect, the test set classification accuracy for each data set is approximately 50 %. Since these data are completely random, we would also expect that the predicted class probabilities for the test set should also be around 0.5. This is true when the number of predictors is small relative to the number of samples. But as the number of predictors grows, the predicted class probabilities become closer to 0 and 1 (Fig. 12.11). At face value, these results seem counterintuitive: test set performance tells us that the model performs as good as a coin toss, but the model is extremely confident about classifying samples into each category.

How can this be? It turns out that these seemingly contradictory conclusions are due to LDA's mathematical construction. Recall that LDA finds an optimal discriminant vector. Geometrically, if the number of samples equals the number of predictors (or dimensions), then we can find at least one vector that perfectly separates the samples. Consider the simplest case where we have two samples and two dimensions. As long as those samples are not in the same location, then we can find one vector (actually infinitely many)

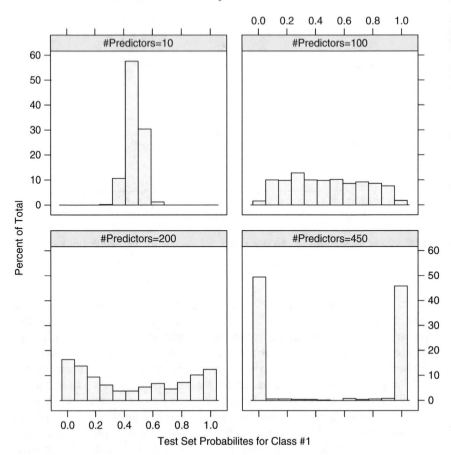

Fig. 12.11: Histograms of test set class probabilities for a simulated two-class example where all predictors are non-informative. As the number of predictors approaches the number of samples (500 in the training set), the class probabilities begin to diverge towards the two extremes (however, the overall accuracy remains near 50 %)

that perfectly separates the two samples. Three samples (two in one class and one in the other) in two dimensions can also be perfectly separated as long as the points are not on a straight line and the single point is not in between the other two from the other class.

Obviously, this data scenario can lead to class probability estimates that are poorly calibrated (as discussed in Sect. 11.3). Due to this inherent problem with LDA, as well as its other fundamental requirements, we recommend that LDA be used on data sets that have at least 5–10 times more samples than predictors. Caution should be applied to LDA results when the ratio dips below 5.

Finally, similar to logistic regression, any predictors used in an LDA model can be transformed and included in the model, like what we observed with the squared numeric value of day of the year in Fig. 12.3. In addition, the practitioner can create cross-product (i.e., interaction) terms among the predictors. Taking this approach is one way to enable LDA to find nonlinear discriminant boundaries. Transforms of or interactions among predictors should only be included, however, if there is good reason to believe that meaningful predictive information exists through these additional predictors. Including additional uninformative predictors will degrade the predictive ability of LDA and could prevent the covariance matrix from being invertible. If the practitioner suspects that nonlinear structure exists between predictors and the classification outcome but is not sure which predictors are involved in this relationship, then we recommend using methods presented in the next chapter.

12.4 Partial Least Squares Discriminant Analysis

As we have noted numerous times throughout the previous chapters, retrospectively or prospectively, measured predictors for any particular problem can be highly correlated or can exceed the number of samples collected. If either of these conditions is true, then the usual LDA approach cannot be directly used to find the optimal discriminant function.

Just like in the regression setting, we can attempt to pre-process our data in a way that removes highly correlated predictors. If more complex correlation structure exist in the data or if the number of predictors still exceeds the number of samples (or the ratio of samples to predictors is too low), then PCA can be used to reduce the predictor-space dimension. However, as previously discussed in Sect. 6.3, PCA may not identify the predictor combinations that optimally separate samples into groups. Recall that Fisher's LDA objective was to find the subspace that maximized the between-to-within group variability. Since PCA does not take into consideration any of the response classification information, we would not expect it to find the optimal subspace for classification. Instead of taking this stepwise approach (PCA-then-LDA) to the overdetermined problem, we recommend using PLS for the purpose of discrimination.

The application of PLS to a classification problem dates back to at least the mid 1980s (Berntsson and Wold 1986). As noted in the regression section, the original NIPALS algorithm was developed and refined in the chemometrics community. Not surprisingly, this community explored and extended the use of PLS to the classification setting and termed this technique PLS discriminant analysis (or PLSDA). Dunn and Wold (1990), for example, illustrated PLSDA on a chemometrics pattern recognition example and showed that it provided a better separation of the samples into groups than the traditional PCA-then-LDA approach.

To build intuition for why PLS would naturally extend to the classification setting, let's briefly return to PLS for regression. Recall that PLS finds latent variables that simultaneously reduce dimension and maximize correlation with a continuous response value (see Fig. 6.9). In the classification setting for a two-group problem, we could naïvely use the samples' class value (represented by 0's and 1's) as the response for this model. Given what we know about PLS for regression, we would then expect that the latent variables would be selected to reduce dimension while optimizing correlation with the categorical response vector. Of course, optimizing correlation isn't the natural objective if classification is the goal—rather, minimizing misclassification error or some other objective related to classification would seem like a better approach. Despite this fact, PLSDA should do better since the group information is being considered while trying to reduce the dimension of the predictor space.

Even though a correlation criterion is being used by PLS for dimension reduction with respect to the response, it turns out that this criterion happens to be doing the right thing. Before getting to the reason why that is true, we first must discuss a practical matter: coding of the response. For a two-group problem, the classes are encoded into a set of 0/1 dummy variables. With C classes, the results would be a set of C dummy variables where each sample has a one in the column representing the corresponding class.[8] As a result, the response in the data is represented by a matrix of dummy variables. Because of this, the problem cannot be solved by the PLS regression approach displayed in Fig. 6.9 and must move to the paradigm for a multivariate response.

Applying PLS in the classification setting with a multivariate response has strong mathematical connections to both canonical correlation analysis and LDA [see Barker and Rayens (2003) for technical details]. Assuming the above coding structure for the outcome, Barker and Rayens (2003) showed that the PLS directions in this context were the eigenvectors of a slightly perturbed between-groups covariance matrix (i.e. **B** from LDA).[9] PLS is, therefore, seeking to find optimal group separation while being guided by between-groups information. In contrast, PCA seeks to reduce dimension using the total variation as directed by the overall covariance matrix of the predictors.

This research provides a clear rationale for choosing PLS over PCA when dimension reduction is required when attempting classification. However, Liu

---

[8] Mathematically, if we know $C - 1$ of the dummy variables, then the value of the last dummy variable is directly implied. Hence, it is also possible to only use $C - 1$ dummy variables.

[9] The perturbed covariance structure is due to the optimality constraints for the response matrix. Barker and Rayens (2003) astutely recognized that the response optimality constraint in this setting did not make sense, removed the constraint, and resolved the problem. Without the response-space constraint, the PLS solution is one that involves exactly the between-group covariance matrix.

Table 12.5: The 2008 holdout set confusion matrix for the PLS model

	Observed class	
	Successful	Unsuccessful
Successful	490	220
Unsuccessful	80	767

This model had an overall accuracy of 80.7 %, a sensitivity of 86 %, and a specificity of 77.7 %. The reduced set of predictors were used to generate this matrix

and Rayens (2007) point out that if dimension reduction is *not* necessary and classification is the goal, then LDA will always provide a lower misclassification rate than PLS. Hence, LDA still has a necessary place in the classification toolbox.

Exactly like PLS for regression, there is one tuning parameter: the number of latent variables to be retained. When performing LDA on the grant data, the reduced set of predictors described on page 278 was used (which eliminated near zero variance predictors and predictors that caused extreme collinearity) with the additional squared term for the day of the year. PLS, however, can produce a model under these conditions. Performance of PLS, as we will shortly see, is affected when including predictors that contain little or no predictive information. Running PLS on the full set of predictors produces an optimal model with an area under the curve ROC of 0.87 based on six components (see Fig. 12.12), a sensitivity of 83.7 %, and a specificity of 77 %. These ROC results are slightly worse than the LDA model, so should we be surprised by this? After all, we included *more* predictors. Actually, including predictors that contain very little or no information about the response degrades the performance of a PLS model. For more details on this phenomenon, see Sect. 19.1.

If PLS performs worse than LDA using a larger set of predictors, then the next logical step would be to examine PLS performance using the reduced set of predictors (also used by LDA).[10] We know from the work of Liu and Rayens (2007) that LDA should outperform PLS in terms of minimizing misclassification errors. For this problem we have chosen to optimize ROC. Using this criterion will LDA still outperform PLS? The optimal number of PLS components with the reduced set of predictors is 4, with a corresponding ROC of 0.89 (Fig. 12.12) and confusion matrix presented in Table 12.5. The smaller set of predictors improves the ROC, uses fewer components to get to that value, and attains a value that is equivalent to the LDA model's performance.

---

[10] As a reminder, the set of predictors is not being selected on the basis of their association with the outcome. This *unsupervised* selection should not produce *selection bias*, which is an issue described in Sect. 19.5.

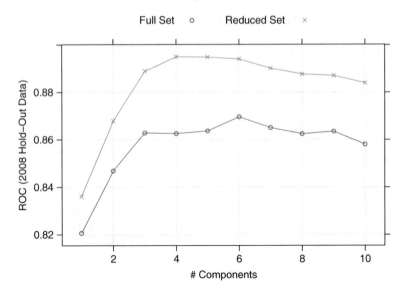

Fig. 12.12: ROC values by component for PLS for the grant data using two sets of predictors. The ROC curve has a maximum area with six components when using all predictors. When using the reduced subset of predictors, the ROC curve has a maximum area with four components

Recall that PLSDA encodes the response as a set of 0/1 dummy variables. Since PLS is a linear model, the predictions for the PLSDA model are not constrained to lie between 0 and 1. The final class is determined by the class with the largest model prediction. However, the raw model predictions require post-processing if class probabilities are required. The *softmax* approach previously described in Sect. 11.1 can be used for this purpose. However, our experience with this technique is that it does not produce meaningful class probabilities—the probabilities are not usually close to 0 or 1 for the most confident predictions. An alternative approach is to use *Bayes' Rule* to convert the original model output into class probabilities (Fig. 12.13). This tends to yield more meaningful class probabilities. One advantage of using Bayes' Rule is that the *prior* probability can be specified. This can be important when the data include one or more rare classes. In this situation, the training set may be artificially balanced and the specification of the prior probability can be used to generate more accurate probabilities. Figure 12.14 shows the class probabilities for the year 2008 grants.[11] While there is overlap between

---

[11] Recall that the models are built on the pre-2008 data and then tuned based on the year 2008 holdout set. These predictions are from the PLSDA model with four components created using only the pre-2008 data.

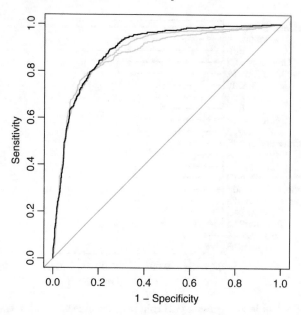

Fig. 12.13: The ROC curve for the 2008 holdout data using PLS (*black*). The AUC is 0.89. The ROC curve for LDA and logistic regression are overlaid (*grey*) for comparison. All three methods perform similarly

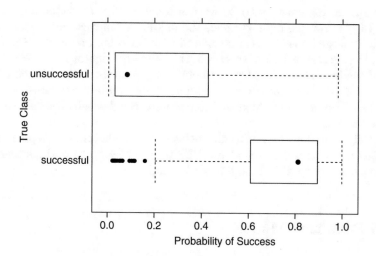

Fig. 12.14: Box plots for the PLSDA class probabilities of the 2008 holdout set calculated using Bayes' Rule

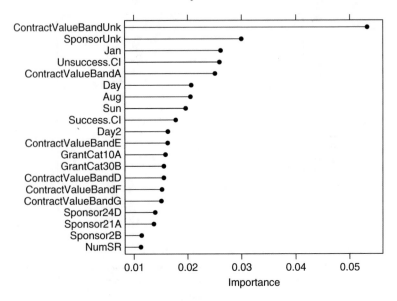

Fig. 12.15: Partial least squares variable importance scores for the grant data

the classes, the distributions are properly shifted; probabilities tend to be higher for the truly successful grants and low for the unsuccessful grants.

As in the regression setting, we can identify PLS predictor importance (Fig. 12.15). For the data at hand, the unknown contract value band has a relatively large importance as compared with the other predictors. Similar to LDA, the success or lack of success of the chief investigator float towards the top of the importance list. Other important predictors to the PLS classification model are contract values, a number of other grant categories, and the months of January and August. Interestingly, Sunday falls towards the top of the list also.

Finally, if nonlinear relationships between the predictors and response exist and the practitioner desires to use PLS to find these relationships then the approaches presented in Sect. 6.3 can be employed.

12.5 Penalized Models

Similar to the regularization methods discussed in Sect. 6.4, many classification models utilize penalties (or regularization) to improve the fit to the data, such as the lasso. In later sections, penalties for inherently nonlinear models, such as support vector machines and neural networks, are discussed.

For example, one might include a penalty term for the logistic regression model in a manner that is very similar to ridge regression. Recall that logistic regression finds parameter values that maximizes the binomial likelihood function, $L(p)$ (see Eq. 12.1). A simple approach to regularizing this model would be to add a squared penalty function to the log likelihood and find parameter estimates that maximize

$$\log L(p) - \lambda \sum_{j=1}^{P} \beta_j^2.$$

Eilers et al. (2001) and Park and Hastie (2008) discuss this model in the context of data where there are a large number of predictors and a small training set sample. In these situations, the penalty term can stabilize the logistic regression model coefficients.[12] As with ridge regression, adding a penalty can also provide a countermeasure against highly correlated predictors.

Recall that another method for regularizing linear regression models is to add a penalty based on the absolute values of the regression coefficients (similar to the lasso model of Sect. 6.4). The glmnet model (Friedman et al. 2010) uses a lasso-like penalty on the binomial (or multinomial) likelihood function. Like the lasso, this results in regression coefficients with values of absolute 0, thus simultaneously accomplishing regularization and feature selection at the same time. The glmnet models uses ridge and lasso penalties simultaneously, like the elastic net, but structures the penalty slightly differently:

$$\log L(p) - \lambda \left[(1-\alpha)\frac{1}{2} \sum_{j=1}^{P} \beta_j^2 + \alpha \sum_{j=1}^{P} |\beta_j| \right].$$

Here, the α value is the "mixing proportion" that toggles between the pure lasso penalty (when $\alpha = 1$) and a pure ridge-regression-like penalty ($\alpha = 0$). The other tuning parameter λ controls the total amount of penalization.

For the grant data, the glmnet model was tuned over seven values of the mixing parameter α and 40 values of the overall amount of penalization. The full set of predictors was used in the model. Figure 12.16 shows a heat map of the area under the ROC curve for these models. The data favor models with a larger mix of the ridge penalty than the lasso penalty, although there are many choices in this grid that are comparable. The bottom row of the heat map indicates that a complete ridge solution is poor regardless of the magnitude of the penalty. In the end, the numerically optimal settings are a mixing percentage of 0.1 and a value of 0.19 for the regularization amount. These settings had the effect of using only 44 predictors out of 1,070 in the final glmnet model, which achieved an area under the ROC curve of

---

[12] Another method for adding this penalty is discussed in the next chapter using neural networks . In this case, a neural network with weight decay and a single hidden unit constitutes a penalized logistic regression model. However, neural networks do not necessarily use the binomial likelihood when determining parameter estimates (see Sect. 13.2).

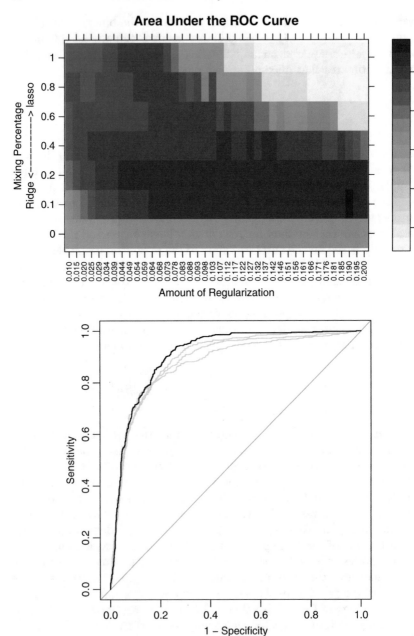

Fig. 12.16: *Top*: A heat map of the area under the ROC curve for the two glmnet tuning parameters. The numerically optimal settings are a mixing percentage of 0.1 and a value of 0.19 for the regularization amount. *Bottom*: The ROC curve for 2008 holdout data using glmnet the model (area under the ROC curve: 0.91)

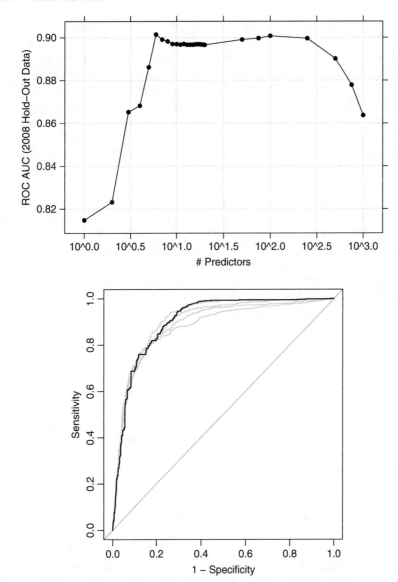

Fig. 12.17: *Top*: The tuning parameter profile for the sparse LDA model *Bottom*: The ROC curve for the model (AUC = 0.901)

0.91. The previous logistic regression model which used the reduced set of predictors resulted in an AUC of 0.87, indicating that the methodical removal of noninformative predictors increased the effectiveness of the model. Other approaches to *supervised* feature selection are discussed in Chap. 19.

Alternatively, penalization strategies can be applied to LDA models. For example, Clemmensen et al. (2011) use this technique with LDA models using the *flexible discriminant analysis (FDA)* framework described in Sects. 13.1 and 13.3. In this model, an elastic-net strategy is used; L_1 penalties have the effect of eliminating predictors while an L_2 penalty shrinks the coefficients of the discriminant functions towards 0. Other approaches to penalizing LDA models are described by Witten and Tibshirani (2009) and Witten and Tibshirani (2011), which contain references to many earlier works. The same lasso penalty has also been applied to PLS discriminant models so that some of the PLS loadings are also eliminated (Chung and Keles 2010).

The penalized LDA model of Clemmensen et al. (2011) was applied to the grant data. The software for this model allows the user to specify the number of retained predictors as a tuning parameter (instead of the value of the L_1 penalty). The model was tuned over this parameter as well as the value of the L_2 penalty. Figure 12.17 shows the results for a single value of the ridge penalty (there was very little difference in performance across a range of values for this penalty). There is moderate performance when the number of predictors is close to the maximum. As the penalty increases and predictors are eliminated, performance improves and remains relatively constant until important factors are removed. At this point, performance falls dramatically. As a result of the tuning process, six predictors were used in the model which is competitive to other models (an AUC of 0.9).

12.6 Nearest Shrunken Centroids

The nearest-shrunken centroid model (also known as PAM, for predictive analysis for microarrays) is a linear classification model that is well suited for high-dimensional problems (Tibshirani et al. 2002, 2003; Guo et al. 2007). For each class, the centroid of the data is found by taking the average value of each predictor (per class) in the training set. The overall centroid is computed using the data from all of the classes.

If a predictor does not contain much information for a particular class, its centroid for that class is likely to be close to the overall centroid. Consider the three class data shown in the left panel of Fig. 12.18. This data set is the famous Fisher/Anderson iris data where four measurements of iris sepals and petals are used to classify flowers into one of three different iris species: setosa, versicolor, and virginica. In this plot, the data for the versicolor and virginica classes overlap but are well separated from the setosa irises. The centroids for the sepal width dimension are shown as grey symbols above the x-axis. The virginica centroid (for sepal width) is very close to the overall centroid, and the versicolor centroid is slightly closer to the overall centroid than the setosa flowers. This indicates that the sepal width predictor is most informative for distinguishing the setosa species from the other two. For sepal length (shown adjacent to the y-axis), the versicolor centroid is very close to the center of the data and the other two species are on the extremes.

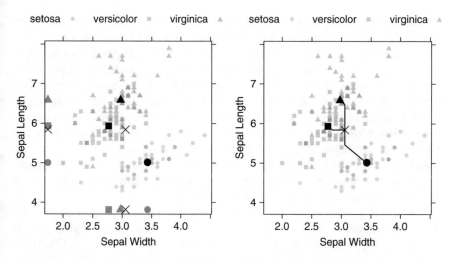

Fig. 12.18: *Left*: An example with three classes, their class-specific centroids (in *black*), and the overall centroid (×). The *grey symbols* along the axes are the centroids projected down into a single dimension. *Right*: The paths of the class centroids when shrunken to the center of the distributions

One approach to classifying unknown samples would be to find the closest class centroid in the full dimensional space and choose that class for prediction (i.e., a "nearest centroid" model). It turns out that this approach would result in linear class boundaries.

The approach taken by Tibshirani et al. (2002) is to shrink the class centroids closer to the overall centroid. In doing this, centroids that start off closer to the overall centroid move to that location before others. For example, in the sepal width dimension, the virginica centroid will reach the center before the other two. For this model, once the class centroid meets the overall centroid, it no longer influences the classification of samples for that class. Again, for sepal width, once the virginica centroid reaches the center, the sepal width can only be used to classify flowers that are versicolor or setosa. With enough shrinkage, it is possible for all the classes to be shrunken to the center. In the case that a predictor reaches the centroid, it has no effect on the model. Consequently, the nearest shrunken centroid model also conducts feature selection during the model training process.

The nearest shrunken centroid method has one tuning parameter: shrinkage. The right panel in Fig. 12.18 shows the path of the centroids over different shrinkage values. Note that each predictor moves diagonally towards the center until one of the class-specific centroids reaches the center. At this point, the classes move in a single dimension towards the center. Centering and scaling the predictors is recommended for this model.

This model works well for problems with a large number of predictors since it has built-in feature selection that is controlled by the shrinkage tuning parameter. Nearest shrunken centroids were originally developed for RNA profiling data, where the number of predictors is large (in the many thousands) and the number of samples is small. Most RNA profiling data sets have less than one or two hundred samples. In this *low n, high P* scenario, the data probably cannot support a highly nonlinear model and linear classification boundaries are a good choice. Also, the prior class probabilities along with the distances between the class centroids and the overall centroid can be used to produce class probabilities. Variable importance scores are calculated using the difference between the class centroids to the overall centroid (larger absolute values implying higher model importance).

For the grant data, the full set of 1,070 predictors was evaluated. The model was tuned over 30 values of the shrinkage parameter, ranging from 0 (implying very little shrinkage and feature selection) to 25 (Fig. 12.19). With large amounts of shrinkage, almost no predictors are retained and the area under the ROC curve is very poor. When the threshold is lowered to approximately 17, five predictors have been added: the number of unsuccessful grants by chief investigators, unknown sponsor, contract value band A, unknown contract value band, and submission month of January. The addition of these predictors clear has a large impact on the model fit. At the curve's apex (a shrinkage value of 2.59), important variables begin to be removed and under-fitting commences as the amount of shrinkage is increased. The sharp peak at a threshold of 8.6 is curious. The increase is associated with the removal of two predictors: sponsor code 2B and contract value band F. However, the next shrinkage value removes three additional predictors (contract value band D, contract value band E, and contract value band G) but this results in a appreciable drop in the area under the ROC curve. This spurious jump in performance is likely due to the fact that only a single holdout is used to measure performance. The true relationship between performance and shrinkage is likely to be more smooth than is demonstrated by this figure. At the best threshold, the area under the ROC curve was 0.87 using 36 predictors. The sensitivity was 83.7 % and the specificity was 77 % for the year 2008 holdout data. The ROC curve is also shown in Fig. 12.19.

12.7 Computing

This section discussed the following R packages: AppliedPredictiveModeling, caret, glmnet, MASS, pamr, pls, pROC, rms, sparseLDA, and subselect.

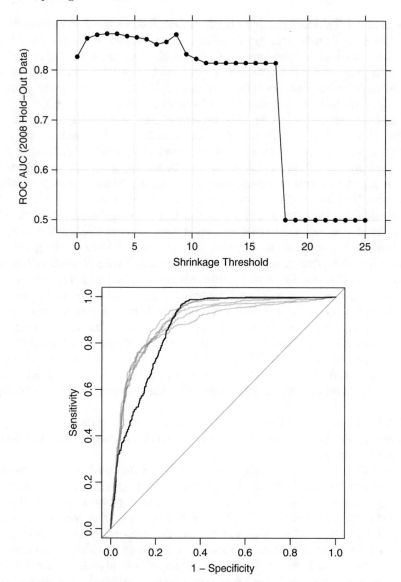

Fig. 12.19: *Top*: The tuning parameter profile for the nearest shrunken centroid model. *Bottom*: The ROC curve for the model (AUC = 0.873)

The grant application data can be found at the Kaggle web site.[13] The R package AppliedPredictiveModeling contains scripts that can be used to reproduce the objects and analyses given here.

---

[13] http://www.kaggle.com/c/unimelb.

Following the data splitting approach described in the first section, there are two data frames with grant data: `training` contains the pre-2008 data and 2008 holdout set used to tune the model while the data frame `testing` has only year 2008 grant data and is not used until a later chapter. A vector called `pre2008` has the row indices of the 6,633 training set grants prior to 2008 (see Table 12.2 for a summary of the data splitting strategy).

Most of the predictors in this set are binary. For example the RFCD codes, SEO codes, sponsors, and contract value band categories are contained in individual binary values with identifying prefixes, such as `RFCD` or `ContractValueBand`.[14] When the value was unknown, a specific dummy variable is created for this situation, such as `SponsorUnk`. Binary dummy variables also exist for the submission month and day of the week.

In addition, there exist count and continuous predictors such as the frequencies of each role associated with the grant. For example, `NumCI` and `NumEA` are the number of chief investigators and external advisors on the grant, respectively. The number of persons with unspecified roles is captured in the predictor `numUnk`. Similar count predictors are also in the data, such as the number of people born within a time frame (e.g., `CI.1925` for chief investigators born between 1925 and 1930), the number born in a certain region (e.g., `HV.Australia`), and their degree status (e.g., `ECI.PhD`). The number of previously successful and unsuccessful grants are enumerated with the predictors `Unsuccess.PS` or `Success.CI`. The publication information is represented in two ways. First, the totals for each role, such as `B.CI` or `Astar.CI`, are available as well as the total counts across all the individuals (`AstarTotal`) or all journal types (`allPub`).

The calendar day of the year is stored as a numeric variable.

Finally, the class outcome is contained in a column called `Class` with levels successful and unsuccessful.

As was illustrated in the regression sections of this book, different models have different constraints on the types of data that can be used. As previously discussed, two general groupings of predictors were created: the set of predictors that contain the full set of binary dummy variables and count data and the reduced set that was filtered for near-zero variance predictors and extremely correlated predictors. For example, the columns `AstarTotal`, `ATotal`, `BTotal`, and `CTotal` all add up to the column `allPub`. In the reduced set, `allPub` was removed. Similarly, one dummy variable for month and one for a day of the week should also be removed from the reduced set. The two columns with the lowest frequencies, `Mar` and `Sun`, were eliminated from the reduced set.

---

[14] In a later chapter, several models are discussed that can represent the categorical predictors in different ways. For example, trees can use the dummy variables in splits but can often create splits based on one or more groupings of categories. In that chapter, factor versions of these predictors are discussed at length.

Two character vectors were created for the purpose of specifying either group: `fullSet` and `reducedSet`:

```
> length(fullSet)
  [1] 1070
> head(fullSet)
  [1] "NumCI"  "NumDR"  "NumEA"  "NumECI" "NumHV"   "NumPS"


> length(reducedSet)
  [1] 252
> head(reducedSet)
  [1] "NumCI"  "NumDR"  "NumECI" "NumPS"  "NumSR"   "NumSCI"
```

How can extreme collinearity problems (such as linear combinations) be diagnosed? The `trim.matrix` function in **subselect** takes a square, symmetric matrix (such as the covariance matrix) and uses an algorithm to eliminate linear combinations. For example, the reduced set has no such issues:

```
> reducedCovMat <- cov(training[, reducedSet])
> library(subselect)
> trimmingResults <- trim.matrix(reducedCovMat)
> names(trimmingResults)
  [1] "trimmedmat"        "numbers.discarded" "names.discarded"
  [4] "size"
> ## See if any predictors were eliminated:
> trimmingResults$names.discarded

  character(0)
```

However, when we apply the same function to the full set, several predictors are identified:

```
> fullCovMat <- cov(training[, fullSet])
> fullSetResults <- trim.matrix(fullCovMat)


> ## A different choices for the day to exclude was
> ## made by this function
> fullSetResults$names.discarded

  [1] "NumDR"       "PS.1955"       "CI.Dept1798" "PS.Dept3268" "PS.Faculty1"
  [6] "DurationUnk" "ATotal"        "Nov"          "Sun"
```

Another function in the **caret** package called `findLinearCombos` follows a similar methodology but does not require a square matrix.

When developing models, `train` is used to tune parameters on the basis of the ROC curve. To do this, a control function is needed to obtain the results of interest. The **caret** function `trainControl` is used for this purpose. First, to compute the area under the ROC curve, the class probabilities must be generated. By default, `train` only generates class predictions. The option `classProbs` can be specified when probabilities are needed. Also by default, overall accuracy and the Kappa statistic are used to evaluate the model. caret contains a built-in function called twoClassSummary that calculates the area under the ROC curve, the sensitivity, and the specificity. To achieve these goals, the syntax would be:

```
> ctrl <- trainControl(summaryFunction = twoClassSummary,
+                         classProbs = TRUE)
```

However, at the start of the chapter, a data splitting scheme was developed that built the model on the pre-2008 data and then used the 2008 holdout data (in the training set) to tune the model. To do this, train must know exactly which samples to use when estimating parameters. The index argument to trainControl identifies these samples. For any resampling method, a set of holdout samples can be exactly specified. For example, with 10-fold cross-validation, the exact samples to be excluded for each of the 10-folds are identified with this option. In this case, index identifies the rows that correspond to the pre-2008 data. The exact syntax should package these row numbers in a list (in case there is more than one holdout). Recall that the vector pre2008 contains the locations of the grants submitted prior to 2008. The call to trainControl is:

```
ctrl <- trainControl(method = "LGOCV",
                     summaryFunction = twoClassSummary,
                     classProbs = TRUE,
                     index = list(TrainSet = pre2008))
```

Note that, once the tuning parameters have been chosen using year 2008 performance estimates, the final model is fit with all the grants in the training set, including those from 2008.

Finally, for illustrative purposes, we need to save the predictions of the year 2008 grants based on the pre-2008 model (i.e., before the final model is re-fit with all of the training data). The savePredictions argument accomplishes this goal:

```
ctrl <- trainControl(method = "LGOCV",
                     summaryFunction = twoClassSummary,
                     classProbs = TRUE,
                     index = list(TrainSet = pre2008),
                     savePredictions = TRUE)
```

Since many of the models described in this text use random numbers, the seed for the random number generator is set prior to running each model so that the computations can be reproduced. A seed value of 476 was randomly chosen for this chapter.

Logistic Regression

The glm function (for GLMs) in base R is commonly used to fit logistic regression models. The syntax is similar to previous modeling functions that work from the formula method. For example, to fit the model shown in the left panel of Fig. 12.3 for the pre-2008 data:

```
> levels(training$Class)
  [1] "successful"   "unsuccessful"
> modelFit <- glm(Class ~ Day,
+                      ## Select the rows for the pre-2008 data:
+                      data = training[pre2008,],
+                      ## 'family' relates to the distribution of the data.
+                      ## A value of 'binomial' is used for logistic regression
+                      family = binomial)
> modelFit
  Call:  glm(formula = Class ~ Day, family = binomial, data = training[pre2008,
    ])

  Coefficients:
  (Intercept)          Day
    -0.91934      0.00424

  Degrees of Freedom: 6632 Total (i.e. Null);  6631 Residual
  Null Deviance:              9190
  Residual Deviance: 8920          AIC: 8920
```

The glm function treats the *second* factor level as the event of interest. Since the slope is positive for the day of the year, it indicates an increase in the rate of unsuccessful grants. To get the probability of a successful grant, we subtract from one:

```
> successProb <- 1 - predict(modelFit,
+                           ## Predict for several days
+                           newdata = data.frame(Day = c(10, 150, 300,
+                                                        350)),
+                           ## glm does not predict the class, but can
+                           ## produce the probability of the event
+                           type = "response")
> successProb
        1       2       3       4
  0.70619 0.57043 0.41287 0.36262
```

To add the nonlinear term for the day of the year, the previous formula is augmented as follows:

```
> daySquaredModel <- glm(Class ~ Day + I(Day^2),
+                        data = training[pre2008,],
+                        family = binomial)
> daySquaredModel
  Call:  glm(formula = Class ~ Day + I(Day^2), family = binomial,
    data = training[pre2008,
    ])

  Coefficients:
  (Intercept)          Day       I(Day^2)
    -1.881341     0.018622     -0.000038
```

```
Degrees of Freedom: 6632 Total (i.e. Null);  6630 Residual
Null Deviance:             9190
Residual Deviance: 8720            AIC: 8730
```

The glm function does not have a non-formula method, so creating models with a large number of predictors takes a little more work. An alternate solution is shown below.

Another R function for logistic model is in the package associated with Harrell (2001), called rms (for Regression Modeling Strategies). The lrm function is very similar to glm and includes helper functions. For example, a *restricted cubic spline* is a tool for fitting flexible nonlinear functions of a predictor. For the day of the year:

```
> library(rms)
> rcsFit <- lrm(Class ~ rcs(Day), data = training[pre2008,])
> rcsFit

Logistic Regression Model

lrm(formula = Class ~ rcs(Day), data = training[pre2008, ])
```

		Model Likelihood Ratio Test		Discrimination Indexes		Rank Discrim. Indexes	
Obs	6633	LR chi2	461.53	R2	0.090	C	0.614
successful	3233	d.f.	4	g	0.538	Dxy	0.229
unsuccessful	3400	Pr(> chi2)	<0.0001	gr	1.713	gamma	0.242
max |deriv|	2e-06			gp	0.122	tau-a	0.114
				Brier	0.234		

	Coef	S.E.	Wald Z	Pr(>|Z|)
Intercept	-1.6833	0.1110	-15.16	<0.0001
Day	0.0124	0.0013	9.24	<0.0001
Day'	-0.0072	0.0023	-3.17	0.0015
Day''	0.0193	0.0367	0.52	0.6001
Day'''	-0.0888	0.1026	-0.87	0.3866

The lrm function, like glm, models the probability of the second factor level. The bottom table in the output shows p-values for the different nonlinear components of the restricted cubic spline. Since the p-values for the first three nonlinear components are small, this indicates that a nonlinear relationship between the class and day should be used. The package contains another function, Predict, which quickly create a prediction profile across one or more variables. For example, the code

```
> dayProfile <- Predict(rcsFit,
+                           ## Specify the range of the plot variable
+                           Day = 0:365,
+                           ## Flip the prediction to get the model for
+                           ## successful grants
+                           fun = function(x) -x)
> plot(dayProfile, ylab = "Log Odds")
```

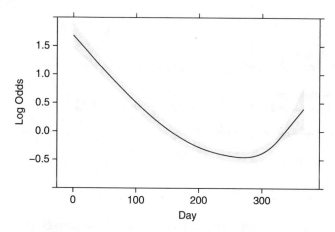

Fig. 12.20: A restricted cubic spline fit for the day of the year produce generated by the rms package. The *grey bands* are confidence limits on the log odds

produces the image in Fig. 12.20. The fun argument changes the signs of the prediction so that the plot reflects the probability of a successful grant. From this plot, it is apparent that a quadratic term for the day of the year would approximate the trends shown by the spline.

The rms package contains many more relevant functions, including resampling techniques for model validation and model visualization functions. See Harrell (2001) for details of the methodologies and R code.

For a large set of predictors, the formula method for specifying models can be cumbersome. As in previous chapters, the train function can efficiently fit and validate models. For logistic regression, train provides an interface to the glm function that bypasses a model formula, directly produces class predictions, and calculates the area under the ROC curve and other metrics.

Prior to fitting the model, we augment the data set and predictor groups with the squared day variable:

```
> training$Day2 <- training$Day^2
> fullSet <- c(fullSet, "Day2")
> reducedSet <- c(reducedSet, "Day2")
```

For the grant data, the code that fits a model with the full predictor set is:

```
> library(caret)
> set.seed(476)
> lrFull <- train(training[,fullSet],
+                 y = training$Class,
+                 method = "glm",
+                 metric = "ROC",
+                 trControl = ctrl)
```

```
> lrFull

  8190 samples
  1071 predictors
     2 classes: 'successful', 'unsuccessful'

  No pre-processing
  Resampling: Repeated Train/Test Splits (1 reps, 0.75%)

  Summary of sample sizes: 6633

  Resampling results

    ROC   Sens  Spec
    0.78  0.77  0.76
```

Note that the top of this output reflects that 8,190 grants were used, but the "Summary of sample sizes" lists a value of 6,633 data points. This latter number reflects the single set of pre-2008 samples (see Table 12.2). The "Resampling Results" is actually the performance estimate of the 2008 holdout set.

To create a model with the smaller predictor set:

```
> set.seed(476)
> lrReduced <- train(training[,reducedSet],
+                    y = training$Class,
+                    method = "glm",
+                    metric = "ROC",
+                    trControl = ctrl)


> lrReduced

  8190 samples
   253 predictors
     2 classes: 'successful', 'unsuccessful'

  No pre-processing
  Resampling: Repeated Train/Test Splits (1 reps, 0.75%)

  Summary of sample sizes: 6633

  Resampling results

    ROC   Sens  Spec
    0.87  0.8   0.82
```

Like the LDA analysis, removal of the near-zero variance predictors has a positive effect on the model fit. The predictions for the holdout set (of year 2008 grants) is contained in the sub-object pred:

```
> head(lrReduced$pred)
          pred        obs successful unsuccessful rowIndex .parameter
6634 successful successful    0.99878    0.0012238     6634       none
6635 successful successful    0.85151    0.1484924     6635       none
6636 successful successful    0.92019    0.0798068     6636       none
6637 successful successful    0.96694    0.0330572     6637       none
6639 successful successful    0.98928    0.0107160     6638       none
6642 successful successful    0.57563    0.4243729     6639       none
          Resample
6634 TrainSet
6635 TrainSet
6636 TrainSet
6637 TrainSet
6639 TrainSet
6642 TrainSet
```

Note the column in the output labeled .parameter. When train saves predictions, it does so for every tuning parameter. This column in the output is used to label which model generated the predictions. This version of logistic regression has no tuning parameters, so .parameter has a single value ("none").

From these data, the confusion matrix can be computed:

```
> confusionMatrix(data = lrReduced$pred$pred,
+                 reference = lrReduced$pred$obs)
Confusion Matrix and Statistics

              Reference
Prediction    successful unsuccessful
  successful         458          176
  unsuccessful       112          811

               Accuracy : 0.815
                 95% CI : (0.795, 0.834)
    No Information Rate : 0.634
    P-Value [Acc > NIR] : < 2e-16

                  Kappa : 0.611
 Mcnemar's Test P-Value : 0.000205

            Sensitivity : 0.804
            Specificity : 0.822
         Pos Pred Value : 0.722
         Neg Pred Value : 0.879
             Prevalence : 0.366
         Detection Rate : 0.294
   Detection Prevalence : 0.407

       'Positive' Class : successful
```

These results match the values shown above for lrReduced. The ROC curve can also be computed and plotted using the **pROC** package:

```
> reducedRoc <- roc(response = lrReduced$pred$obs,
+                    predictor = lrReduced$pred$successful,
+                    levels = rev(levels(lrReduced$pred$obs)))
> plot(reducedRoc, legacy.axes = TRUE)

> auc(reducedRoc)
  Area under the curve: 0.872
```

Linear Discriminant Analysis

A popular function for creating LDA models is lda in the **MASS** package. The input to this function can either be a formula and data frame or a matrix of predictors and a grouping variable as a factor which contains the class membership information. We can fit the LDA model as follows:

```
> library(MASS)
> ## First, center and scale the data
> grantPreProcess <- preProcess(training[pre2008, reducedSet])
> grantPreProcess

  Call:
  preProcess.default(x = training[pre2008, reducedSet])

  Created from 6,633 samples and 253 variables
  Pre-processing: centered, scaled
> scaledPre2008 <- predict(grantPreProcess,
+                          newdata = training[pre2008, reducedSet])
> scaled2008HoldOut <- predict(grantPreProcess,
+                              newdata = training[-pre2008, reducedSet])

> ldaModel <- lda(x = scaledPre2008,
+                 grouping = training$Class[pre2008])
```

Recall that because these data involve two classes, only one discriminant vector can be obtained. This discriminant vector is contained in the object ldaModel$scaling; the first six entries of this matrix are:

```
> head(ldaModel$scaling)

              LD1
  NumCI    0.1301673
  NumDR    0.0017275
  NumECI   0.1219478
  NumPS    0.0042669
  NumSR   -0.0642209
  NumSCI  -0.0655663
```

This information provides an interpretation about the predictors, relationships among predictors, and, if the data have been centered and scaled, then relative importance values. The discriminant vector is involved in the prediction of samples, and the MASS package simplifies this process through the predict function. For the grant data test set, the predictions are produced with the syntax:

```
> ldaHoldOutPredictions <- predict(ldaModel, scaled2008HoldOut)
```

The predicted class, posterior probability, and linear discriminant value are all contained in this object, thus enabling the user to create (1) a confusion matrix of the observed versus predicted values, (2) the distribution of posterior probabilities, and/or (3) the distribution of linear discriminant values.

A direct implication of the two-class setting is that there is no training over the number of discriminant vectors to retain for prediction. When working with data that contain more than two classes, the optimal number of linear discriminant vectors can be determined through the usual validation process. Through the lda function, the number of linear discriminants to retain for prediction can be set with the dimen option of the predict function. Conveniently, this optimization process is automated with the train function in the caret package:

```
> set.seed(476)
> ldaFit1 <- train(x = training[, reducedSet],
+                  y = training$Class,
+                  method = "lda",
+                  preProc = c("center","scale"),
+                  metric = "ROC",
+                  ## Defined above
+                  trControl = ctrl)

> ldaFit1

  8190 samples
   253 predictors
     2 classes: 'successful', 'unsuccessful'

Pre-processing: centered, scaled
Resampling: Repeated Train/Test Splits (1 reps, 0.75%)

Summary of sample sizes: 6633

Resampling results

  ROC   Sens  Spec
  0.89  0.8   0.82
```

No formal tuning occurs because there are only two classes and thus only one discriminant vector. We can generate predicted classes and probabilities for the test set in the usual manner:

```
> ldaTestClasses <- predict(ldaFit1,
+                           newdata = testing[,reducedSet])
> ldaTestProbs <- predict(ldaFit1,
+                         newdata = testing[,reducedSet],
+                         type = "prob")
```

When the problem involves more than two classes and we desire to optimize over the number of discriminant vectors, then the train function can still be used with method set to "lda2" and tuneLength set to the maximum number of dimensions that the practitioner desires to evaluate.

Partial Least Squares Discriminant Analysis

PLSDA can be performed using the plsr function within the pls package by using a categorical matrix which defines the response categories. We refer the reader to Sect. 6.3 for a description of the algorithmic variations of PLS, which directly extend to the classification setting.

The caret package contains a function (plsda) that can create the appropriate dummy variable PLS model for the data and then post-process the raw model predictions to return class probabilities. The syntax is very similar to the regression model code for PLS given in Sect. 6.3. The main difference is a factor variable is used for the outcome.

For example, to fit the model with the reduced predictor set:

```
> plsdaModel <- plsda(x = training[pre2008,reducedSet],
+                     y = training[pre2008, "Class"],
+                     ## The data should be on the same scale for PLS. The
+                     ## 'scale' option applies this pre-processing step
+                     scale = TRUE,
+                     ## Use Bayes method to compute the probabilities
+                     probMethod = "Bayes",
+                     ## Specify the number of components to model
+                     ncomp = 4)
> ## Predict the 2008 hold-out set
> plsPred <- predict(plsdaModel,
+                    newdata = training[-pre2008, reducedSet])
> head(plsPred)
  [1] successful successful successful successful successful successful
  Levels: successful unsuccessful
> plsProbs <- predict(plsdaModel,
+                     newdata = training[-pre2008, reducedSet],
+                     type = "prob")
> head(plsProbs)
  [1] 0.98842 0.88724 0.83455 0.88144 0.94848 0.53991
```

The plsdaModel object inherits all of the same functions that would have resulted from the object coming directly from the plsr function. Because of this, other functions from the pls package can be used, such as loadings or scoreplot.

The `train` function can also be used with PLS in the classification setting. The following code evaluates the first ten PLS components with respect to the area under the ROC curve as well as automatically centers and scales the predictors prior to model fitting and sample prediction:

```
> set.seed(476)
> plsFit2 <- train(x = training[, reducedSet],
+                  y = training$Class,
+                  method = "pls",
+                  tuneGrid = expand.grid(.ncomp = 1:10),
+                  preProc = c("center","scale"),
+                  metric = "ROC",
+                  trControl = ctrl)
```

The basic `predict` call evaluates new samples, and `type = "prob"` returns the class probabilities. Computing variable importance as illustrated in Fig. 12.15 can be done with the following code:

```
> plsImpGrant <- varImp(plsFit2, scale = FALSE)
> plsImpGrant

pls variable importance

  only 20 most important variables shown (out of 253)

                     Overall
ContractValueBandUnk  0.0662
SponsorUnk            0.0383
Jan                   0.0338
Unsuccess.CI          0.0329
ContractValueBandA    0.0316
Day                   0.0266
Aug                   0.0257
Success.CI            0.0219
GrantCat10A           0.0211
Day2                  0.0209
GrantCat30B           0.0202
ContractValueBandE    0.0199
ContractValueBandD    0.0193
ContractValueBandF    0.0188
ContractValueBandG    0.0184
Sponsor24D            0.0172
Sponsor21A            0.0169
Sponsor2B             0.0147
NumSR                 0.0144
Jul                   0.0124
> plot(plsImpGrant, top = 20, scales = list(y = list(cex = .95)))
```

Penalized Models

The primary package for penalized logistic regression is glmnet (although the next chapter describes how to fit similar models using neural networks). The glmnet function is very similar to the enet function described previously in Sect. 6.5. The main arguments correspond to the data: x is a *matrix* of predictors and y is a factor of classes (for logistic regression). Additionally, the family argument is related to the distribution of the outcome. For two classes, using family="binomial" corresponds to logistic regression, and, when there are three or more classes, family="multinomial" is appropriate.

The function will automatically select a sequence of values for the amount of regularization, although the user can select their own values with the lambda option. Recall that the type of regularization is determined by the mixing parameter α. glmnet defaults this parameter to alpha = 1, corresponding to a complete lasso penalty.

The predict function for glmnet predicts different types of values, including: the predicted class, which predictors are used in the model, and/or the regression parameter estimates. For example:

```
> library(glmnet)
> glmnetModel <- glmnet(x = as.matrix(training[,fullSet]),
+                       y = training$Class,
+                       family = "binomial")


> ## Compute predictions for three difference levels of regularization.
> ## Note that the results are not factors
> predict(glmnetModel,
+         newx = as.matrix(training[1:5,fullSet]),
+         s = c(0.05, 0.1, 0.2),
+         type = "class")
      1              2              3
1 "successful"   "successful"   "unsuccessful"
2 "successful"   "successful"   "unsuccessful"
3 "successful"   "successful"   "unsuccessful"
4 "successful"   "successful"   "unsuccessful"
5 "successful"   "successful"   "unsuccessful"
> ## Which predictors were used in the model?
> predict(glmnetModel,
+         newx = as.matrix(training[1:5,fullSet]),
+         s = c(0.05, 0.1, 0.2),
+         type = "nonzero")
$`1`
[1]    71    72   973 1027 1040 1045 1055

$`2`
[1] 1027 1040

$`3`
[1] 1040
```

As a side note, the glmnet package has a function named auc. If the pROC package is loaded prior to loading glmnet, this message will appear: "The following object(s) are masked from 'package:pROC': auc." If this function is invoked at this point, R will be unclear on which to use. There are two different approaches to dealing with this issue:

- If one of the packages is no longer needed, it can be detached using detach(package:pROC).
- The appropriate function can be called using the *namespace* convention when invoking the function. For example, pROC:::auc and glmnet:::auc would reference the specific functions.

Another potential instance of this issue is described below.

Tuning the model using the area under the ROC curve can be accomplished with train. For the grant data:

```
> ## Specify the tuning values:
> glmnGrid <- expand.grid(.alpha = c(0,   .1,   .2, .4, .6, .8, 1),
+                         .lambda = seq(.01, .2, length = 40))
> set.seed(476)
> glmnTuned <- train(training[,fullSet],
+                    y = training$Class,
+                    method = "glmnet",
+                    tuneGrid = glmnGrid,
+                    preProc = c("center", "scale"),
+                    metric = "ROC",
+                    trControl = ctrl)
```

The heat map in the top panel of Fig. 12.16 was produced using the code plot(glmnTuned, plotType = "level"). Penalized LDA functions can be found in the sparseLDA and PenalizedLDA packages. The main function in the sparseLDA package is called sda.[15] This function has an argument for the ridge parameter called lambda. The lasso penalty can be stated in two possible ways with the argument stop. The magnitude of the lasso penalty is controlled using a positive number (e.g., stop = 0.01) or, alternatively, the number of retained predictors can be chosen using a *negative* integer (e.g., stop = -6 for six predictors). For example:

```
> library(sparseLDA)
> sparseLdaModel <- sda(x = as.matrix(training[,fullSet]),
+                       y = training$Class,
+                       lambda = 0.01,
+                       stop = -6)
```

The argument method = "sparseLDA" can be used with train. In this case, train will tune the model over lambda and the number of retained predictors.

---

[15] Another duplicate naming issue may occur here. A function called sda in the sda package (for shrinkage discriminant analysis) may cause confusion. If both packages are loaded, using sparseLDA:::sda and sda:::sda will mitigate the issue.

Nearest Shrunken Centroids

The original R implementation for this model is found in the **pamr** package (for "*P*redictive *A*nalysis of *M*icroarrays in R"). Another package, rda, contains extensions to the model described in Guo et al. (2007).

The syntax of the functions in the **pamr** package is somewhat nonstandard. The function to train the model is pamr.train, which takes the input data in a single list object with components x and y. The usual convention for data sets is to have samples in rows and different columns for the predictors. pamr.train requires the training set predictors to be encoded in the opposite format where rows are predictors and columns are samples.[16] For the grant data, the input data would be in the format shown below:

```
> ## Switch dimensions using the t() function to transpose the data.
> ## This also implicitly converts the training data frame to a matrix.
> inputData <- list(x = t(training[, fullSet]), y = training$Class)
```

The basic syntax to create the model is:

```
> library(pamr)
> nscModel <- pamr.train(data = inputData)
```

By default, the function chooses 30 appropriate shrinkage values to evaluate. There are options to use specific values for the shrinkage amount, the prior probabilities and other aspects of the model. The function pamr.predict generates predictions on new samples as well as determines which specific predictors were used in the model for a given shrinkage value. For example, to specify a shrinkage value of 5:

```
> exampleData <- t(training[1:5, fullSet])
> pamr.predict(nscModel, newx = exampleData, threshold = 5)
   [1] successful   unsuccessful successful   unsuccessful successful
   Levels: successful unsuccessful
> ## Which predictors were used at this threshold? The predict
> ## function shows the column numbers for the retained predictors.
> thresh17Vars <- pamr.predict(nscModel, newx = exampleData,
+                                 threshold = 17, type = "nonzero")
> fullSet[thresh17Vars]
   [1] "Unsuccess.CI"        "SponsorUnk"           "ContractValueBandA"
   [4] "ContractValueBandUnk" "Jan"
```

The package also contains functions for *K*-fold cross-validation to choose an appropriate amount of shrinkage but is restricted to a single type of resampling and tunes the model with overall accuracy. The train syntax is:

---

[16] In microarray data, the number of predictors is usually much larger than the number of samples. Because of this, and the limited number of columns in popular spreadsheet software, the convention is reversed.

```
>  ## We chose the specific range of tuning parameters here:
> nscGrid <- data.frame(.threshold = 0:25)
> set.seed(476)
> nscTuned <- train(x = training[,fullSet],
+                   y = training$Class,
+                   method = "pam",
+                   preProc = c("center", "scale"),
+                   tuneGrid = nscGrid,
+                   metric = "ROC",
+                   trControl = ctrl)
```

This approach provides more options for model tuning (e.g., using the area under the ROC curve) as well as a consistent syntax. The `predict` function for `train` does not require the user to manually specify the shrinkage amount (the optimal value determined by the function is automatically used).

The `predictors` function will list the predictors used in the prediction equation (at the optimal threshold determined by `train`). In the tuned model, 36 were selected:

```
> predictors(nscTuned)
 [1] "NumSR"               "Success.CI"             "Unsuccess.CI"
 [4] "CI.Faculty13"        "CI.Faculty25"           "CI.Faculty58"
 [7] "DurationGT15"        "Astar.CI"               "AstarTotal"
[10] "allPub"              "Sponsor21A"             "Sponsor24D"
[13] "Sponsor2B"           "Sponsor34B"             "Sponsor4D"
[16] "Sponsor62B"          "Sponsor6B"              "Sponsor89A"
[19] "SponsorUnk"          "ContractValueBandA"     "ContractValueBandC"
[22] "ContractValueBandD"  "ContractValueBandE"     "ContractValueBandF"
[25] "ContractValueBandG"  "ContractValueBandUnk"   "GrantCat10A"
[28] "GrantCat30B"         "Aug"                    "Dec"
[31] "Jan"                 "Jul"                    "Fri"
[34] "Sun"                 "Day"                    "Day2"
```

Also, the function `varImp` will return the variable importance based on the distance between the class centroid and the overall centroid:

```
> varImp(nscTuned, scale = FALSE)

pam variable importance

   only 20 most important variables shown (out of 1071)

                      Importance
ContractValueBandUnk    -0.2260
SponsorUnk               0.1061
Jan                      0.0979
ContractValueBandA       0.0948
Unsuccess.CI            -0.0787
Day                     -0.0691
Aug                     -0.0669
Sun                      0.0660
GrantCat10A             -0.0501
Success.CI               0.0413
```

```
Day2                     -0.0397
ContractValueBandE        0.0380
GrantCat30B              -0.0379
ContractValueBandD        0.0344
Sponsor21A                0.0340
ContractValueBandF        0.0333
ContractValueBandG        0.0329
Sponsor24D               -0.0299
Sponsor2B                -0.0233
NumSR                     0.0224
```

In these data, the sign of the difference indicates the direction of the impact of the predictor. For example, when the contractor band is unknown, only a small percentage of grants are successful (19.4 % versus the baseline success rate of 46.4 %). The negative sign for this predictor indicates a drop in the event rate. Conversely, when the sponsor is unknown, the success rate is high (82.2 %; see Table 12.1). The distance for this predictor is positive, indicating an increase in the event rate.

Exercises

12.1. The hepatic injury data set was described in the introductory chapter and contains 281 unique compounds, each of which has been classified as causing no liver damage, mild damage, or severe damage (Fig. 1.2). These compounds were analyzed with 184 biological screens (i.e., experiments) to assess each compound's effect on a particular biologically relevant target in the body. The larger the value of each of these predictors, the higher the activity of the compound. In addition to biological screens, 192 chemical fingerprint predictors were determined for these compounds. Each of these predictors represent a substructure (i.e., an atom or combination of atoms within the compound) and are either counts of the number of substructures or an indicator of presence or absence of the particular substructure. The objective of this data set is to build a predictive model for hepatic injury so that other compounds can be screened for the likelihood of causing hepatic injury. Start R and use these commands to load the data:

```
> library(caret)
> data(AppliedPredictiveModeling)
> # use ?hepatic to see more details
```

The matrices `bio` and `chem` contain the biological assay and chemical fingerprint predictors for the 281 compounds, while the vector `injury` contains the liver damage classification for each compound.

(a) Given the classification imbalance in hepatic injury status, describe how you would create a training and testing set.

(b) Which classification statistic would you choose to optimize for this exercise and why?

(c) Split the data into a training and a testing set, pre-process the data, and build models described in this chapter for the biological predictors and separately for the chemical fingerprint predictors. Which model has the best predictive ability for the biological predictors and what is the optimal performance? Which model has the best predictive ability for the chemical predictors and what is the optimal performance? Based on these results, which set of predictors contains the most information about hepatic toxicity?

(d) For the optimal models for both the biological and chemical predictors, what are the top five important predictors?

(e) Now combine the biological and chemical fingerprint predictors into one predictor set. Retrain the same set of predictive models you built from part (c). Which model yields best predictive performance? Is the model performance better than either of the best models from part (c)? What are the top five important predictors for the optimal model? How do these compare with the optimal predictors from each individual predictor set?

(f) Which model (either model of individual biology or chemical fingerprints or the combined predictor model), if any, would you recommend using to predict compounds' hepatic toxicity? Explain.

12.2. In Exercise 4.4, we described a data set which contained 96 oil samples each from one of seven types of oils (pumpkin, sunflower, peanut, olive, soybean, rapeseed, and corn). Gas chromatography was performed on each sample and the percentage of each type of 7 fatty acids was determined. We would like to use these data to build a model that predicts the type of oil based on a sample's fatty acid percentages.

(a) Like the hepatic injury data, these data suffer from extreme imbalance. Given this imbalance, should the data be split into training and test sets?

(b) Which classification statistic would you choose to optimize for this exercise and why?

(c) Of the models presented in this chapter, which performs best on these data? Which oil type does the model most accurately predict? Least accurately predict?

12.3. The web site[17] for the MLC++ software package contains a number of machine learning data sets. The "churn" data set was developed to predict telecom customer churn based on information about their account. The data files state that the data are "artificial based on claims similar to real world."

The data consist of 19 predictors related to the customer account, such as the number of customer service calls, the area code, and the number of minutes. The outcome is whether the customer churned.

---

[17] http://www.sgi.com/tech/mlc.

The data are contained in the C50 package and can be loaded using:

```
> library(C50)
> data(churn)
> ## Two objects are loaded: churnTrain and churnTest
> str(churnTrain)
> table(churnTrain$Class)
```

(a) Explore the data by visualizing the relationship between the predictors and the outcome. Are there important features of the predictor data themselves, such as between-predictor correlations or degenerate distributions? Can functions of more than one predictor be used to model the data more effectively?

(b) Fit some basic models to the training set and tune them via resampling. What criteria should be used to evaluate the effectiveness of the models?

(c) Use lift charts to compare models. If you wanted to identify 80% of the churning customers, how many other customers would also be identified?

Chapter 13
Nonlinear Classification Models

The previous chapter described models that were intrinsically linear—the structure of the model would produce linear class boundaries unless nonlinear functions of the predictors were manually specified. This chapter deals with some intrinsically nonlinear models. As in the regression sections, there are other nonlinear models that use trees or rules for modeling the data. These are discussed in the next chapter.

With a few exceptions (such as FDA models, Sect. 13.3), the techniques described in this chapter can be adversely affected when a large number of non-informative predictors are used as inputs. As such, combining these models with feature selection tools (described in Chap. 19) can significantly increase performance. The analyses shown in this chapter are conducted without supervised removal of non-informative predictors, so performance is likely to be less than what could be achieved with a more comprehensive approach.

13.1 Nonlinear Discriminant Analysis

We saw in the previous chapter that the linear boundaries of linear discriminant analysis came about by making some very specific assumptions for the underlying distributions of the predictors. In this section, we will explore ways that linear discriminant methods as described in the previous chapter are modified in order to handle data that are best separated by nonlinear structures. These methods include quadratic discriminant analysis (QDA), regularized discriminant analysis (RDA), and mixture discriminant analysis (MDA).

M. Kuhn and K. Johnson, *Applied Predictive Modeling*,
DOI 10.1007/978-1-4614-6849-3_13,
© Springer Science+Business Media New York 2013

Quadratic and Regularized Discriminant Analysis

Recall that linear discriminant analysis could be formulated such that the trained model minimized the total probability of misclassification. The consequence of the assumption that the predictors in each class shared a common covariance structure was that the class boundaries were linear functions of the predictors.

In quadratic discriminant models, this assumption is relaxed so that a class-specific covariance structure can be accommodated. The primary repercussion of this change is that the decision boundaries now become quadratically curvilinear in the predictor space. The increased discriminant function complexity may improve model performance for many problems. However, another repercussion of this generalization is that the data requirements become more stringent. Since class-specific covariance matrices are utilized, the inverse of the matrices must exist. This means that the number of predictors must be less than the number of cases within each class. Also, the predictors within each class must not have pathological levels of collinearity. Additionally, if the majority of the predictors in the data are indicators for discrete categories, QDA will only to able to model these as linear functions, thus limiting the effectiveness of the model.

In pure mathematical optimization terms, LDA and QDA each minimize the total probability of misclassification assuming that the data can truly be separated by hyperplanes or quadratic surfaces. Reality may be, however, that the data are best separated by structures somewhere between linear and quadratic class boundaries. RDA, proposed by Friedman (1989), is one way to bridge the separating surfaces between LDA and QDA. In this approach, Friedman advocated the following covariance matrix:

$$\widetilde{\Sigma}_\ell(\lambda) = \lambda\Sigma_\ell + (1 - \lambda)\Sigma, \tag{13.1}$$

where Σ_ℓ is the covariance matrix of the ℓth class and Σ is the pooled covariance matrix across all classes. It is easy to see that the tuning parameter, λ, enables the method to flex the covariance matrix between LDA (when $\lambda = 0$) and QDA (when $\lambda = 1$). If a model is tuned over λ, a data-driven approach can be used to choose between linear or quadratic boundaries as well as boundaries that fall between the two.

RDA makes another generalization of the data: the pooled covariance matrix can be allowed to morph from its observed value to one where the predictors are assumed to be independent (as represented by an identity matrix):

$$\Sigma(\gamma) = \gamma\Sigma + (1 - \gamma)\sigma^2\mathbf{I}, \tag{13.2}$$

where σ^2 is the common variance of all predictors and $\mathbf{I}$ is the identity matrix (i.e., the diagonal entries of the matrix are 1 and all other entries are 0), which forces the model to assume that all of the predictors are independent. Recall the familiar two-class example with two predictors, last seen in Chap. 4

(p. 69). There is a high correlation between these predictors indicating that γ values near 1 are most likely to be appropriate. However, in higher dimensions, it becomes increasingly more difficult to visually recognize such patterns, so tuning an RDA model over λ and γ enables the training set data to decide the most appropriate assumptions for the model. Note, however, that unless γ is one or λ is zero, the more stringent data standards of QDA must be applied.

Mixture Discriminant Analysis

MDA was developed by Hastie and Tibshirani (1996) as an extension of LDA. LDA assumes a distribution of the predictor data such that the class-specific means are different (but the covariance structure is independent of the classes). MDA generalizes LDA in a different manner; it allows each class to be represented by *multiple* multivariate normal distributions. These distributions can have different means but, like LDA, the covariance structures are assumed to be the same. Figure 13.1 presents this idea with a single predictor. Here, each class is represented by three normal distributions with different means and common variances. These are effectively sub-classes of the data. The modeler would specify how many different distributions should be used and the MDA model would determine their optimal locations in the predictor space.

How are the distributions aggregated so that a class prediction can be calculated? In the context of Bayes' Rule (Eq. 12.4), MDA modifies $Pr[X|Y = C_\ell]$. The class-specific distributions are combined into a single multivariate normal distribution by creating a per-class mixture. Suppose $D_{\ell k}(x)$ is the discriminant function for the kth subclass in the ℓth class, the overall discriminant function for the ℓth class would be proportional to

$$D_\ell(x) \propto \sum_{k=1}^{L_\ell} \phi_{\ell k} D_{\ell k}(x),$$

where L_ℓ is the number of distributions being used for the ℓth class and the $\phi_{\ell k}$ are the mixing proportions that are estimated during training. This overall discriminant function can then produce class probabilities and predictions.

For this model, the number of distributions per class is the tuning parameter for the model (they need not be equal per class). Hastie and Tibshirani (1996) describe algorithms for determining starting values for the class-specific means required for each distribution, along with numerical optimization routines to solve the nontrivial equations. Also, similar to LDA, Clemmensen et al. (2011) describe using ridge- and lasso-like penalties to MDA, which would integrate feature selection into the MDA model.

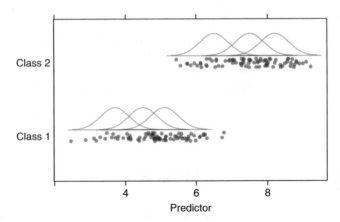

Fig. 13.1: For a single predictor, three distinct subclasses are determined within each class using mixture discriminant analysis

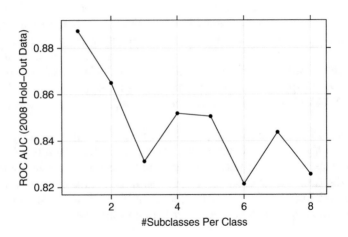

Fig. 13.2: The tuning parameter profile for the MDA model for the grants data. The optimal number of subclasses is 1, which is identical to performing LDA

For the grant data, MDA was tuned over the number of subclasses per group with possible values ranging from 1 to 8 (Fig. 13.2). The areas under the ROC curve was optimized using one subclass per group, which is the same as performing LDA. MDA may be adverse to more complex discriminant boundaries in these data due to the large number of binary predictors.

13.2 Neural Networks

As we have seen with other classification methods, such as partial least squares discriminant analysis, the C classes can be encoded into C binary columns of dummy variables and then used as the outcomes for the model. Although the previous discussion on neural networks for regression used a single response, the model can easily handle multiple outputs for both regression and classification. For neural network classification, this is the approach discussed here.

Figure 13.3 shows a diagram of the model architecture for classification. Instead of a single output (as in Fig. 7.1 for regression), the bottom layer has multiple nodes for each class. Note that, unlike neural networks for regression, an additional nonlinear transformation is used on the combination of hidden units. Each class is predicted by a linear combination of the hidden units that have been transformed to be between zero and one (usually by a sigmoidal function). However, even though the predictions are between zero and one (due the extra sigmoidal function), they aren't "probability-like" since they do not add up to one. The *softmax* transformation described in Sect. 11.1 is used here to ensure that the outputs of the neural network comply with this extra constraint:

$$f_{i\ell}^*(x) = \frac{e^{f_{i\ell}(x)}}{\sum_l e^{f_{il}(x)}},$$

where $f_{i\ell}(x)$ is the model prediction of the ℓth class and the ith sample.

What should the neural network optimize to find appropriate parameter estimates? For regression, the sum of the squared errors was the focus and, for this case, it would be altered to handle multiple outputs by accumulating the errors across samples *and* the classes:

$$\sum_{\ell=1}^{C} \sum_{i=1}^{n} (y_{i\ell} - f_{i\ell}^*(x))^2,$$

where $y_{i\ell}$ is the 0/1 indicator for class ℓ. For classification, this can be effective method for determining parameter values. The class with the largest predicted value would be used to classify the sample.

Alternatively, parameter estimates can be found that can maximize the likelihood of the Bernoulli distribution, which corresponds to a binomial likelihood function (Eq. 12.1) with a sample size of $n = 1$:

$$\sum_{\ell=1}^{C} \sum_{i=1}^{n} y_{i\ell} \ln f_{i\ell}^*(x). \tag{13.3}$$

This function also goes by then names *entropy* or *cross-entropy*, which is used in some of the tree-based models discussed in the next chapter (Sect. 14). The likelihood has more theoretical validity than the squared error approach,

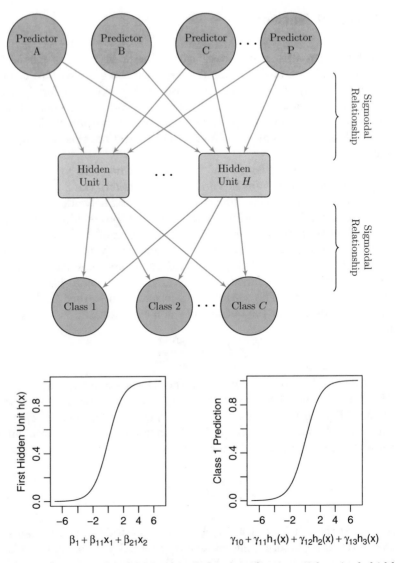

Fig. 13.3: A diagram of a neural network for classification with a single hidden layer. The hidden units are linear combinations of the predictors that have been transformed by a sigmoidal function. The output is also modeled by a sigmoidal function

although studies have shown that differences in performance tend to be negligible (Kline and Berardi 2005). However, Bishop (1995) suggests that the entropy function should more accurately estimate small probabilities than those generated by the squared-error function.

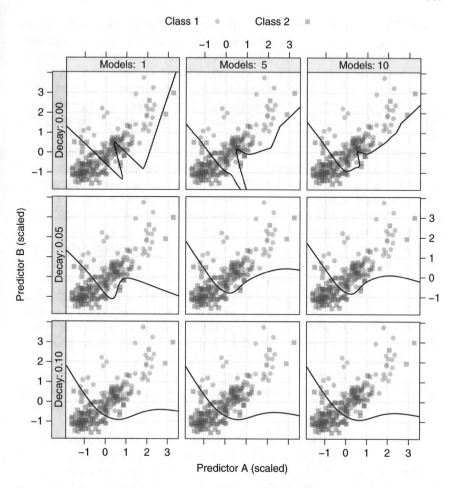

Fig. 13.4: Classification boundaries for neural networks with varying levels of smoothing and regularization. As weight decay and number of models increase, the boundaries become smoother

Like their regression counterparts, neural networks for classification have a significant potential for over-fitting. When optimizing the sums of squares error or entropy, weight decay attenuates the size of the parameter estimates. This can lead to much smoother classification boundaries. Also, as previously discussed, model averaging helps reduce over-fitting. In this case, the class probability estimates $(f_{i\ell}^*(x))$ would be averaged across networks and these average values would be used to classify samples.

Figure 13.4 shows examples of models fit with different amounts of weight decay and model averaging. Each model was initiated with the same random seed, used three hidden units, and was optimized for the sums of squared errors. The first row of models without weight decay shows significant over-fitting, and, in these cases, model averaging has a marginal impact. The small amount of decay shown in the second row shows an improvement (as does the model averaging) but is still over-adapting to the training data when a single network is used. The highest amount of weight decay showed the best results with virtually no impact of model averaging. For these data, a single model with weight decay is probably the best choice since it is computationally least expensive.

Many other aspects of neural network classification models mirror their regression counterparts. Increasing the number of predictors or hidden units will still give rise to a large number of parameters in the model and the same numerical routines, such as back-propagation, can be used to estimate these parameters. Collinearity and non-informative predictors will have a comparable impact on model performance.

Several types of neural networks were fit to the grant data. First, single network models (i.e., no model averaging) were fit using entropy to estimate the model coefficients. The models were tuned over the number of units in the hidden layer (ranging from 1 to 10), as well as the amount of weight decay ($\lambda = 0$, 0.1, 1, 2). The best model used eight hidden units with $\lambda = 2$ and had an area under the ROC curve of 0.884. The tuning parameter profiles show a significant amount of variation, with no clear trend across the tuning parameters.

To counter this variation, the same tuning process was repeated, but 10 networks were fit to the data and their results averaged. Here, the best model had six hidden units with $\lambda = 2$ and had an area under the ROC curve of 0.884.

To increase the effectiveness of the model, various transformations of the data were evaluated. One in particular, the spatial sign transformation, had a significant positive impact on the performance of the neural networks for these data. When combined with a single network model, the area under the curve was 0.903. When model averaging was used, the area under the ROC curve was 0.911.

Figure 13.5 visualizes the tuning parameter profiles across the various models. When no data transformations are used, model averaging increases the performance of the models across all of the tuning parameters. It also has the effect of smoothing out differences between the models; the profile curves are much closer together. When the spatial sign transformation is used with the single network model, it shows an improvement over the model without the transformation. However, performance appears to be optimized when using both model averaging and the spatial sign.

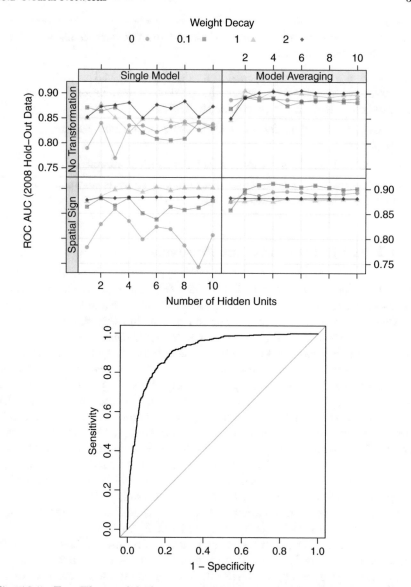

Fig. 13.5: *Top*: The models for grant success were tuned under four different conditions: with and without a transformation on the predictors and with and without model averaging. *Bottom*: The ROC curve for the 2008 holdout set when a model averaged network is used with the spatial sign transformation (area under the curve: 0.911)

---

1 Create a new response matrix of binary dummy variable columns for each of the C classes

2 Create a multivariate regression model using any method that generates slopes and intercepts for predictors or functions of the predictors (e.g. linear regression, MARS, etc)

3 Post-process the model parameters using the optimal scoring technique

4 Use the adjusted regression coefficients as discriminant values

---

Algorithm 13.1: The flexible discriminant analysis algorithm for generalizing LDA model (Hastie et al. 1994)

13.3 Flexible Discriminant Analysis

In the last chapter, the motivation for classical linear discriminant analysis was based on minimizing the total probability of misclassification. It turns out that the same model can be derived in a completely different manner. Hastie et al. (1994) describe a process where, for C classes, a set of C linear regression models can be fit to binary class indicators and show that the regression coefficients from these models can be post-processed to derive the discriminant coefficients (see Algorithm 13.1). This allows the idea of linear discriminant analysis to be extended in a number of ways. First, many of the models in Chaps. 6 and 7, such as the lasso, ridge regression, or MARS, can be extended to create discriminant variables. For example, MARS can be used to create a set of hinge functions that result in discriminant functions that are nonlinear combinations of the original predictors. As another example, the lasso can create discriminant functions with feature selection. This conceptual framework is referred to as *flexible discriminant analysis* (FDA).

We can illustrate the nonlinear nature of the flexible discriminant algorithm using MARS with the example data in Fig. 4.1 (p. 63). Recall that MARS has two tuning parameters: the number of retained terms and the degree of predictors involved in the hinge functions. If we use an additive model (i.e., a first-degree model), constrain the maximum number of retained terms to 2 and have a binary response of class membership, then discriminant function is

$$D(A, B) = 0.911 - 19.1 \times h(0.2295 - B)$$

In this equation, $h(\cdot)$ is the hinge function described in Eq. 7.1 on p. 146. If the discriminant function is greater than zero, the sample would be predicted to be the first class. In this model, the prediction equation only used the one variable, and the left-hand panel in Fig. 13.6 shows the resulting class boundaries. The class boundary is a horizontal line since predictor B is the only predictor in the split.

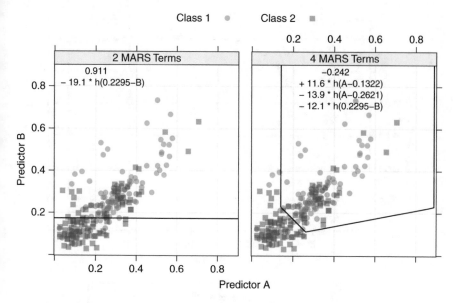

Fig. 13.6: Classification boundaries for two FDA models of different complexities

The effectiveness of FDA is not apparent when MARS is so severely restricted. If the maximum number of retained terms is relaxed to 4, then the discriminant equation is estimated to be

$$
\begin{aligned}
D(A, B) = -\,& 0.242 \\
+\,& 11.6 \times h(A - 0.1322) \\
-\,& 13.9 \times h(A - 0.2621) \\
-\,& 12.1 \times h(0.2295 - B).
\end{aligned}
$$

This FDA model uses both predictors and its class boundary is shown in the right-hand panel of Fig. 13.6. Recall that the MARS hinge function h sets one side of the breakpoint to zero. Because of this, the hinge functions isolate certain regions of the data. For example, if $A < 0.1322$ and $B > 0.2295$, none of the hinge functions affect the prediction and the negative intercept in the model indicates that all points in this region correspond to the second class. However, if $A > 0.2621$ and $B < 0.2295$, the prediction is a function of all three hinge functions. Essentially, the MARS features isolate multidimensional polytopal regions of the predictor space and predict a common class within these regions.

An FDA model was tuned and trained for the grant application model. First-degree MARS hinge functions were evaluated where the number of retained terms ranged from 2 to 25. Performance increases as the number of

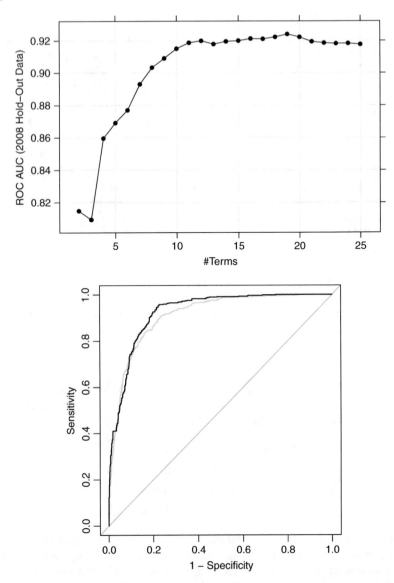

Fig. 13.7: *Top*: The parameter tuning profile for the FDA model. *Bottom*: The FDA ROC curve (area under the curve: 0.924) is shown in relation to the curve for the previous neural network model (in *grey*)

terms increases and plateaus around 15 terms (see Fig. 13.7). The numerically optimal value was 19 although there is clearly some flexibility in this parameter. For this model, the area under the ROC curve for the 2008 data was estimated to be 0.924, with a sensitivity of 82.5 % and a specificity of

86.4 %. Although the FDA model contained 19 terms, 14 unique predictors were used (of a possible 1,070). Also, nine of the model terms were simple linear functions of binary categorical predictors. The discriminant equation for the model is

$$
\begin{aligned}
D(x) = {} & 0.85 \\
& - 0.53 \times h(1 - \text{number of chief investigators}) \\
& + 0.11 \times h(\text{number of successful grants by chief investigators} - 1) \\
& - 1.1 \times h(1 - \text{number of successful grants by chief investigators}) \\
& - 0.23 \times h(\text{number of unsuccessful grants by chief investigators} - 1) \\
& + 1.4 \times h(1 - \text{number of unsuccessful grants by chief investigators}) \\
& + 0.18 \times h(\text{number of unsuccessful grants by chief investigators} - 4) \\
& - 0.035 \times h(8 - \text{number of A journal papers by all investigators}) \\
& - 0.79 \times \text{sponsor code 24D} \\
& - 1 \times \text{sponsor code 59C} \\
& - 0.98 \times \text{sponsor code 62B} \\
& - 1.4 \times \text{sponsor code 6B} \\
& + 1.2 \times \text{unknown sponsor} \\
& - 0.34 \times \text{contract value band B} \\
& - 1.5 \times \text{unknown contract value band} \\
& - 0.34 \times \text{grant category code 30B} \\
& + 0.3 \times \text{submission day of Saturday} \\
& + 0.022 \times h(54 - \text{numeric day of the year}) \\
& + 0.076 \times h(\text{numeric day of the year} - 338).
\end{aligned}
$$

From this equation, the exact effect of the predictors on the model can be elucidated. For example, as the number of chief investigators increases from zero to one, the probability of a successful grant increases. Having more than one chief investigator does not affect the model since the opposite hinge function was eliminated. Also, the probability of success increases with the number of successful grants by chief investigators and decreases with the number of unsuccessful grants by chief investigators; this is a similar result to what was found with previous models. For the day of the year, the probability of a successful grant decreases as the year proceeds and has no affect on the model until late in the year when the probability of success increases.

The discriminant function shown above can be additionally transformed to produce class probability estimates. Visually, the probability trends for the continuous predictors are shown in Fig. 13.8. Recall that since an additive model was used, the probability profile for each variable can be considered independently of the others. Here, the terms for the number of chief investigators and the number of publications in A-level journals only affect the prediction up to a point. This is the result of the pruning algorithm elimi-

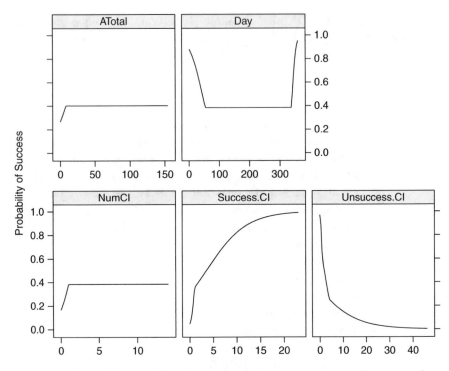

Fig. 13.8: Probability profiles for each of the continuous predictors used in the additive FDA model

nating one of each predictor's reflective pairs. The profile for the day of the year has two terms that remain from two different reflected pairs. As a result, this predictor only affects the model in the early and late periods of the year. In the last chapter, there was good evidence that this predictor had a nonlinear relationship with the outcome that was approximated by adding a quadratic function of the predictor. Here, FDA also tries to approximate the same relationship. One predictor, the number of unsuccessful grants by chief investigators, has multiple terms in the model, which is reflected in the smoother probability profile. Of the binary terms, the predictors for contract value band B, unknown contract value band, grant category code 30B, sponsor code 24D, sponsor code 59C, sponsor code 62B, and sponsor code 6B had a positive effect on the probability of success while the terms for submission day of Saturday and unknown sponsor were associated with a decrease in the success rate.

Bagging the model coerces FDA to produce smoother relationships between the predictors and the outcome. MARS models are moderately unstable predictors since they use exhaustive searches of the data and the splits are based on specific data points in the training set.[1] Bagging the FDA model will have the effect of adding more splits for the important predictors, leading to a better approximation. However, our experience is that bagging MARS or FDA models has a marginal impact on model performance and increased number of terms diminishes the interpretation of the discriminant equation (similar to the trend shown in Fig. 8.16).

Since many of the predictors in the FDA model are on different scales, it is difficult to use the discriminant function to uncover which variables have the most impact on the outcome. The same method of measuring variable importance described in Sect. 7.2 can be employed here. The five most important predictors are, in order: unknown contract value band, the number of unsuccessful grants by chief investigators, the number of successful grants by chief investigators, unknown sponsor, and numeric day of the year.

As an alternative to using MARS within the FDA framework, Milborrow (2012) describes a two-phase approach with logistic regression when there are two classes. Here, an initial MARS model is created to predict the binary dummy response variable (i.e., the first two steps in Algorithm 13.1). After this, a logistic regression model is created with the MARS features produced by the original dummy variable model. Our preliminary experiences with this approach are that it yields results very similar to the FDA model.

13.4 Support Vector Machines

Support vector machines are a class of statistical models first developed in the mid-1960s by Vladimir Vapnik. In later years, the model has evolved considerably into one of the most flexible and effective machine learning tools available, and Vapnik (2010) provides a comprehensive treatment. The regression version of these models was previously discussed in Sect. 7.3, which was an extension of the model from its original development in the classification setting. Here we touch on similar concepts from SVM for regression and layout the case for classification.

Consider the enviable problem shown in the left panel of Fig. 13.9 where two variables are used to predict two classes of samples that are completely separable. As shown on the left, there are a multitude (in fact an infinite) number of linear boundaries that perfectly classify these data. Given this, how would we choose an appropriate class boundary? Many performance measures, such as accuracy, are insufficient since all the curves would be deemed equivalent. What would a more appropriate metric be for judging the efficacy of a model?

Vapnik defined an alternate metric called the *margin*. Loosely speaking, the margin is the distance between the classification boundary and the closest

---

[1] However, MARS and FDA models tend to be more stable than tree-based models since they use linear regression to estimate the model parameters.

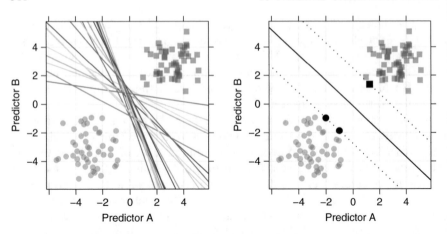

Fig. 13.9: *Left*: A data set with completely separable classes. An infinite number of linear class boundaries would produce zero errors. *Right*: The class boundary associated with the linear maximum margin classifier. The solid black points indicate the support vectors

training set point. For example, the right-hand panel of Fig. 13.9 shows one possible classification boundary as a solid line. The dashed lines on both sides of the boundary are at the maximum distance from the line to the closest training set data (equidistant from the boundary line). In this example the three data points are equally closest to the classification boundary and are highlighted with solid black symbols. The margin defined by these data points can be quantified and used to evaluate possible models. In SVM terminology, the slope and intercept of the boundary that maximize the buffer between the boundary and the data is known as the maximum margin classifier.

Let's explore a few of the mathematical constructs of SVM in the context of a simple example in order to better understand the inner workings of the method. Suppose we have a two-class problem and we code the class #1 samples with a value of 1 and the class #2 samples with -1. Also, let the vectors $\mathbf{x}_i$ contain the predictor data for a training set sample. The maximum margin classifier creates a decision value $D(\mathbf{x})$ that classifies samples such that if $D(\mathbf{x}) > 0$ we would predict a sample to be class #1, otherwise class #2. For an unknown sample $\mathbf{u}$, the decision equation can be written in a similar form as a linear discriminant function that is parameterized in terms of an intercept and slopes as

$$D(\mathbf{u}) = \beta_0 + \boldsymbol{\beta}'\mathbf{u}$$

$$= \beta_0 + \sum_{j=1}^{P} \beta_j u_j.$$

Notice that this equation works from the viewpoint of the predictors. This equation can be transformed so that the maximum margin classifier can be written in terms of each data point in the sample. This changes the equation to

$$D(\mathbf{u}) = \beta_0 + \sum_{j=1}^{P} \beta_j u_j$$

$$= \beta_0 + \sum_{i=1}^{n} y_i \alpha_i \mathbf{x}_i' \mathbf{u} \qquad (13.4)$$

with $\alpha_i \geq 0$ (similar to Eq. 7.2). It turns out that, in the completely separable case, the α parameters are exactly zero for all samples that are not on the margin. Conversely, the set of nonzero α values are the points that fall on the boundary of the margin (i.e., the solid black points in Fig. 13.9). Because of this, the predictor equation is a function of only a subset of the training set points and these are referred to as the *support vectors*. Interestingly, the prediction function is only a function of the training set samples that are closest to the boundary and are predicted with the least amount of certainty.[2] Since the prediction equation is *supported* solely by these data points, the maximum margin classifier is the usually called the *support vector machine*.

On first examination, Eq. 13.4 may appear somewhat arcane. However, it can shed some light on how support vector machines classify new samples. Consider Fig. 13.10 where a new sample, shown as a solid grey circle, is predicted by the model. The distances between each of the support vectors and the new sample are as grey dotted lines.

For these data, there are three support vectors, and therefore contain the only information necessary for classifying the new sample. The meat of Eq. 13.4 is the summation of the product of: the sign of the class, the model parameter, and the dot product between the new sample and the support vector predictor values. The following table shows the components of this sum, broken down for each of the three support vectors:

	True class	Dot product	y_i	α_i	Product
SV 1	Class 2	−2.4	−1	1.00	2.40
SV 2	Class 1	5.1	1	0.34	1.72
SV 3	Class 1	1.2	1	0.66	0.79

The dot product, $\mathbf{x}_i' \mathbf{u}$, can be written as a product of the distance of $\mathbf{x}_i$ from the origin, the distance of $\mathbf{u}$ from the origin, and the cosine of the angle between $\mathbf{x}_i$ and $\mathbf{u}$ (Dillon and Goldstein 1984).

---

[2] Recall a similar situation with support vector regression models where the prediction function was determined by the samples with the largest residuals.

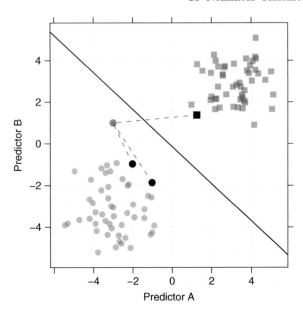

Fig. 13.10: Prediction of a new sample using a support vector machine. The final value of the decision equation is $D(u) = 0.583$. The grey lines indicate the distance of the new sample to the support vectors

Based on the parameter estimates α_i, the first support vector has the largest single effect on the prediction equation (all other things being equal) and it has a negative slope. For our new sample, the dot product is negative, so the total contribution of this point is positive and pushes the prediction towards the first class (i.e., a positive value of the decision function $D(u)$). The remaining two support vectors have positive dot products and an overall product that increases the decision function value for this sample. For this model, the intercept is -4.372; $D(u)$ for the new sample is therefore 0.583. Since this value is greater than zero, the new sample has the highest association with the first class.

What happens when the classes are not completely separable? Cortes and Vapnik (1995) develop extensions to the early maximum margin classifier to accommodate this situation. Their formulation puts a cost on the sum of the training set points that are on the boundary or on the wrong side of the boundary. When determining the estimates of the α values, the margin is penalized when data points are on the wrong side of the class boundary or inside the margin. The cost value would be a tuning parameter for the model and is the primary mechanism to control the complexity of the boundary. For example, as the cost of errors increases, the classification boundary will shift and contort itself so that it correctly classifies as many of the training set points as possible. Figure 4.2 in Chap. 4 demonstrated this; the panel on the right-hand side of this figure used an inappropriately high cost value, resulting in severe over-fitting.

Echoing the comments in Sect. 7.3, most of the regularization models discussed in this book add penalties to the coefficients, to prevent over-fitting. Large penalties, similar to costs, impose limits on the model complexity. For support vector machines, cost values are used to penalize number of *errors*; as a consequence, larger cost values induce higher model complexity rather than restrain it.

Thus far, we have considered linear classification boundaries for these models. In Eq. 13.4, note the dot product $\mathbf{x}'_i\mathbf{u}$. Since the predictors enter into this equation in a linear manner, the decision boundary is correspondingly linear. Boser et al. (1992) extended the linear nature of the model to nonlinear classification boundaries by substituting the kernel function instead of the simple linear cross product:

$$D(\mathbf{u}) = \beta_0 + \sum_{i=1}^{n} y_i\alpha_i\mathbf{x}'_i\mathbf{u}$$
$$= \beta_0 + \sum_{i=1}^{n} y_i\alpha_i K(\mathbf{x}_i, \mathbf{u}),$$

where $K(\cdot, \cdot)$ is a *kernel function* of the two vectors. For the linear case, the kernel function is the same inner product $\mathbf{x}'_i\mathbf{u}$. However, just as in regression SVMs, other nonlinear transformations can be applied, including:

$$\text{polynomial} = (scale\,(\mathbf{x}'\mathbf{u}) + 1)^{degree}$$
$$\text{radial basis function} = \exp(-\sigma\|\mathbf{x} - \mathbf{u}\|^2)$$
$$\text{hyperbolic tangent} = \tanh\,(scale\,(\mathbf{x}'\mathbf{u}) + 1)\,.$$

Note that, due to the dot product, the predictor data should be centered and scaled prior to fitting so that attributes whose values are large in magnitude do not dominate the calculations.

The *kernel trick* allows the SVM model produce extremely flexible decision boundaries. The choice of the kernel function parameters and the cost value control the complexity and should be tuned appropriately so that the model does not over-fit the training data. Figure 13.11 shows examples of the classification boundaries produced by several models using different combinations of the cost and tuning parameter values. When the cost value is low, the models clearly underfit the data. Conversely, when the cost is relatively high (say a value of 16), the model can over-fit the data, especially if the kernel parameter has a large value. Using resampling to find appropriate estimates of these parameters tends to find a reasonable balance between under- and over-fitting. Section 4.6 used the radial basis function support vector machine as an example for model tuning.

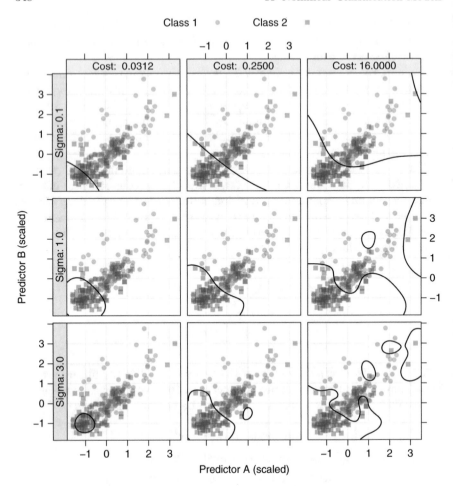

Fig. 13.11: Classification boundaries for nine radial basis function support vector machine models varied over the cost parameter and the kernel parameter (σ)

Support vector machines fall into a more general category of *kernel methods* and this has been an extremely active area of research for some time. Here, we have discussed extensions to the original model to allow for misclassified samples and nonlinear class boundaries. Still more extensions have been developed for support vector machines, such as handling more than two classes (Hsu and Lin 2002; Duan and Keerthi 2005). Also, the original motivation of the model is to create a hard decision boundary for the purpose of classifying samples, as opposed to estimating class probabilities. However, Platt (2000) describes methods of post-processing the output of the SVM model to estimate class probabilities. Alternate versions of the support vector machine model also exist, such as least squares support vector machines (Suykens and Vandewalle 1999), relevance vector machines (Tipping 2001), and import vector machines (Zhu and Hastie 2005).

Specialized kernels have also been developed. For example, the QSAR application discussed in Sect. 6.1 and used throughout the regression chapters used chemical descriptors as predictors. Figure 6.1 shows the chemical formula of aspirin. Rather than deriving descriptors from a molecular formula, the formula can be converted to a graph (or network) representation. A specialized class of kernel functions, called *graph kernels*, can directly relate the content of the chemical formula to the model without deriving descriptor variables (Mahé et al. 2005; Mahé and Vert 2009). Similarly, there are different kernels that can be employed in text mining problems. The "bag-of-words" approach summarizes a body of text by calculating frequencies of specific words. These counts are treated as predictor variables in classification models. There are a few issues with this approach. First, the additional computational burden of deriving the predictor variables can be taxing. Secondly, this term-based approach does not consider the ordering of the text. For example, the text "Miranda ate the bear" and "the bear ate Miranda" would score the same in the bag-of-words model but have very different meanings. *String kernels* (Lodhi et al. 2002; Cancedda et al. 2003) can use the entire text of a document directly and has more potential to find important relationships than the bag-of-words approach.

For the grant data, there are several approaches to using SVMs. We evaluated the radial basis function kernel as well as the polynomial kernel (configured to be either linear or quadratic). Also, both the full and reduced predictor sets were evaluated. As will be shown in Chap. 19, support vector machines can be negatively affected by including non-informative predictors in the model.

For the radial basis function kernel, the analytical approach for determining the radial basis function parameter was assessed. For the full set of predictors, the estimate was $\sigma = 0.000559$ and for the reduced set, the value was calculated to be $\sigma = 0.00226$. However, these models did not show good performance, so this parameter was varied over values that were smaller than analytical estimates. Figure 13.12 shows the results of these models. The smaller predictor set yields better results than the more comprehensive set, with an optimal area under the ROC curve of 0.895, a sensitivity of 84 %, and a specificity of 80.4 %. Also, for the reduced set, smaller values of σ produced better results, although values below 0.001167 did not improve the model fit.

For the polynomial models, a fair amount of trial and error was used to determine appropriate values for this kernel's scaling factor. Inappropriate values would result in numerical difficulties for the models and feasible values of this parameter depended on the polynomial degree and the cost parameter. Figure 13.13 shows the results for the holdout set. Models built with the reduced set of predictors did uniformly better than those utilizing the full set. Also, the optimal performance for linear and quadratic models was about

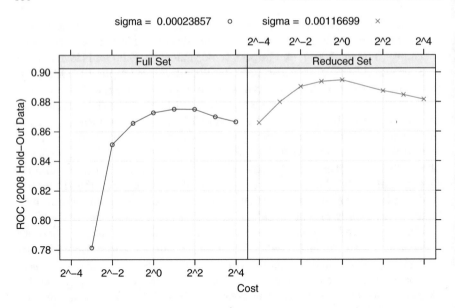

Fig. 13.12: Tuning parameter profile of the radial basis function SVM model for the grant data

the same. This suggests that the models are mostly picking up on linear relationships in the data. Given that many of the predictors are binary, this makes sense. Of these models, the best area under the ROC curve was 0.898.

Overall, the support vector machine models did not have competitive performance in comparison to models created thus far. Many of the linear models shown in Chap. 12 had similar (or better) performance; the FDA model in this chapter, so far, is more effective. However, in our experience, SVM models tend to be very competitive for most problems.

13.5 *K*-Nearest Neighbors

We first met the *K*-nearest neighbors (*K*NNs) model for classification in Sect. 4.2 when discussing model tuning and the problem of over-fitting. We have also learned extensively about *K*NN in the context of regression in Sect. 7.4. While many of the ideas from *K*NN for regression directly apply here, we will highlight the unique aspects of how this method applies to classification.

The classification methods discussed thus far search for linear or nonlinear boundaries that optimally separate the data. These boundaries are then used to predict the classification of new samples. *K*NN takes a different approach

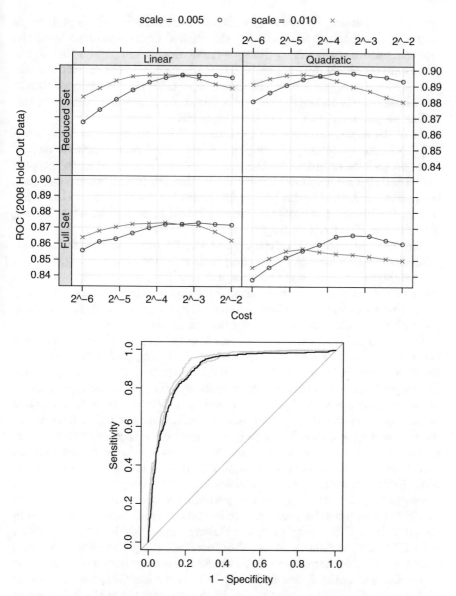

Fig. 13.13: *Top*: Performance profiles for the quadratic SVM model. *Bottom*: The ROC curve for the optimal model (area under the curve: 0.895)

by using a sample's geographic neighborhood to predict the sample's classification. Similar to the regression context, *K*NN for classification predicts a new sample using the *K*-closest samples from the training set. "Closeness" is determined by a distance metric, like Euclidean and Minkowski (Sect. 7.4), and choice of metric depends on predictor characteristics. For any distance metric, it is important to recall that the original measurement scales of the predictors affect the resulting distance calculations. This implies that if predictors are on widely different scales, the distance value between samples will be biased towards predictors with larger scales. To allow each predictor to contribute equally to the distance calculation, we recommend centering and scaling all predictors prior to performing KNN.

As in the regression context, to determine the classification of a new sample, the K-closest training set samples are determined via the distance metric. Class probability estimates for the new sample are calculated as the proportion of training set neighbors in each class. The new sample's predicted class is the class with the highest probability estimate; if two or more classes are tied for the highest estimate, then the tie is broken at random or by looking ahead to the $K + 1$ closest neighbor.

Any method with tuning parameters can be prone to over-fitting, and KNN is especially susceptible to this problem as was shown in Fig. 4.2. Too few neighbors leads to highly localized fitting (i.e., over-fitting), while too many neighbors leads to boundaries that may not locate necessary separating structure in the data. Therefore, we must take the usual cross-validation or resampling approach for determining the optimal value of K.

For the grant data the neighborhood range evaluated for tuning was between 1 and 451. Figure 13.14 illustrates the tuning profile for area under the ROC curve for the 2008 holdout data. There is a distinct jump in predictive performance from 1 to 5 neighbors and a continued steady increase in performance through the range of tuning. The initial jump in predictive performance indicates that local geographic information is highly informative for categorizing samples. The steady incremental increase in predictive performance furthermore implies that neighborhoods of informative information for categorizing samples are quite large. This pattern is somewhat unusual for KNN in that as the number of neighbors increases we begin to underfit and a corresponding decrease in predictive performance occurs like was illustrated by Fig. 7.10. In most data sets, we are unlikely to use this many neighbors in the prediction. This example helps to identify a numerical instability problem with KNN: as the number of neighbor increases, the probability of ties also increases. For this example, a neighborhood size greater than 451 leads to too many ties. The optimal area under the ROC curve was 0.81, which occurred at $K = 451$. The bottom plot in Fig. 13.14 compares the KNN ROC profile with those of SVM and FDA. For these data, the predictive ability of KNN is inferior to the other tuned nonlinear models. While geographic information is predictive, it is not as useful as models that seek to find global optimal separating boundaries.

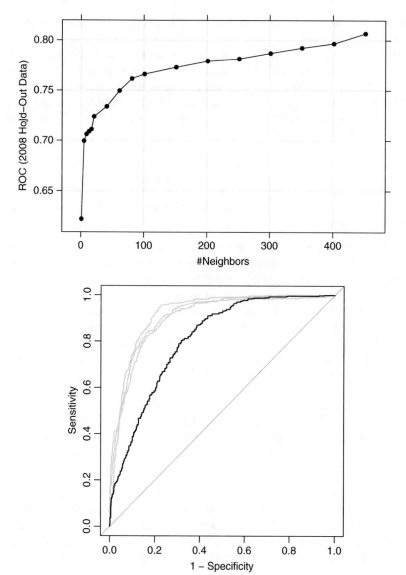

Fig. 13.14: *Top*: The parameter tuning profile for the *K*NN model. *Bottom*: The ROC curve for the test set data. The area under the curve was 0.81

13.6 Naïve Bayes

Bayes' Rule was previously discussed in the context of linear discriminant analysis in a previous chapter. This section expands on that discussion and focuses on a specific classification model that, like the previous LDA, QDA, and RDA models, is defined in terms of how the multivariate probability densities are created.

Bayes' Rule answers the question "based on the predictors that we have observed, what is the probability that the outcome is class C_ℓ?" More mathematically, let Y be the class variable and X represent the collection of predictor variables. We are trying to estimate $Pr[Y = C_\ell | X]$, which is "given X, what is the probability that the outcome is the ℓth class?" Bayes' Rule provides the machinery to answer this:

$$Pr[Y = C_\ell | X] = \frac{Pr[Y]Pr[X|Y = C_\ell]}{Pr[X]} \tag{13.5}$$

$Pr[Y = C_\ell | X]$ is typically referred to as the *posterior probability* of the class. The components are:

- $Pr[Y]$ is the *prior* probability of the outcome. Essentially, based on what we know about the problem, what would we expect the probability of the class to be? For example, when predicting customer churn, companies typically have a good idea of the overall turnover rate of customers. For problems related to diseases, this prior would be the disease prevalence rate in the population (see Sect. 11.2 on p. 254 for a discussion).
- $Pr[X]$ is the probability of the predictor values. For example, if a new sample is being predicted, how likely is this pattern in comparison to the training data? Formally, this probability is calculated using a multivariate probability distribution. In practice, significant assumptions are usually made to reduce the complexity of this calculation.
- $Pr[X|Y = C_\ell]$ is the *conditional probability*. For the data associated with class C_ℓ, what is the probability of observing the predictor values? Similar to $Pr[X]$, this can be a complex calculation unless strict assumptions are made.

The naïve Bayes model simplifies the probabilities of the predictor values by assuming that all of the predictors are independent of the others. This is an extremely strong assumption. For most of the case studies and illustrative examples in this text, it would be difficult to claim that this assumption were realistic. However, the assumption of independence yields a significant reduction in the complexity of the calculations.

For example, to calculate the conditional probability $Pr[X|Y = C_\ell]$, we would use a product of the probability densities for each individual predictor:

$$Pr[X|Y = C_\ell] = \prod_{j=1}^{P} Pr[X_j|Y = C_\ell]$$

The unconditional probability $Pr[X]$ results in a similar formula when assuming independence. To estimate the individual probabilities, an assumption of

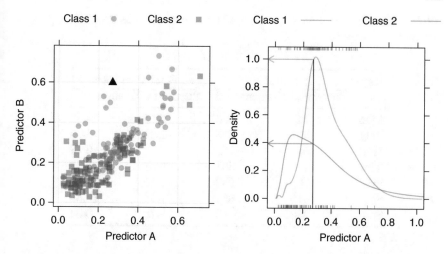

Fig. 13.15: *Left*: A plot of two class illustrative data where a new sample (the *solid triangle*) is being predicted. *Right*: Conditional density plots of predictor A created using a nonparametric density estimate. The value of predictor A for the new sample is shown by the *vertical black line*

normality might be made for continuous predictors (using the sample mean and variance from the training set). Other methods, such as nonparametric kernel density estimators (Hardle et al. 2004), can more flexibly estimate the probability densities. For categorical predictors, the probability distribution can be determined with the observed frequencies in the training set data.

For example, Fig. 13.15 shows the familiar two-class illustrative example. In the left panel, the training data are shown. Clearly, the two predictors are unlikely to be independent (their correlation is 0.78). Suppose a new sample (shown as a solid black triangle) requires prediction. To compute the overall conditional probability $Pr[X|Y = C_\ell]$, each predictor is considered separately. For predictor A, the two conditional densities are shown in the right panel of Fig. 13.15 with a vertical black line indicating the value of the new sample for this predictor. For the training set data, using this predictor alone, the first class appears to be much more likely.

To produce the class probability $Pr[X|Y = C_\ell]$ for the first class, two conditional probability values are determined for predictors A and B then multiplied together to calculate the overall conditional probability for the class.

For $Pr[X]$ a similar procedure would occur except the probabilities for predictors A and B would be determined from the entire training set (i.e., both classes). For the example in Fig. 13.15, the correlation between the predictors is fairly strong, which indicates that the new sample is highly unlikely.

Table 13.1: The frequencies and conditional probabilities $Pr[X|Y = C_\ell]$ for the day of the week

Day	Count		Percent of total	
	Successful	Unsuccessful	Successful	Unsuccessful
Mon	749	803	9.15	9.80
Tues	597	658	7.29	8.03
Wed	588	752	7.18	9.18
Thurs	416	358	5.08	4.37
Fri	606	952	7.40	11.62
Sat	619	861	7.56	10.51
Sun	228	3	2.78	0.04

However, using the assumption of independence, this probability is likely to be overestimated.

The prior probability allows the modeler to *tilt* the final probability towards one or more classes. For example, when modeling a rare event, it is common to selectively sample the data so that the class distribution in the training set is more balanced. However, the modeler may wish to specify that the event is indeed rare by assigning it a low prior probability. If no prior is explicitly given, the convention is to use the observed proportions from the training set to estimate the prior.

Given such a severe and unrealistic assumption, why would one consider this model? First, the naïve Bayes model can be computed quickly, even for large training sets. For example, when the predictors are all categorical, simple lookup tables with the training set frequency distributions are all that are required. Secondly, despite such a strong assumption, the model performs competitively in many cases.

Bayes' Rule is essentially a probability statement. Class probabilities are created and the predicted class is the one associated with the largest class probability. The meat of the model is the determination of the conditional and unconditional probabilities associated with the predictors. For continuous predictors, one might choose simple distributional assumptions, such as normality. The nonparametric densities (such as those shown in Fig. 13.16) can produce more flexible probability estimates. For the grant application data, the predictor for the numeric day of the year has several time frames where an inordinate number of grants were submitted. In this figure, the black curve for the normal distribution is extremely broad and does not capture the nuances of the data. The red curve is the nonparametric estimate and appears produce the trends in the data with higher fidelity.

For categorical predictors, the frequency distribution of the predictor in the training set is used to estimate $Pr[X]$ and $Pr[X|Y = C_\ell]$. Table 13.1

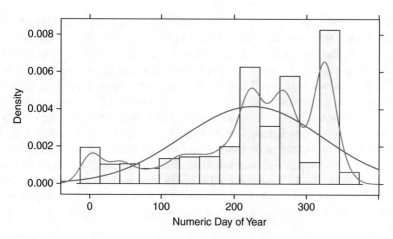

Fig. 13.16: Two approaches to estimating the density function $Pr[X]$ for the day of the year. The *blue line* is based on a normal distribution while the *red line* is generated using a nonparametric density estimator

shows the observed frequencies for the day of the week in which the grant was submitted. The columns showing the percent of total are the estimates of $Pr[X|Y = C_\ell]$ for each class. When a new sample is predicted, a simple lookup on this table is used to estimate the probabilities.

An obvious issue, especially for small samples sizes, occurs when one or more frequencies are zero. If a predictor has no training set samples for a specific class, the conditional probability would be zero and, since the probabilities are multiplied together, one predictor would coerce the posterior probability to be zero. One method for avoiding this issue is to use a *Laplace correction* or *Laplace smoothing* (Niblett 1987; Zadrozny and Elkan 2001; Provost and Domingos 2003) where the same correction factor, usually between one and two, is added to the numerator. For the denominator, the frequencies are increase by the correction factor times the number of values of the predictor. For example, there are very low frequencies for grants submitted on Sunday. To correct for the extreme probabilities, a correction factor of one would changes the observed frequencies to 229 and 4, but the denominator would be increased by seven. Given the large sample size for the training set, this correction only has a small impact (the estimated success rate on Sunday is increased from 2.78 % to 2.79 %). However, all of the three unsuccessful grants in the table were submitted after 2008. Training on pre-2008 data would generate zero probabilities. In this case, a correction of value of one would change the probability for grants to 0.02 % while a correction factor of two would increase the value to 0.03 %. For smaller training set sizes, the correction can have a substantial positive effect on the missing cells in the table.

For the grant data, many of the predictors were counts. Although these are numbers, they are discrete values and could be treated as categories. In many cases, the observed frequency distribution is compact. For example, in the training set, the number of chief investigators in department 2,678 takes on the four values between 0 and 3 and has a very right-skewed distribution. Treating such a granular predictor as if it was generated by a symmetric normal distribution may produce poor probability estimates. For this analysis, the reduced set of predictors was evaluated such that all predictors with less than 15 possible values were treated as discrete and their probabilities were calculated using their frequency distribution (such as the day of the week shown in Table 13.1. There were 14 predictors with more than 15 unique values, including the number of successful grants by chief investigators, the number of A* journal papers by chief investigators, and numeric day of the year.

These predictors were modeled using either a normal distribution or a nonparametric density (the density type was treated as a tuning parameter), and a Laplace correction of 2 was used. When using a normal distribution for the continuous predictors, the area under the curve was estimated to be 0.78, a sensitivity of 58.8 %, and a specificity of 79.6 %. Using nonparametric estimation of the probability densities, the area under the ROC curve improves to 0.81, which corresponding increases in sensitivity (64.4 %) and specificity (82.4 %). Unfortunately, the performance for this model is on par with KNNs, which is substantially below the results of the other models in this chapter.

Section 11.1 showed that Bayes' Rule can be used to calibrate class probability estimates. To do this, the true classes are used as Y, but the class probability values for the training set are used as the "predictor" and $Pr[X|Y = C_\ell]$ is determined from the model predictions on the training set. When new samples are predicted, the class probabilities that are generated by the model are post-processed using Bayes' Rule to improve the calibration. Ironically, class probabilities created by apply Bayes' Rule in the normal fashion tend not to be well-calibrated themselves. As the number of predictors increases (relative to the sample size), the posterior probabilities will become more extreme (similar to the observation related to linear discriminant analysis shown in Fig. 12.11). Recall that QDA is based on Bayes' Rule (using multivariate normality for the predictors) and the QDA results shown in Fig. 11.1 showed poor calibration with two predictor variables (but was improved by recalibrating using another application of Bayes' Rule).

13.7 Computing

The following R packages are discussed in this chapter: caret, earth, kernlab, klaR, MASS, mda, nnet, and rrcov. This section also uses the same R objects created in the last chapter that contain the data (such as the data frame training).

Nonlinear Discriminant Analysis

A number of packages are available to perform the varieties of nonlinear discriminant analysis described earlier in this chapter. QDA is implemented in the qda function in the MASS as well as an outlier-resistant version in the QdaCov function in the rrcov package. RDA is available in the rda function in the klaR package, and MDA can be found in the mda package. The syntax for these models is very similar and we will demonstrate their usage by fitting an MDA model to the grant data.

The mda function has a model formula interface. The tuning parameter is the number of subclasses per class, which do not have to be the same for each class. For example, to fit an MDA model to the grant data with three subpopulations per class:

```
> library(mda)
> mdaModel <- mda(Class ~ .,
+                 ## Reduce the data to the relevant predictors and the
+                 ## class variable to use the formula shortcut above
+                 data = training[pre2008, c("Class", reducedSet)],
+                 subclasses = 3)
> mdaModel
   Call:
   mda(formula = Class ~ ., data = training[pre2008, c("Class",
       reducedSet)], subclasses = 3)

   Dimension: 5

   Percent Between-Group Variance Explained:
       v1      v2      v3      v4      v5
    72.50   92.57   96.10   98.66  100.00

   Degrees of Freedom (per dimension): 253

   Training Misclassification Error: 0.18709 ( N = 6633 )

   Deviance: 6429.499
> predict(mdaModel,
+         newdata = head(training[-pre2008, reducedSet]))
   [1] successful successful successful successful successful successful
   Levels: successful unsuccessful
```

Each of these nonlinear discriminant models can be built and optimal tuning parameters can be found using the caret package. The trControl option for the grants data is set as described in Sect. 12.7 and will be used here:

```
> set.seed(476)
> mdaFit <- train(training[,reducedSet], training$Class,
+                 method = "mda",
+                 metric = "ROC",
+                 tuneGrid = expand.grid(.subclasses = 1:8),
+                 trControl = ctrl)
```

Similar syntax can be used for RDA (using `method = "rda"`) and QDA (method values of either `"rda"` or `"QdaCov"` for the outlier-resistant version in the **rrcov** package).

A penalized version of MDA is also available in the **sparseLDA** package with the `smda` function. See Clemmensen et al. (2011) for more details.

Neural Networks

There are many R packages for neural networks, including **nnet**, **RSNNS**, **qrnn**, and **neuralnet**. Two resources for using neural networks in R are Venables and Ripley (2002) and Sect. 7 of Bergmeir and Benitez (2012).

The analyses here focus on the **nnet** package. The syntax is extremely similar to that of the regression models with a few exceptions. The `linout` argument should be set to FALSE since most classification models use a sigmoidal transformation to relate the hidden units to the outputs. The sums of squared errors or entropy estimates model parameters and the logical arguments `softmax` and `entropy` toggle between the two.

The package has both a formula interface and an interface for passing matrices or data frames for the predictors and the outcome. For the latter, the outcome cannot be a factor variable and must be converted to a set of C binary indicators. The package contains a function, `class.ind`, that is useful in making this conversion:

```
> head(class.ind(training$Class))
     successful unsuccessful
[1,]          1            0
[2,]          1            0
[3,]          1            0
[4,]          1            0
[5,]          0            1
[6,]          1            0
```

Using the formula interface to fit a simple model:

```
> set.seed(800)
> nnetMod <- nnet(Class ~ NumCI + CI.1960,
+                 data = training[pre2008,],
+                 size = 3, decay = .1)
  # weights:  13
  initial  value 4802.892391
  iter  10 value 4595.629073
  iter  20 value 4584.893054
  iter  30 value 4582.614616
  iter  40 value 4581.010289
  iter  50 value 4580.866146
  iter  60 value 4580.781092
  iter  70 value 4580.756342
```

```
final   value 4580.756133
converged
> nnetMod

a 2-3-1 network with 13 weights
inputs: NumCI CI.1960
output(s): Class
options were - entropy fitting  decay=0.1
> predict(nnetMod, newdata = head(testing))
          [,1]
6641 0.5178744
6647 0.5178744
6649 0.5138892
6650 0.5837029
6655 0.4899851
6659 0.5701479
> predict(nnetMod, newdata = head(testing), type = "class")

[1] "unsuccessful" "unsuccessful" "unsuccessful" "unsuccessful"
[5] "successful"   "unsuccessful"
```

When three or more classes are modeled, the basic call to `predict` produces columns for each class.

As before, `train` provides a wrapper to this function to tune the model over the amount of weight decay and the number of hidden units. The same model code is used (`method = "nnet"`) and either model interface is available, although `train` does allow factor vectors for the classes (using `class.ind` internally do encode the dummy variables). Also, as in regression, model averaging can be used via the stand-alone `avNNet` function or using `train` (with `method = "avNNet"`).

The final model for the grant data has the following syntax:

```
> nnetGrid <- expand.grid(.size = 1:10,
+                         .decay = c(0, .1, 1, 2))
> maxSize <- max(nnetGrid$.size)
> numWts <- 1*(maxSize * (length(reducedSet) + 1) + maxSize + 1)
> set.seed(476)
> nnetFit <- train(x = training[,reducedSet],
+                  y = training$Class,
+                  method = "nnet",
+                  metric = "ROC",
+                  preProc = c("center", "scale", "spatialSign"),
+                  tuneGrid = nnetGrid,
+                  trace = FALSE,
+                  maxit = 2000,
+                  MaxNWts = numWts,
+                  ## ctrl was defined in the previous chapter
+                  trControl = ctrl)
```

Flexible Discriminant Analysis

The mda package contains a function (fda) for building this model. The model accepts the formula interface and has an option (method) that specifies the exact method for estimating the regression parameters. To use FDA with MARS, there are two approaches. method = mars uses the MARS implementation in the mda package. However, the earth package, previously described in Sect. 7.5, fits the MARS model with a wider range of options. Here, load the earth package and then specify method = earth. For example, a simple FDA model for the grant application data could be created as

```
> library(mda)
> library(earth)
> fdaModel <- fda(Class ~ Day + NumCI, data = training[pre2008,],
+                 method = earth)
```

Arguments to the earth function, such as nprune, can be specified when calling fda and are passed through to earth. The MARS model is contained in a sub-object called fit:

```
> summary(fdaModel$fit)
  Call: earth(x=x, y=Theta, weights=weights)

                coefficients
  (Intercept)    1.41053449
  h(Day-91)     -0.01348332
  h(Day-202)     0.03259400
  h(Day-228)    -0.02660477
  h(228-Day)    -0.00997109
  h(Day-282)    -0.00831905
  h(Day-319)     0.17945773
  h(Day-328)    -0.51574151
  h(Day-332)     0.50725158
  h(Day-336)    -0.20323060
  h(1-NumCI)     0.11782107

  Selected 11 of 12 terms, and 2 of 2 predictors
  Importance: Day, NumCI
  Number of terms at each degree of interaction: 1 10 (additive model)
  GCV 0.8660403    RSS 5708.129    GRSq 0.1342208    RSq 0.1394347
```

Note that the model coefficients shown here have not been post-processed. The final model coefficients can be found with coef(fdaModel). To predict:

```
> predict(fdaModel, head(training[-pre2008,]))
  [1] successful successful successful successful successful successful
  Levels: successful unsuccessful
```

The train function can be used with method = "fda" to tune this model over the number of retained terms. Additionally, the varImp function from this package determines predictor importance in the same manner as for MARS models (described in Sect. 7.2).

Support Vector Machines

As discussed in the regression chapter, there are a number of R packages with implementations for support vector machine and other kernel methods, including e1071, kernlab, klaR, and svmPath. The most comprehensive of these is the kernlab package.

The syntax for SVM classification models is largely the same as the regression case. Although the epsilon parameter is only relevant for regression, a few other parameters are useful for classification:

- The logical prob.model argument triggers ksvm to estimate an additional set of parameters for a sigmoidal function to translate the SVM decision values to class probabilities using the method of Platt (2000). If this option is not set to TRUE, class probabilities cannot be predicted.
- The class.weights argument assigns asymmetric costs to each class (Osuna et al. 1997). This can be especially important when one or more specific types of errors are more harmful than others or when there is a severe class imbalance that biases the model to the majority class (see Chap. 16). The syntax here is to use a *named* vector of weights or costs. For example, if there was a desire to bias the grant model to detect unsuccessful grants, then the syntax would be

```
class.weights = c(successful = 1, unsuccessful = 5)
```

This makes a false-negative error five times more costly than a false-positive error. Note that the implementation of class weights in ksvm affects the predicted class, but the class probability model is unaffected by the weights (in this implementation). This feature is utilized in Chap. 17.

The following code fits a radial basis function to the reduced set of predictors in the grant data:

```
> set.seed(202)
> sigmaRangeReduced <- sigest(as.matrix(training[,reducedSet]))
> svmRGridReduced <- expand.grid(.sigma = sigmaRangeReduced[1],
+                                .C = 2^(seq(-4, 4)))
> set.seed(476)
> svmRModel <- train(training[,reducedSet], training$Class,
+                    method = "svmRadial",
+                    metric = "ROC",
+                    preProc = c("center", "scale"),
+                    tuneGrid = svmRGridReduced,
+                    fit = FALSE,
+                    trControl = ctrl)

> svmRModel

8190 samples
 252 predictors
   2 classes: 'successful', 'unsuccessful'
```

```
Pre-processing: centered, scaled
Resampling: Repeated Train/Test Splits (1 reps, 0.75%)

Summary of sample sizes: 6633

Resampling results across tuning parameters:

  C       ROC    Sens   Spec
  0.0625  0.866  0.775  0.787
  0.125   0.88   0.842  0.776
  0.25    0.89   0.867  0.772
  0.5     0.894  0.851  0.784
  1       0.895  0.84   0.804
  2       NaN    0.814  0.814
  4       0.887  0.814  0.812
  8       0.885  0.804  0.814
  16      0.882  0.805  0.818


Tuning parameter 'sigma' was held constant at a value of 0.00117
ROC was used to select the optimal model using  the largest value.
The final values used for the model were C = 1 and sigma = 0.00117.
```

When the outcome is a factor, the function automatically uses prob.model =
TRUE.

Other kernel functions can be defined via the kernel and kpar arguments.
Prediction of new samples follows the same pattern as other functions:

```
> library(kernlab)
> predict(svmRModel, newdata = head(training[-pre2008, reducedSet]))
  [1] successful successful successful successful successful successful
  Levels: successful unsuccessful
> predict(svmRModel, newdata = head(training[-pre2008, reducedSet]),
+         type = "prob")

    successful unsuccessful
  1  0.9522587   0.04774130
  2  0.8510325   0.14896755
  3  0.8488238   0.15117620
  4  0.9453771   0.05462293
  5  0.9537204   0.04627964
  6  0.5009338   0.49906620
```

K-Nearest Neighbors

Fitting a KNN classification model has similar syntax to fitting a regression
model. In this setting, the **caret** package with method set to "knn" generates
the model. The syntax used to produce the top of Fig. 13.14 is

```
> set.seed(476)
> knnFit <- train(training[,reducedSet], training$Class,
```

```
+                       method = "knn",
+                       metric = "ROC",
+                       preProc = c("center", "scale"),
+                       tuneGrid = data.frame(.k = c(4*(0:5)+1,
+                                                    20*(1:5)+1,
+                                                    50*(2:9)+1)),
+                   trControl = ctrl)
```

The following code predicts the test set data and the corresponding ROC curve:

```
> knnFit$pred <- merge(knnFit$pred,  knnFit$bestTune)
> knnRoc <- roc(response = knnFit$pred$obs,
+               predictor = knnFit$pred$successful,
+               levels = rev(levels(knnFit$pred$obs)))
> plot(knnRoc, legacy.axes = TRUE)
```

Naïve Bayes

The two main functions for fitting the naïve Bayes models in R are naiveBayes in the e1071 package and NaiveBayes in the klaR package. Both offer Laplace corrections, but the version in the klaR package has the option of using conditional density estimates that are more flexible.

Both functions accept the formula and non-formula approaches to specifying the model terms. However, feeding these models binary dummy variables (instead of a factor variable) is problematic since the individual categories will be treated as numerical data and the model will estimate the probability density function (i.e., $Pr[X]$) from a continuous distribution, such as the Gaussian.

To follow the strategy described above where many of the predictors are converted to factor variables, we create alternate versions of the training and test sets:

```
> ## Some predictors are already stored as factors
> factors <- c("SponsorCode", "ContractValueBand", "Month", "Weekday")
> ## Get the other predictors from the reduced set
> nbPredictors <- factorPredictors[factorPredictors %in% reducedSet]
> nbPredictors <- c(nbPredictors, factors)

> ## Leek only those that are needed
> nbTraining <- training[, c("Class", nbPredictors)]
> nbTesting <- testing[, c("Class", nbPredictors)]

> ## Loop through the predictors and convert some to factors
> for(i in nbPredictors)
+   {
+     varLevels <- sort(unique(training[,i]))
```

```
+      if(length(varLevels) <= 15)
+        {
+          nbTraining[, i] <- factor(nbTraining[,i],
+                                    levels = paste(varLevels))
+          nbTesting[, i] <- factor(nbTesting[,i],
+                                    levels = paste(varLevels))
+        }
+    }
```

Now, we can use the NaiveBayes function's formula interface to create a model:

```
> library(klaR)
> nBayesFit <- NaiveBayes(Class ~ .,
+                         data = nbTraining[pre2008,],
+                         ## Should the non-parametric estimate
+                         ## be used?
+                         usekernel = TRUE,
+                         ## Laplace correction value
+                         fL = 2)
> predict(nBayesFit, newdata = head(nbTesting))

  $class
        6641       6647       6649       6650       6655       6659
  successful successful successful successful successful successful
  Levels: successful unsuccessful

  $posterior
        successful unsuccessful
  6641   0.9937862 6.213817e-03
  6647   0.8143309 1.856691e-01
  6649   0.9999078 9.222923e-05
  6650   0.9992232 7.768286e-04
  6655   0.9967181 3.281949e-03
  6659   0.9922326 7.767364e-03
```

In some cases, a warning appears: "Numerical 0 probability for all classes with observation 1." The predict function for this model has an argument called threshold that replaces the zero values with a small, nonzero number (0.001 by default).

The train function treats the density estimate method (i.e., usekernel) and the Laplace correction as tuning parameters. By default, the function evaluates probabilities with the normal distribution and the nonparametric method (and no Laplace correction).

Exercises

13.1. Use the hepatic injury data from the previous exercise set (Exercise 12.1). Recall that the matrices bio and chem contain the biological assay and chemical fingerprint predictors for the 281 compounds, while the vector injury contains the liver damage classification for each compound.

(a) Work with the same training and testing sets as well as pre-processing steps as you did in your previous work on these data. Using the same classification statistic as before, build models described in this chapter for the biological predictors and separately for the chemical fingerprint predictors. Which model has the best predictive ability for the biological predictors and what is the optimal performance? Which model has the best predictive ability for the chemical predictors and what is the optimal performance? Does the nonlinear structure of these models help to improve the classification performance?

(b) For the optimal models for both the biological and chemical predictors, what are the top five important predictors?

(c) Now combine the biological and chemical fingerprint predictors into one predictor set. Re-train the same set of predictive models you built from part (a). Which model yields best predictive performance? Is the model performance better than either of the best models from part (a)? What are the top 5 important predictors for the optimal model? How do these compare with the optimal predictors from each individual predictor set? How do these important predictors compare the predictors from the linear models?

(d) Which model (either model of individual biology or chemical fingerprints or the combined predictor model), if any, would you recommend using to predict compounds' hepatic toxicity? Explain.

13.2. Use the fatty acid data from the previous exercise set (Exercise 12.2).

(a) Use the same data splitting approach (if any) and pre-processing steps that you did in the previous chapter. Using the same classification statistic as before, build models described in this chapter for these data. Which model has the best predictive ability? How does this optimal model's performance compare to the best linear model's performance? Would you infer that the data have nonlinear separation boundaries based on this comparison?

(b) Which oil type does the optimal model most accurately predict? Least accurately predict?

Chapter 14
Classification Trees and Rule-Based Models

Classification trees fall within the family of tree-based models and, similar to regression trees, consist of nested `if-then` statements. For the familiar two-class problem shown in the last two chapters, a simple classification tree might be

```
if Predictor B >= 0.197 then
|   if Predictor A >= 0.13 then Class = 1
|   else Class = 2
else Class = 2
```

In this case, two-dimensional predictor space is cut into three regions (or terminal nodes) and, within each region, the outcome categorized into either "Class 1" or "Class 2." Figure 14.1 presents the tree in the predictor space. Just like in the regression setting, the nested `if-then` statements could be collapsed into rules such as

```
if Predictor A >= 0.13 and Predictor B >= 0.197 then Class = 1
if Predictor A >= 0.13 and Predictor B <  0.197 then Class = 2
if Predictor A <  0.13 then Class = 2
```

Clearly, the structure of trees and rules is similar to the structure we saw in the regression setting. And the benefits and weaknesses of trees in the classification setting are likewise similar: they can be highly interpretable, can handle many types of predictors as well as missing data, but suffer from model instability and may not produce optimal predictive performance. The process for finding the optimal splits and rules, however, is slightly different due to a change in the optimization criteria, which will be described below.

Random forests, boosting, and other ensemble methodologies using classification trees or rules are likewise extended to this setting and are discussed in Sects. 14.3 through 14.6.

M. Kuhn and K. Johnson, *Applied Predictive Modeling*,
DOI 10.1007/978-1-4614-6849-3_14,
© Springer Science+Business Media New York 2013

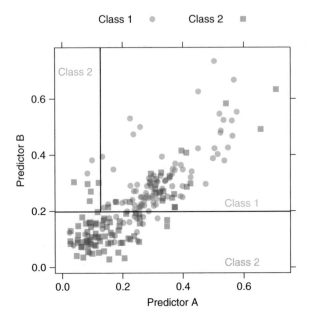

Fig. 14.1: An example of the predicted classes within regions defined by a tree-based model

14.1 Basic Classification Trees

As with regression trees, the aim of classification trees is to partition the data into smaller, more homogeneous groups. Homogeneity in this context means that the nodes of the split are more pure (i.e., contain a larger proportion of one class in each node). A simple way to define purity in classification is by maximizing accuracy or equivalently by minimizing misclassification error. Accuracy as a measure of purity, however, is a bit misleading since the measure's focus is on partitioning the data in a way that minimizes misclassification rather than a focus on partitioning the data in a way that place samples primarily in one class.

Two alternative measures, the Gini index (Breiman et al. 1984) and cross entropy, which is also referred to as deviance or information (defined later in this section), shift the focus from accuracy to purity. For the two-class problem, the Gini index for a given node is defined as

$$p_1 \left(1 - p_1\right) + p_2 \left(1 - p_2\right), \tag{14.1}$$

where p_1 and p_2 are the Class 1 and Class 2 probabilities, respectively. Since this is a two-class problem $p_1 + p_2 = 1$, and therefore Eq. 14.1 can equivalently be written as $2p_1p_2$. It is easy to see that the Gini index is minimized when either of the class probabilities is driven towards zero, meaning that the node is pure with respect to one of the classes. Conversely, the Gini index is maximized when $p_1 = p_2$, the case in which the node is least pure.

When working with a continuous predictor and a categorical response, the process for finding the optimal split point is similar to the process we saw in Sect. 8.1. First, the samples are sorted based on their predictor values. The split points are then the midpoints between each unique predictor value. If the response is binary, then this process generates a 2×2 contingency table at each split point. This table can be generally represented as

	Class 1	Class 2	
> split	n_{11}	n_{12}	n_{+1}
≤ split	n_{21}	n_{22}	n_{+2}
	n_{1+}	n_{2+}	n

The Gini index prior to the split would be

$$Gini(\text{prior to split}) = 2\left(\frac{n_{1+}}{n}\right)\left(\frac{n_{2+}}{n}\right).$$

And the Gini index can be calculated after the split within each of the new nodes with values $2\left(\frac{n_{11}}{n_{+1}}\right)\left(\frac{n_{12}}{n_{+1}}\right)$ and $2\left(\frac{n_{21}}{n_{+2}}\right)\left(\frac{n_{22}}{n_{+2}}\right)$ for greater than and less than or equal to the split, respectively. These values are combined using the proportion of samples in each part of the split as weights with $\left(\frac{n_{+1}}{n}\right)$ and $\left(\frac{n_{+2}}{n}\right)$ representing the respective weights for greater than and less than or equal to the split. After some simplification, the Gini index to evaluate the split would be:

$$Gini(\text{after split}) = 2\left[\left(\frac{n_{11}}{n}\right)\left(\frac{n_{12}}{n_{+1}}\right) + \left(\frac{n_{21}}{n}\right)\left(\frac{n_{22}}{n_{+2}}\right)\right].$$

Now consider the simple example presented in Fig. 14.1, where the contingency table for the Predictor B split is as follows:

	Class 1	Class 2	
$B > 0.197$	91	30	121
$B \leq 0.197$	20	67	87

The Gini index for the samples in the $B > 0.197$ split would be 0.373 and for the samples with $B \leq 0.197$ would be 0.354. To determine if this is a good overall split, these values must be combined which is done by weighting each purity value by the proportion of samples in the node relative to the total number of samples in the parent node. In this case, the weight for the $B > 0.197$ split would be 0.582 and 0.418 when $B \leq 0.197$. The overall Gini index measure for this split would then be $(0.582)(0.373) + (0.418)(0.354) = 0.365$.

Here we have evaluated just one possible split point; partitioning algorithms, however, evaluate nearly all split points[1] and select the split point value that minimizes the purity criterion. The splitting process continues within each newly created partition, therefore increasing the depth of the tree, until the stopping criteria is met (such as the minimum number of samples in a node or the maximum tree depth).

Trees that are constructed to have the maximum depth are notorious for over-fitting the training data. A more generalizable tree is one that is a pruned version of the initial tree and can be determined by cost-complexity tuning, in which the purity criterion is penalized by a factor of the total number of terminal nodes in the tree. The cost-complexity factor is called the complexity parameter and can be incorporated into the tuning process so that an optimal value can be estimated. More details about this process can be found in Sect. 8.1.

After the tree has been pruned, it can be used for prediction. In classification, each terminal node produces a vector of class probabilities based on the training set which is then used as the prediction for a new sample. In the simple example above, if a new sample has a value of Predictor $B = 0.10$, then predicted class probability vector would be $(0.23, 0.77)$ for Class 1 and Class 2, respectively.

Similar to regression trees, classification trees can handle missing data. In tree construction, only samples with non-missing information are considered for creating the split. In prediction, surrogate splits can be used in place of the split for which there are missing data. Likewise, variable importance can be computed for classification trees by assessing the overall improvement in the optimization criteria for each predictor. See Sect. 8.1 for the parallel explanation in regression.

When the predictor is continuous, the partitioning process for determining the optimal split point is straightforward. When the predictor is categorical, the process can take a couple of equally justifiable paths, one of which differs from the traditional statistical modeling approach. For example, consider a logistic regression model which estimates slopes and intercepts associated with the predictors. For categorical predictors, a set of binary dummy variables (Sect. 3.6) is created that decomposes the categories to independent bits of information. Each of these dummy variables is then included separately in the model. Tree models can also bin categorical predictors. Evaluating purity for each of these new predictors is then simple, since each predictor has exactly one split point.

For tree models, the splitting procedure may be able to make more dynamic splits of the data, such as groups of two or more categories on either side of the split. However, to do this, the algorithm must treat the categorical predictors as an ordered set of bits. Therefore, when fitting trees and rule-based models, the practitioner must make a choice regarding the treatment of categorical predictor data:

---

[1] See Breiman (1996c) for a discussion of the technical nuances of splitting algorithms.

1. Each categorical predictor can be entered into the model as a single entity so that the model decides how to group or split the values. In the text, this will be referred to as using *grouped categories*.
2. Categorical predictors are first decomposed into binary dummy variables. In this way, the resulting dummy variables are considered independently, forcing binary splits for the categories. In effect, splitting on a binary dummy variable prior to modeling imposes a "one-versus-all" split of the categories. This approach will be labelled as using *independent categories*.

Which approach is more appropriate depends on the data and the model. For example, if a subset of the categories are highly predictive of the outcome, the first approach is probably best. However, as we will see later, this choice can have a significant effect on the complexity of the model and, as a consequence, the performance. In the following sections, models will be created using *both* approaches described above to assess which approach is model advantageous. A summary of the differences in the two approaches are summarized in Fig. 14.14 on p. 402 of this chapter.

To illustrate the partitioning process for a categorical predictor, consider the CART model of the grant data illustrated in Fig. 14.3. The first split for these data is on contract value band, which has 17 possible categories, and places values I, J, P, and Unknown into one partition and the remaining categories in the other. From a combinatorial standpoint, as the number of possible categories increase, the number of possible category orderings increases factorially. The algorithmic approach must therefore take a rational but greedy path to ordering the categories prior to determining the optimal split. One approach is to order the categories based on the proportion of samples in a selected class. The top plot in Fig. 14.2 displays the probability of successful grant application within each contract value band, ordered from least successful to most successful. To calculate the Gini index, the split points are the divisions between each of the ordered categories, with the categories to the left placed into one group and the categories to the right placed into the other group. The results from these sequential partitions are presented in the bottom plot. Clearly, adding samples from the Unknown category to the samples from categories P and J greatly reduces the Gini index. While it is difficult to see from the figure, the minimum value occurs at the split point between categories I and M. Therefore, the algorithm chooses to place samples from contract value band I, J, P, and Unknown into one partition and the remaining samples into the other. Using only this split, the model would classify a new sample as unsuccessful if it had a contract value band of I, J, P, or Unknown and successful otherwise.

Continuing the tree building process treating the predictors as grouped categories and pruning via cost complexity produces the tree in Fig. 14.3. Because the predictors are encoded, it is difficult to interpret the tree without an in-depth knowledge of the data. However, it is still possible to use the tree structure to gain insight to the relevance of the predictors to the response. We can also see that grouped category variables such as sponsor

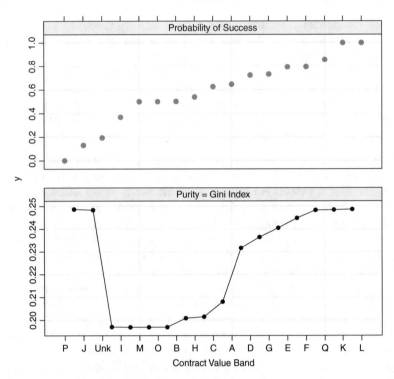

Fig. 14.2: *Top*: A scatter plot of the ordered probability of success (*y*-axis) for each contract value band. *Bottom*: The Gini index profile across each ordered split. The Gini index for the split points between categories Unknown, I, M, O, and B are nearly equivalent, with the minimum occurring between categories I and M

code, weekday, and month are relevant to the success of grant funding. The grouped categories model has an area under the ROC curve of 0.91 using 16 terminal nodes.

A CART model was also built using independent category predictors. Because this approach creates many more predictors, we would expect that the pruned tree would have more terminal nodes. Counter to intuition, the final pruned tree has 16 nodes and is illustrated in Fig. 14.4. This tree has an AUC of 0.912, and Fig. 14.5 compares its performance with the grouped category predictors. For classification trees using CART, there is no practical difference in predictive performance when using grouped categories or independent categories predictors for the grant data.

A comparison of Figs. 14.3 and 14.4 highlights a few interesting similarities and differences between how a tree model handles grouped category versus independent predictors. First, notice that the upper levels of the trees are generally the same with each selecting contract value band, sponsor code, and

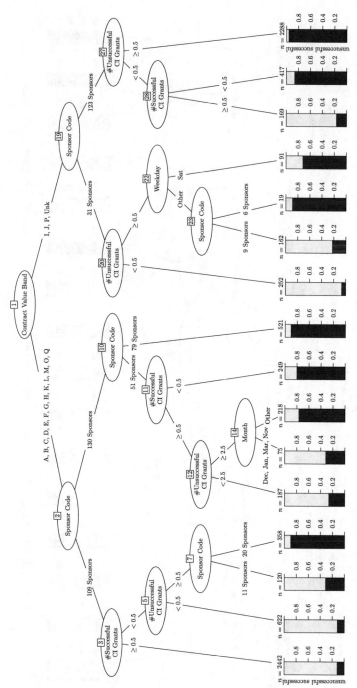

Fig. 14.3: The final CART model for the grant data using grouped category predictors

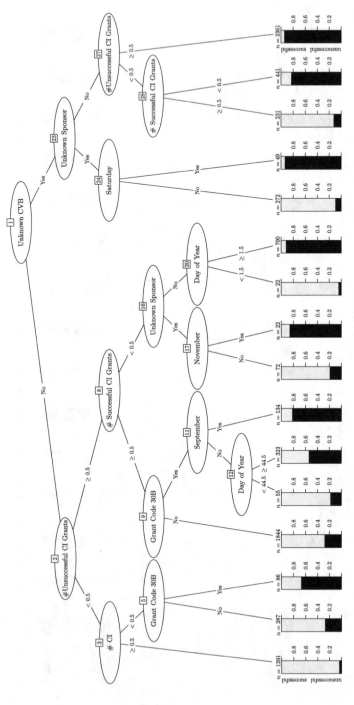

Fig. 14.4: The final CART model for the grant data using independent category predictors

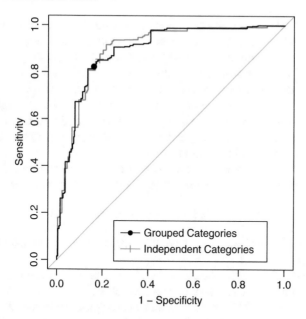

Fig. 14.5: The CART ROC curves for the holdout data. When using grouped categories, the area under the curve was 0.89. With independent categories, the AUC was also 0.89

number of unsuccessful and successful grants by chief investigators within the first four levels. Although the trees are identifying similarly important information, the independent category tree is much easier to interpret than the grouped category tree. For example, while the contract value band predictor is chosen as the first split in each tree, the independent category tree indicates that the value of Unknown is most critical for creating subsequent nodes that are more pure. Without producing a purity plot of the ordered categories, the importance of the Unknown band is masked within the grouping of bands I, J, P, and Unknown for the grouped category tree. Similar contrasts can be made with predictors of Month and Weekday, where the independent category tree provides further insight into the importance of specific months and weekdays. In the case of trees, therefore, creating independent category predictors may provide valuable interpretation about the relationship between predictors and the response that is not readily available when treating predictors as grouped categories.

Another approach for classification trees is the C4.5 model (Quinlan 1993b). Here, the splitting criteria is based on information theory (Wallace 2005; Cover and Thomas 2006). Suppose we want to communicate some piece of information, such as the probability distribution of the classes in the terminal node of a tree, in a series of messages. If the probability distribution is extremely unbalanced, there is a high likelihood of the sample belonging to the majority class, thus less uncertainty when guessing. However, if the class probabilities in the node were even, there is high uncertainty of a sample's true class. If we were trying to communicate the content of the probability distribution in a series of messages, on average, more information needs to be conveyed when there is a high degree of uncertainty in the message. Shannon (1948) and others developed a theory for the communication of information. The quantity that they call the *information statistic* represents the average number of bits needed to communicate in a message.

In our context, suppose there are $C = 2$ classes and the probability of the first class is p. The formal definition of the information statistic is

$$info = -[p \, log_2 p + (1 - p) \, log_2(1 - p)].$$

When $p = 0$, it is customary to have $0 \, log_2(0) = 0$. As previously mentioned, the units are called *bits*.

For the two class data shown in Fig. 14.1, the classes are almost even. If p is the proportion of samples in the first class, then $p = 0.53$. From this, the average number of bits of information to guess the true class (i.e., the information) would be 0.997. Now consider an unbalanced situation where fewer of the samples were in class 1 ($p = 0.10$). In this case, the information would be 0.46 bits, which is smaller because the class imbalance makes it easier to randomly guess the true class.[2] This metric has been previously discussed twice: as an objective function for neural networks (Eq. 13.3) and logistic regression (in Eq. 12.1 with a single data point).

How does this relate to determining splits? Using the general contingency table notation from above, the total information content of the data prior to splitting would be

$$info(\text{prior to split}) = -\left[\frac{n_{1+}}{n} \times log2\left(\frac{n_{1+}}{n}\right)\right] - \left[\frac{n_{2+}}{n} \times log2\left(\frac{n_{2+}}{n}\right)\right].$$

Again, when $n_{1+} = 0$ or $n_{2+} = 0$, it is traditional to set the terms inside the brackets to zero.

We can measure the improvement in the information criteria that would be induced by creating splits in a classification tree. The *information gain*[3] (or simply the *gain*) would be

$$gain(split) = info(\text{prior to split}) - info(\text{after split}).$$

---

[2] An alternate way to think of this is in terms of *entropy*, a measure of uncertainty. When the classes are balanced 50/50, we have no real ability to guess the outcome: it is as uncertain as possible. However, if ten samples were in class 1, we would have less uncertainty since it is more likely that a random data point would be in class 1.

[3] Also known as the *mutual information* statistic. This statistic is discussed again in Chap. 18.

Splits with larger information gains are more attractive than those with smaller gains.

For the binary split shown in the table above, the information after the split would be the sum of the information values from each of the resulting partitions. For example, the information for the data with values greater than the split value is

$$info(\text{greater}) = -\left[\frac{n_{11}}{n_{+1}} \times log2\left(\frac{n_{11}}{n_{+1}}\right)\right] - \left[\frac{n_{12}}{n_{+1}} \times log2\left(\frac{n_{12}}{n_{+1}}\right)\right].$$

The formula for the data on the other side of the split is analogous. The total information after the split is a weighted average of these values where the weights are related to the number of samples in the leaves of the split

$$info(\text{after split}) = \frac{n_{+1}}{n} info(\text{greater}) + \frac{n_{+2}}{n} info(\text{less than}).$$

Going back to the two class data, consider the predictor B split at a value of 0.197. The information when $B > 0.197$ is 0.808 and, on the other side of the split, the value is 0.778 when weighted by the proportion of samples on each side of the split, the total information is 0.795, a gain of $0.997 - 0.795 = 0.201$ Suppose, on the other hand, another split chosen that was completely non-informative, the information after the split would be the same as prior to the split, so the gain would be zero.

For continuous predictors, a tree could be constructed by searching for the predictor and single split that maximizes the information gain.[4] For these data, this gain is the largest when splitting predictor B at 0.197 and this is the split shown in Fig. 14.1. It also turns out that this split is also the best split for the Gini criterion used by CART.

There is one issue with this strategy. Since the predictors might have different numbers of possible values, the information gain criteria is biased against predictors that have a large number of possible outcomes (i.e., would favor categorical predictors with only a few distinct values over continuous predictors). This phenomenon is similar to the previously discussed bias for regression trees in Sect. 8.1. In this case, the bias is related to the ability of the algorithm to split the categorical predictors many ways (instead of a binary split on continuous predictors). The multi-way splits are likely to have larger gains. To correct for the bias, the *gain ratio* is used, which divides the gain by a measure of the amount of information in the split itself. Quinlan (1993b) shows additional examples of these calculations while Quinlan (1996b) describes refinements to this procedure for continuous predictors using the minimum description length (MDL) principle.

---

[4] By default, C4.5 uses simple binary split of continuous predictors. However, Quinlan (1993b) also describes a technique called *soft thresholding* that treats values near the split point differently. For brevity, this is not discussed further here.

When evaluating splits of categorical predictors, one strategy is to represent the predictor using multi-way splits such that there is a separate split for each category. When a predictor has a large number of possible values, this can lead to overly complex trees. For example, the sponsor code predictor in the grant data have 298 unique values. If this predictor were considered important, an initial 298-way split of the data would be created (prior to pruning). After the pruning process described below, some of these splits are likely to be combined and simplified.

Chapter 7 of Quinlan (1993b) describes a modified approach for creating multi-way splits that have the ability to group two or more categories. Prior to evaluating a categorical predictor as a split variable, the model first enumerates the gain ratio when the predictor is represented as:

- A multi-way split with as many splits as distinct values (i.e., the default approach where each category is a separate split).
- Multi-way splits for all possible combinations when two categories are grouped together and the others are split separately.

Based on the results of these representations of the predictor, a greedy algorithm is used to find the best categories to merge. As a result, there are many possible representations of the categorical predictor. Once the model constructs the final groupings, the gain ratio is calculated for this configuration. The ratio is compared to the other predictors when searching for the best split variable. This process is repeated each time the model conducts a search for a new split variable. This option is computationally expensive and may have a minimal impact on the tree if the categorical predictors have only a few possible levels. Unfortunately, this option is not available in the implementation of C4.5 that is currently available (in the Weka software suite under the name J48). The effect of this option on the data cannot be directly demonstrated here, but will be shown later when describing C5.0 (the descendent of C4.5). Since this can have a profound impact on the model, we will label this version of C4.5 as J48 to differentiate the versions.

When constructing trees with training sets containing missing predictor values, C4.5 makes several adjustments to the training process:

- When calculating the information gain, the information statistics are calculated using the non-missing data then scaled by the fraction of non-missing data at the split.
- Recall that C4.5 deals with selection bias by adjusting the gain statistic by the information value for the predictor. When the predictor contains missing values, the number of branches is increased by one; missing data are treated as an "extra" category or value of the predictor.
- Finally, when the class distribution is determined for the resulting splits, missing predictor values contribute *fractionally* to each class. The fractional contribution of the data points are based on the class distribution of the non-missing values. For example, suppose 11 samples are being split and one value was missing. If three samples are Class #1 and the rest are

Class #2, the missing value would contribute 0.30 to Class #1 and 0.70 to Class #2 (on both sides of the split).

Because of this accounting, the class frequency distribution in each node may not contain whole numbers. Also, the number of errors in the terminal node can be fractional.

Like CART, C4.5 builds a large tree that is likely to over-fit the data then prunes the tree back with two different strategies:

- Simple elimination of a sub-tree.
- *Raising* a sub-tree so that it replaces a node further up the tree.

Whereas CART uses cost complexity pruning, *pessimistic pruning* evaluates whether the tree should be simplified. Consider the case where a sub-tree is a candidate for removal. Pessimistic pruning estimates the number of errors with and without the sub-tree. However, it is well-known that the apparent error rate is extremely optimistic. To counteract this, pessimistic pruning calculates an upper confidence bound on the number of errors—this is the *pessimistic estimate* of the number of errors. This is computed with and without the sub-tree. If the estimated number of errors without the sub-tree is lower than the tree that includes it, the sub-tree is pruned from the model.

When determining the estimated error rate, C4.5 uses a default confidence level for the interval of 0.25 (called the *confidence factor*). This can be considered a tuning parameter for the model, as increasing the confidence factor leads larger trees. While intuitive, this approach stands on shaky statistical grounds, Quinlan (1993b) acknowledges this, saying that the approach

> "does violence to statistical notions of sampling and confidence limits, so the reasoning should be taken with a grain of salt."

That said, this technique can be very effective and is more computationally efficient than using cross-validation to determine the appropriate size of the tree.

Once the tree has been grown and pruned, a new sample is classified by moving down the appropriate path until it reaches the terminal node. Here, the majority class for the training set data falling into the terminal node is used to predict a new sample. A *confidence value*, similar to a class probability, can also be calculated on the basis of the class frequencies associated with the terminal nodes. Quinlan (1993b) describes how upper and lower ranges for the confidence factors can be derived from calculations similar to the pessimistic pruning algorithm described above.

When *predicting* a sample with one or more missing values, the sample is again treated fractionally. When a split is encountered for a variable that is missing in the data, each possible path down the tree is determined. Ordinarily, the predicted class would be based on the class with the largest frequency from a single terminal node. Since the missing value could have possibly landed in more than one terminal node, each class receives a weighted vote to determine the final predicted class. The class weights for all the relevant

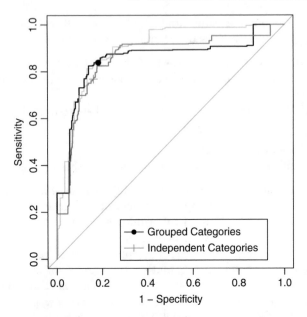

Fig. 14.6: The J48 ROC curves for the holdout data using two different approaches for handling categorical predictors. The symbols (*filled circle* and *plus*) represent the 50% probability cutoff. The areas under the curves were 0.835 when using grouped categories and 0.842 when using independent categories. The *grey line* corresponds to the previous CART model

terminal nodes are aggregated and the class associated with the largest total weight is used to predict the sample. In this way, each terminal node with possible associations with the sample contributes to the overall prediction.

J48 trees were created for the grant application data. Although the confidence factor could be treated as a tuning parameter, our experience is that the default value (0.25) works well. Two models were fit using the two different approaches for representing the categorical predictors. Based on the prior discussion, there is the expectation that treating the categories as a cohesive set will results in a much larger tree than one using independent categories. This is exactly the case for these data. Grouping the categories resulted in a pruned tree with 2,918 terminal nodes. This was primarily due to a large number of splits using the sponsor code; 2,384 splits out of 2,918 (82%) involve this predictor. When using independent categories, the tree was much smaller (821 terminal nodes).

The area under the ROC curve for the large model was 0.835, compared to 0.842 when using independent categories. Figure 14.6 shows the two ROC curves and the points on each curve corresponding to the default 50% probability cutoff. From this, it is clear that the specificities are about the same for each approach (81.7% for the larger model vs. 83.8%), but there is a significant difference in the sensitivity of the models; the more complex model resulted in a sensitivity of 83.9 % while the independent category model had relatively poor ability to predict successful grants (with a sensitivity of 76.8 %). However, these statistics are based on the nominal 50 % cutoff for success. The curves overlap considerably and alternate cutoffs would produce almost identical results (see Sect. 16.4).

While CART and C4.5 classification trees are the most widely used, there has been extensive research in this area and many other proposals for tree-based models. For example, as discussed in the section on regression trees, conditional inference trees (Hothorn et al. 2006) avoid selection bias during splitting. Also, several techniques exist (Frank et al. 1998; Loh 2002; Chan and Loh 2004; Zeileis et al. 2008) that use more complex models in the terminal nodes, similar to M5 and Cubist. Other types of splits can be employed. For example, Breiman et al. (1984) introduced the idea of splitting on a linear combination of the predictors. These *oblique trees* may be beneficial when the classes are linearly separable, which traditional splits have a difficult time approximating. Menze et al. (2011) discusses tree ensemble models with oblique trees.

14.2 Rule-Based Models

As previously discussed, rule-based models consist of one or more independent conditional statements. Unlike trees, a sample may be predicted from a set of rules. Rules have a long history as classifiers and this section will discuss approaches for creating classification rules.

C4.5Rules

There are several different philosophies and algorithms for creating rule-based models from classification trees. Some of the first were described by Quinlan (1987) and Quinlan (1993b). This model, called C4.5Rules, builds on the C4.5 tree methodology described in the last section. To start, an unpruned tree is created, then each path through the tree is collapsed into an individual rule.

Given this initial set, each rule is evaluated individually to assess whether it can be generalized by eliminating terms in the conditional statement. The pruning process here is similar to the one used to prune C4.5 trees. For a rule, the model first calculates a baseline pessimistic error rate, then removes each condition in the rule in isolation. Once a condition is removed, the pessimistic error rate is recomputed. If any error rate is smaller than the baseline, the condition associated with the smallest error rate is removed. The process is repeated until all conditions are above the baseline rate or all conditions are removed. In the latter case, the rule is completely pruned from the model. The table below shows the pruning process with a five condition rule for the grant data:

	Pessimistic error rate		
Condition	Pass 1	Pass 2	Pass 3
Baseline	*14.9*	*5.8*	*5.2*
First day of year	12.9	**5.2**	
Zero unsuccessful grants (CI)	77.3	53.5	50.7
Number of CI	42.0	21.6	19.7
Number of SCI	18.0	8.1	7.3
Zero successful grants (CI)	**5.8**		

On the first pass, removing the condition associated with zero successful grants by a chief investigator has the least impact on the error rate, so this condition is deleted from the rule. Three passes of pruning were needed until none of the error rates were below the baseline rate. Also, note that the pessimistic error rate decreases with each iteration. Finally, the condition related to zero unsuccessful grants for a chief investigator appears to have the most importance to the rule since the error rate is the largest when the condition is removed from the rule.

After the conditions have been pruned *within* each rule, the set of rules associated with each class are processed separately to reduce and order the rules. First, redundant or ineffective rules are removed using the MDL principle [see Quinlan and Rivest (1989) and Chap. 5 of Quinlan (1993b)]. An MDL metric is created that encapsulates a ruleset's performance and complexity— for two rulesets with equivalent performance, the simpler collection of rules is favored by the metric. Within each class, an initial group of groups is assembled such that every training set sample is covered by at least one rule. These are combined into the initial ruleset. Starting with this set, search methods (such as greedy hill climbing or simulated annealing) are used to add and remove rules until no further improvements can be made on the ruleset. The second major operation within a class is to order the rules from most to least accurate.

Once the rulesets within each class have been finalized, the classes are ordered based on accuracy and a default class is chosen for samples that have no relevant rules. When predicting a new sample, each rule is evaluated in order until one is satisfied. The predicted class corresponds to the class for the first active rule.

1 **repeat**
2   Create a pruned classification tree
3   Determine the path through the tree with the largest coverage
4   Add this path as a rule to the rule set
5   Remove the training set samples covered by the rule
6 **until** *all training set samples are covered by a rule*

Algorithm 14.1: The PART algorithm for constructing rule-based models (Frank and Witten 1998)

PART

C4.5Rules follows the philosophy that the initial set of candidate rules are developed simultaneously then post-processed into an improved model. Alternatively, rules can be created incrementally. In this way, a new rule can adapt to the previous set of rules and may more effectively capture important trends in the data.

Frank and Witten (1998) describe another rule model called PART shown in Algorithm 14.1. Here, a pruned C4.5 tree is created from the data and the path through the tree that covers the most samples is retained as a rule. The samples covered by the rule are discarded from the data set and the process is repeated until all samples are covered by at least one rule. Although the model uses trees to create the rules, each rule is created separately and has more potential freedom to adapt to the data.

The PART model for the grant data slightly favored the grouped category model. For this model, the results do not show an improvement above and beyond the previous models: the estimated sensitivity was 77.9 %, the specificity was 80.2 %, and the area under the ROC curve (not shown) was 0.809. The model contained 360 rules. Of these, 181 classify grants as successful while the other 179 classify grants as unsuccessful. Here, the five most prolific predictors were sponsor code (332 rules), contract value band (30 rules), the number of unsuccessful grants by chief investigators (27 rules), the number of successful grants by chief investigators (26 rules), and the number of chief investigators (23 rules).

14.3 Bagged Trees

Bagging for classification is a simple modification to bagging for regression (Sect. 8.4). Specifically, the regression tree in Algorithm 8.1 is replaced with an unpruned classification tree for modeling C classes. Like the regression

Table 14.1: The 2008 holdout set confusion matrix for the random forest model

	Observed class	
	Successful	Unsuccessful
Successful	491	144
Unsuccessful	79	843

This model had an overall accuracy of 85.7%, a sensitivity of 86.1%, and a specificity of 85.4%

setting, each model in the ensemble is used to predict the class of the new sample. Since each model has equal weight in the ensemble, each model can be thought of as casting a vote for the class it thinks the new sample belongs to. The total number of votes within each class are then divided by the total number of models in the ensemble (M) to produce a predicted probability vector for the sample. The new sample is then classified into the group that has the most votes, and therefore the highest probability.

For the grant data, bagging models were built using both strategies for categorical predictors. As discussed in the regression trees chapter, bagging performance often plateaus with about 50 trees, so 50 was selected as the number of trees for each of these models. Figure 14.7 illustrates the bagging ensemble performance using either independent or grouped categories. Both of these ROC curves are smoother than curves produced with classification trees or J48, which is an indication of bagging's ability to reduce variance via the ensemble. Additionally, both bagging models have better AUCs (0.92 for both) than either of the previous models. For these data, there seems to be no obvious difference in performance for bagging when using either independent or grouped categories; the ROC curves, sensitivities, and specificities are all nearly identical. The holdout set performance in Fig. 14.7 shows an improvement over the J48 results (Fig. 14.6).

Similar to the regression setting, variable importance measures can be calculated by aggregating variable importance values from the individual trees in the ensemble. Variable importance of the top 16 predictors for both the independent and grouped category bagged models set are presented in Fig. 14.15, and a comparison of these results is left to the reader in Exercise 14.1.

14.4 Random Forests

Random forests for classification requires a simple tweak to the random forest regression algorithm (Algorithm 8.2): a classification tree is used in place of

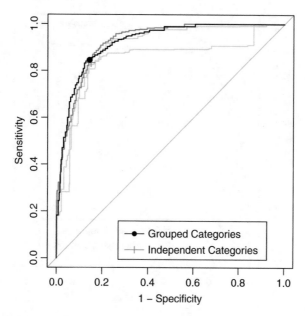

Fig. 14.7: The ROC curves for the bagged classification tree model. The area under the curves for both models was 0.92. The sensitivities and specificities were 82.98 and 85.71, respectively

a regression tree. As with bagging, each tree in the forest casts a vote for the classification of a new sample, and the proportion of votes in each class across the ensemble is the predicted probability vector.

While the type of tree changes in the algorithm, the tuning parameter of number of randomly selected predictors to choose from at each split is the same (denoted as m_{try}). As in regression, the idea behind randomly sampling predictors during training is to de-correlate the trees in the forest. For classification problems, Breiman (2001) recommends setting m_{try} to the square root of the number of predictors. To tune m_{try}, we recommend starting with five values that are somewhat evenly spaced across the range from 2 to P, where P is the number of predictors. We likewise recommend starting with an ensemble of 1,000 trees and increasing that number if performance is not yet close to a plateau.

For the most part, random forest for classification has very similar properties to the regression analog discussed previously, including:

- The model is relatively insensitive to values of m_{try}.
- As with most trees, the data pre-processing requirements are minimal.
- Out-of-bag measures of performance can be calculated, including accuracy, sensitivity, specificity, and confusion matrices.

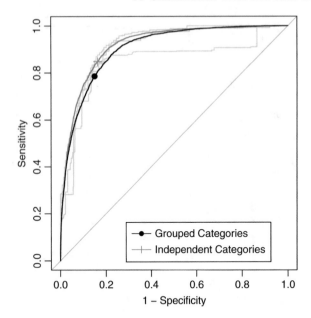

Fig. 14.8: The ROC curves for the random forest model. The area under the curve for independent categories was 0.92 and for the grouped category model the AUC was 0.9

One difference is the ability to weight classes differentially. This aspect of the model is discussed more in Chap. 16.

Random forest models were built on both independent and grouped category models. The tuning parameter, m_{try}, was evaluated at values ranging from 5 to 1,000. For independent categories, the optimal tuned value of m_{try} was 100, and for grouped categories the value was also 250. Figure 14.8 presents the results, and in this case the independent categories have a slightly higher AUC (0.92) than the grouped category approach (0.9). The binary predictor model also has better sensitivity (86.1 % vs. 84.7 %) but slightly worse specificity (85.4 % vs. 87.2 %).

For single trees, variable importance can be determined by aggregating the improvement in the optimization objective for each predictor. For random forests, the improvement criteria (default is typically the Gini index) is aggregated across the ensemble to generate an overall variable importance measure. Alternatively, predictors' impact on the ensemble can be calculated using a permutation approach (Breiman 2000) as discussed in Sect. 8.5. Variable importance values based on aggregated improvement have been computed for the grant data for both types of predictors and the most important predictors are presented in Fig. 14.15. The interpretation is left to the reader in Exercise 14.1.

Conditional inference trees can also be used as the base learner for random forests. But current implementations of the methodology are computationally burdensome for problems that are the relative size of the grant data. A comparison of the performance of random forests using CART trees and conditional inference trees is explored in Exercise 14.3.

14.5 Boosting

Although we have already discussed boosting in the regression setting, the method was originally developed for classification problems (Valiant 1984; Kearns and Valiant 1989), in which many weak classifiers (e.g., a classifier that predicts marginally better than random) were combined into a strong classifier. There are many species of boosting algorithms, and here we discuss the major ones.

AdaBoost

In the early 1990s several boosting algorithms appeared (Schapire 1990; Freund 1995) to implement the original theory. Freund and Schapire (1996) finally provided the first practical implementation of boosting theory in their famous AdaBoost algorithm; an intuitive version is provided in Algorithm 14.2.

To summarize the algorithm, AdaBoost generates a sequence of weak classifiers, where at each iteration the algorithm finds the best classifier based on the current sample weights. Samples that are incorrectly classified in the kth iteration receive more weight in the $(k + 1)$st iteration, while samples that are correctly classified receive less weight in the subsequent iteration. This means that samples that are difficult to classify receive increasingly larger weights until the algorithm identifies a model that correctly classifies these samples. Therefore, each iteration of the algorithm is required to learn a different aspect of the data, focusing on regions that contain difficult-to-classify samples. At each iteration, a *stage weight* is computed based on the error rate at that iteration. The nature of the stage weight described in Algorithm 14.2 implies that more accurate models have higher positive values and less accurate models have lower negative values.[5] The overall sequence of weighted classifiers is then combined into an ensemble and has a strong potential to classify better than any of the individual classifiers.

---

[5] Because a weak classifier is used, the stage values are often close to zero.

1	Let one class be represented with a value of +1 and the other with a value of -1
2	Let each sample have the same starting weight $(1/n)$
3	**for** $k = 1$ *to* K **do**
4	Fit a weak classifier using the weighted samples and compute the kth model's misclassification error (err_k)
5	Compute the kth stage value as $\ln\left((1 - err_k)/err_k\right)$.
6	Update the sample weights giving more weight to incorrectly predicted samples and less weight to correctly predicted samples
7	**end**
8	Compute the boosted classifier's prediction for each sample by multiplying the kth stage value by the kth model prediction and adding these quantities across k. If this sum is positive, then classify the sample in the +1 class, otherwise the -1 class.

Algorithm 14.2: AdaBoost algorithm for two-class problems

Boosting can be applied to any classification technique, but classification trees are a popular method for boosting since these can be made into weak learners by restricting the tree depth to create trees with few splits (also known as stumps). Breiman (1998) gives an explanation for why classification trees work particularly well for boosting. Since classification trees are a low bias/high variance technique, the ensemble of trees helps to drive down variance, producing a result that has low bias and low variance. Working through the lens of the AdaBoost algorithm, Johnson and Rayens (2007) showed that low variance methods cannot be greatly improved through boosting. Therefore, boosting methods such as LDA or KNN will not show as much improvement as boosting methods such as neural networks (Freund and Schapire 1996) or naïve Bayes (Bauer and Kohavi 1999).

Stochastic Gradient Boosting

As mentioned in Sect. 8.6, Friedman et al. (2000) worked to provide statistical insight of the AdaBoost algorithm. For the classification problem, they showed that it could be interpreted as a forward stagewise additive model that minimizes an exponential loss function. This framework led to algorithmic generalizations such as Real AdaBoost, Gentle AdaBoost, and LogitBoost. Subsequently, these generalizations were put into a unifying framework called gradient boosting machines which was previously discussed in the regression trees chapter.

---

1 Initialized all predictions to the sample log-odds: $f_i^{(0)} = \log \frac{\widehat{p}}{1-\widehat{p}}$.

2 for *iteration* $j = 1 \ldots M$ **do**

3   Compute the residual (i.e. gradient) $z_i = y_i - \widehat{p}_i$

4   Randomly sample the training data

5   Train a tree model on the random subset using the residuals as the outcome

6   Compute the terminal node estimates of the Pearson residuals:
$r_i = \frac{1/n \sum_i^n (y_i - \widehat{p}_i)}{1/n \sum_i^n \widehat{p}_i (1 - \widehat{p}_i)}$

7   Update the current model using $f_i = f_i + \lambda f_i^{(j)}$

8 end

Algorithm 14.3: Simple gradient boosting for classification (2-class)

Akin to the regression setting, when trees are used as the base learner, basic gradient boosting has two tuning parameters: tree depth (or *interaction depth*) and number of iterations. One formulation of stochastic gradient boosting models an event probability, similar to what we saw in logistic regression, by

$$\widehat{p}_i = \frac{1}{1 + exp\left[-f(x)\right]},$$

where $f(x)$ is a model prediction in the range of $[-\infty, \infty]$. For example, an initial estimate of the model could be the sample log odds, $f_i^{(0)} = \log \frac{\widehat{p}}{1-\widehat{p}}$, where p is the sample proportion of one class from the training set.

Using the Bernoulli distribution, the algorithm for stochastic gradient boosting for two classes is shown in Algorithm 14.3.

The user can tailor the algorithm more specifically by selecting an appropriate loss function and corresponding gradient (Hastie et al. 2008). Shrinkage can be implemented in the final step of Algorithm 14.3. Furthermore, this algorithm can be placed into the stochastic gradient boosting framework by adding a random sampling scheme prior to the first step in the inner **For** loop. Details about this process can be found in Sect. 8.6.

For the grant data a tuning parameter grid was constructed where interaction depth ranged from 1 to 9, number of trees ranged from 100 to 2,000, and shrinkage ranged from 0.01 to 0.1. This grid was applied to constructing a boosting model where the categorical variables were treated as independent categories and separately as grouped categories. For the independent category model, the optimal area under the ROC curve was 0.94, with an interaction depth of 9, number of trees 1,300, and shrinkage 0.01. For the grouped category model, the optimal area under the ROC curve was 0.92, with an interaction depth of 7, number of trees 100, and shrinkage 0.01 (see

Fig. 14.9). In this case, the independent category model performs better than the grouped category model on the basis of ROC. However, the number of trees in each model was substantially different, which logically follows since the binary predictor set is larger than the grouped categories.

An examination of the tuning parameter profiles for the grouped category and independent category predictors displayed in Figs. 14.10 and 14.11 reveals some interesting contrasts. First, boosting independent category predictors has almost uniformly better predictive performance across tuning parameter settings relative to boosting grouped category predictors. This pattern is likely because only one value for many of the important grouped category predictors contains meaningful predictive information. Therefore, trees using the independent category predictors are more easily able to find that information quickly which then drives the boosting process. Within the grouped category predictors, increasing the shrinkage parameter almost uniformly degrades predictive performance across tree depth. These results imply that for the grouped category predictors, boosting obtains most of its predictive information from a moderately sized initial tree, which is evidenced by comparable AUCs between a single tree (0.89) and the optimal boosted tree (0.92).

Boosting independent category predictors shows that as the number of trees increases, model performance improves for low values of shrinkage and degrades for higher values of shrinkage. But, whether a lower or higher value of shrinkage is selected, each approach finds peak predictive performance at an ROC of approximately 0.94. This result implies, for these data, that boosting can find an optimal setting fairly quickly without the need for too much shrinkage.

Variable importance for boosting in the classification setting is calculated in a similar manner to the regression setting: within each tree in the ensemble, the improvement based on the splitting criteria for each predictor is aggregated. These importance values are then averaged across the entire boosting ensemble.

14.6 C5.0

C5.0 is a more advanced version of Quinlan's C4.5 classification model that has additional features, such as boosting and unequal costs for different types of errors. Like C4.5, it has tree- and rule-based versions and shares much of its core algorithms with its predecessor. Unlike C4.5 or Cubist, there is very little literature on the improvements and our description comes largely from evaluating the program source code, which was made available to the public in 2011.

The model has many features and options and our discussion is broken down into four separate areas: creating a single classification tree, the cor-

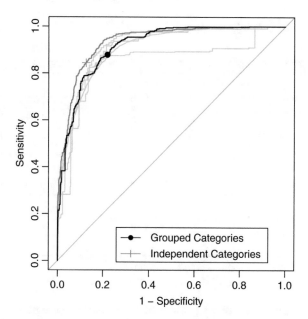

Fig. 14.9: The ROC curves for the boosted tree model. The area under the curve for independent categories was 0.936 and for the grouped category model the AUC was 0.916

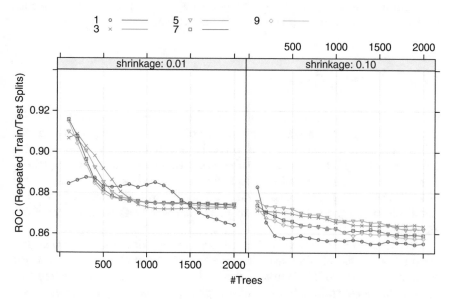

Fig. 14.10: Tuning parameter profiles for the boosted tree model using grouped categories

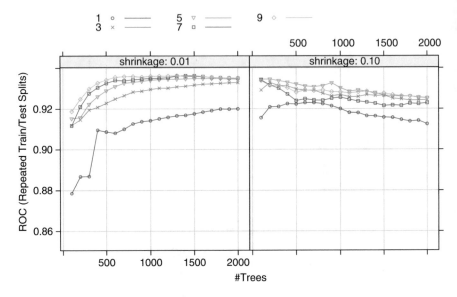

Fig. 14.11: Tuning parameter profiles for the boosted tree model using independent categories

responding rule-based model, C5.0's boosting procedure, and miscellaneous features of the algorithm (e.g., variable importance etc).

Classification Trees

C5.0 trees have several basic improvements that are likely to generate smaller trees. For example, the algorithm will combine nonoccurring conditions for splits with several categories. It also conducts a final global pruning procedure that attempts to remove the sub-trees with a cost-complexity approach. Here, sub-trees are removed until the error rate exceeds one standard error of the baseline rate (i.e., no pruning). Initial experimentation suggests that these additional procedures tend to create simpler trees than the previous algorithm.

The nominal C5.0 tree was fit to the grant data with the categorical predictors treated as cohesive sets. The tree had 86 terminal nodes and resulted in an area under the ROC curve of 0.685. The five most prolific predictors in the tree were contract value band (six splits), numeric day of the year (six splits), sponsor code (five splits), category code (four splits), and day of the week (four splits). Recall that the analogous J48 tree had many more terminal nodes (2,918), which was primarily due to how splits were made on categorical variables with many possible values, such as the sponsor code. The C5.0 tree avoids this issue using the heuristic algorithm described in Sect. 14.1 that attempts to consolidate the categories into two or more smaller groups. If this option is turned off in C5.0, the tree is much larger (213 terminal nodes) due to the categorical predictors. However, the area under the ROC curve for the larger tree (0.685) is nearly the same as the smaller tree.

Neither C5.0 model approaches the size of the previously described J48 tree. For J48 and C5.0 (without grouping), categorical predictors with many values are used in more splits, and, at each split, they tend to result in more than two branches when the grouping option is not used.

Classification Rules

The process used for creating rules is similar to C4.5; an initial tree is grown, collapsed into rules, then the individual rules are simplified via pruning and a global procedure is used on the entire set to potentially reduce the number of constituent rules. The process for pruning conditions within a rule and simplifying the ruleset follows C4.5, but C5.0 does not order the rules. Instead, when predicting new samples, C5.0 uses *all* active rules, each of which votes for the most likely class. The votes for each class are weighted by the confidence values and the class associated with the highest vote is used. However, the predicted confidence value is the one associated with the most specific active rule. Recall that C4.5 sorts the rules, and uses the first active rule for prediction.

The grant data were analyzed with this algorithm. The rule-based model consists of 22 rules with an estimated area under the ROC curve of 0.675. The complexity of the model is much simpler than PART. When ordered by the confidence value of the rule, the top three rules to predict a successful grant are:

1. (First day of the year)
2. (The number of chief investigators > 0) and (the number of principal supervisors ≤ 0) and (the number of student chief investigators ≤ 0) and (the number of unsuccessful grants by chief investigators ≤ 0) and (SEO code ≠ 730106) and (numeric day of the year ≤ 209)
3. (The number of external chief investigators ≤ 0) and (the number of chief investigators born around 1975 ≤ 0) and (the number of successful grants by chief investigators ≤ 0) and (numeric day of the year > 109) and (unknown category code) and (day of the week in Tues, Fri, Mon, Wed, Thurs)

Similarly, the top three rules for unsuccessful grants are:

1. (The number of unsuccessful grants by chief investigators > 0) and (numeric day of the year > 327) and (sponsor code in 2B, 4D, 24D, 60D,

90B, 32D, 176D, 7C, 173A, 269A) and (contract value band in Unk, J) and (CategoryCode in 10A, 30B, 30D, 30C)

2. (The number of chief investigators $\leq$ 1) and (the number of unsuccessful grants by chief investigators $>$ 0) and (the number of B journal papers by chief investigators $>$ 3) and (sponsor code $=$ 4D) and (contract value band in B, Unk, J) and (Month in Nov, Dec, Feb, Mar, May, Jun)

3. (The number of chief investigators $>$ 0) and (the number of chief investigators born around 1945 $\leq$ 0) and (the number of successful grants by chief investigators $\leq$ 0) and (numeric day of the year $>$ 209) and (sponsor code in 21A, 60D, 172D, 53A, 103C, 150B, 175C, 93A, 207C, 294B)

There were 11 rules to predict successful grants and 11 for unsuccessful outcomes. The predictors involved in the most rules were the number of unsuccessful grants by chief investigators (11 rules), contract value band (9 rules), category code (8 rules), numeric day of the year (8 rules), and Month (5 rules).

C5.0 has other features for rule-based models. For example, the model can create *utility bands*. Here, the utility is measured as the increase in error that occurs when the rule is removed from the set. The rules are ordered with an iterative algorithm: the model removes the rule with the smallest utility and recomputes the utilities for the other rules. The sequence in which the rules are removed defines their importance. For example, the first rule that is removed is associated with the lowest utility and the last rule with the highest utility. The bands are groups of rules of roughly equal size based on the utility order (highest to smallest). The relationship between the cumulative error rate can be profiled as the groups of rules are added to the model.

Boosting

C5.0's boosting procedure is similar to the previously described AdaBoost algorithm in the basic sense: models are fit sequentially and each iteration adjusts the case weights based on the accuracy of a sample's prediction. There are, however, some notable differences. First, C5.0 attempts to create trees that are about the same size as the first tree by coercing the trees to have about the same number of terminal nodes per case as the initial tree. Previous boosting techniques treated the tree complexity as a tuning parameter. Secondly, the model combines the predictions from the constituent trees differently than AdaBoost. Each boosted model calculates the confidence values for each class as described above and a simple average of these values is calculated. The class with the largest confidence value is selected. Stage weights are not calculated during the model training process. Third, C5.0 conducts two sorts of "futility analysis" during model training. The model will automatically stop boosting if the model is very effective (i.e., the sum of the

weights for the misclassified samples is less than 0.10) or if it is highly ineffective (e.g., the average weight of incorrect samples is greater than 50 %).
Also, after half of the requested boosting iterations, each sample is assessed
to determine if a correct prediction is possible. If it is not, the case is dropped
from further computations.

Finally, C5.0 uses a different weighting scheme during model training.
First, some notation:

$$N = \text{training set size}$$
$$N_- = \text{number of incorrectly classified samples}$$
$$w_k = \text{case weight for sample at the } k\text{th boosting iteration}$$
$$S_+ = \text{sum of weights for correctly classified samples}$$
$$S_- = \text{sum of weights for incorrectly classified samples}$$

The algorithm begins by determining the midpoint between the sum of the
weights for misclassified samples and half of the overall sum of the weights

$$midpoint = \frac{1}{2}\left[\frac{1}{2}(S_- + S_+) - S_-\right] = \frac{1}{4}(S_+ - S_-).$$

From this, the correctly classified samples are adjusted with the equation

$$w_k = w_{k-1} \times \frac{S_+ - midpoint}{S_+}$$

and the misclassified samples are updated using

$$w_k = w_{k-1} + \frac{midpoint}{N_-}.$$

This updating scheme gives a large positive jump in the weights when a
sample is incorrectly predicted. When a sample is correctly predicted, the
multiplicative nature of the equation makes the weights drop more slowly
and with a decreasing rate as the sample continues to be correctly predicted.
Figure 14.12 shows an example of the change in weights for a single sample
over several boosting iterations.

Quinlan (1996a) describes several experiments with boosting and bagging
tree-based models including several where boosting C4.5 resulted in a less
effective model.

Other Aspects of the Model

C5.0 measures predictor importance by determining the percentage of
training set samples that fall into all the terminal nodes after the split. For

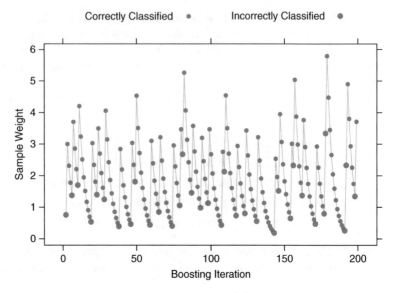

Fig. 14.12: An example of the sample weighting scheme using C5.0 when boosting

example, the predictor in the first split automatically has an importance measurement of 100 % since all samples are affected by this split. Other predictors may be used frequently in splits, but if the terminal nodes cover only a handful of training set samples, the importance scores may be close to zero. The same strategy is applied to rule-based models and boosted versions of the model.

C5.0 also has an option to *winnow* or remove predictors: an initial algorithm uncovers which predictors have a relationship with the outcome, and the final model is created from only the important predictors. To do this, the training set is randomly split in half and a tree is created for the purpose of evaluating the utility of the predictors (call this the "winnowing tree"). Two procedures characterize the importance of each predictor to the model:

1. Predictors are considered unimportant if they are not in any split in the winnowing tree.
2. The half of the training set samples not included to create the winnowing tree are used to estimate the error rate of the tree. The error rate is also estimated without each predictor and compared to the error rate when all the predictors are used. If the error rate improves without the predictor, it is deemed to be irrelevant and is provisionally removed.

Once the tentative list of non-informative predictors is established, C5.0 recreates the tree. If the error rate has become worse, the winnowing process is disabled and no predictors are excluded.

After the important predictors are established (if any), the conventional C5.0 training process is used with the full training set but with *only* the predictors that survived the winnowing procedure.

For example, C5.0 split the grant data into roughly equal parts, built a tree on one-half of the data, and used the second half to estimate the error rate to be about 14.6 %. When the predictor related to the number of student chief investigators was excluded, the error rate decreased slightly to 14.2 %. Given this, the number of student chief investigators was excluded from further consideration. Conversely, when the contract value band was excluded, the error rate rose to 24.8 %. This predictor was retained for subsequent C5.0 models.

Grant Data

For the grant data, several variations of the C5.0 model were evaluated:

- Single tree- and rule-based models
- Tree and rules with boosting (up to 100 iterations)
- All predictors and the winnowed set
- The two previously described approaches for handling categorical predictors

For the last set of model conditions, there was very little difference in the models. Figure 14.13 shows the ROC curves for the two methods of encoding the categorical predictors. The curves are almost identical.

The top panel of Fig. 14.13 shows the tuning profile for the C5.0 models with grouped categories. There was a slight decrease in performance when the winnowing algorithm was applied, although this is likely to be within the experimental noise of the data. Boosting clearly had a positive effect for these models and there is marginal improvement after about 50 iterations. Although single rules did worse than single trees, boosting showed the largest impact on the rule-based models, which ended up having superior performance. The optimal area under the ROC curve for this model was 0.942, the best seen among the models.

What predictors were used in the model? First, it may be helpful to know how often each predictor was used in a rule across all iterations of boosting. The vast majority of the predictors were used rarely; 99 % of the predictors were used in less than 0.71 % of the rules. The ten most frequent predictors were: contract value band (9.2 %), the number of unsuccessful grants by chief investigators (8.3 %), the number of successful grants by chief investigators (7.1 %), numeric day of the year (6.3 %), category code (6 %), Month (3.5 %), day of the week (3.1 %), sponsor code (2.8 %), the number of external chief investigators (1.1 %), and the number of C journal papers by chief investigators (0.9 %). As previously described, the predictors can be ranked by their importance values, as measured by the aggregate percentage of samples covered by the predictor. With boosting, this metric is less informative since the predictor in the first split is calculated to have 100 % importance. In this model, where a significant number of boosting iterations were used, 40 predictors had importance values of 100 %. This model only used 357 predictors (24 %).

14.7 Comparing Two Encodings of Categorical Predictors

All of the models fit in this chapter used two methods for encoding categorical predictors. Figure 14.14 shows the results of the holdout set for each model and approach. In general, large differences in the area under the ROC curve were not seen between the two encodings. J48 saw a loss in sensitivity with separate binary dummy variables, while stochastic gradient boosting and PART have losses in specificity when using grouped variables. In some cases, the encodings did have an effect on the complexity of the model. For the boosted trees, the choice of encodings resulted in very different tuning profiles, as demonstrated in Figs. 14.10 and 14.11. It is difficult to extrapolate these findings to other models and other data sets, and, for this reason, it may be worthwhile to try both encodings during the model training phase.

14.8 Computing

This section uses functions from the following packages: C50, caret, gbm, ipred, partykit, pROC, randomForest, and RWeka. This section also uses the same R objects created in Sect. 12.7 that contain the Grant Applications data (such as the data frame `training`).

In addition to the sets of dummy variables described in Sect. 12.7, several of the categorical predictors are encoded as R factors: `SponsorCode`, `ContractValueBand`, `CategoryCode`, and `Weekday`. When fitting models with independent categories for these predictors, the character vector `fullSet` is used. When treating the categorical predictors as a cohesive set, an alternate list of predictors is contained in the vector `factorPredictors`, which contains the factor versions of the relevant data. Additionally, the character string `factorForm` is an R formula created using all the predictors contained in `factorPredictors` (and is quite long).

A good deal of the syntax shown in this section is similar to other computing sections, especially the previous one related to regression trees. The focus here will be on the nuances of individual model functions and interpreting their output. Some code is shown to recreate the analyses in this chapter.

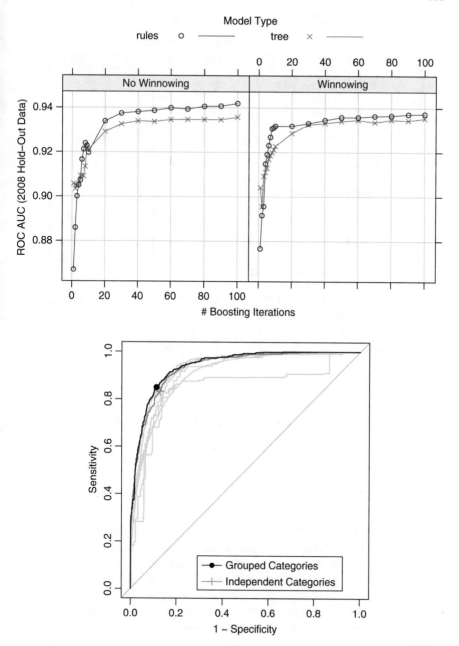

Fig. 14.13: *Top*: The parameter tuning profile for the C5.0 model using grouped categories. *Bottom*: The ROC curves for the boosted C5.0 models. The grouped and independent categories versions of the model are almost identical, with an area under the ROC curve of 0.942

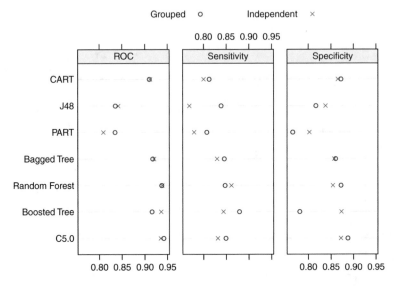

Fig. 14.14: The effect of different methods of representing categorical predictors in tree- and rule-based models. "Grouped" indicates that the categories for a predictor were treated as a cohesive set, while "independent" indicates that the categories were converted to independent dummy variables prior to modeling

A comprehensive program for the models shown is contained in the Chapter directory of the AppliedPredictiveModeling package.

Classification Trees

There are a number of R packages to build single classification trees. The primary package is rpart. As discussed in regression, the function takes only the formula method for specifying the exact form of the model.

There are a large number of predictors for the grant data, and, as previously mentioned, an R formula was created programmatically to model the classes for grouped categories. The following syntax fits a CART model to these predictors with our data splitting strategy:

```
> library(rpart)
> cartModel <- rpart(factorForm, data = training[pre2008,])
```

This automatically grows and prunes the tree using the internal cross-validation procedure. One important argument for classification is parms. Here, several alterations to the model training process can be declared, such as the prior probabilities of the outcome and the type of splitting (either the Gini coefficient or the information statistic). These values should be in a list.[6] See ?rpart for the details. Also, the control argument can customize the fitting procedure in terms of the numerical methods (such as the tree depth).

The model output is somewhat different than in regression trees. To show this we generate a smaller model with two predictors:

```
> rpart(Class ~ NumCI + Weekday, data = training[pre2008,])
  n= 6633

node), split, n, loss, yval, (yprob)
      * denotes terminal node

  1) root 6633 3200 unsuccessful (0.49 0.51)
    2) Weekday=Sun 223    0 successful (1.00 0.00) *
    3) Weekday=Fri,Mon,Sat,Thurs,Tues,Wed 6410 3000 unsuccessful (0.47 0.53)
      6) Weekday=Mon,Thurs,Tues 2342 1000 successful (0.57 0.43) *
      7) Weekday=Fri,Sat,Wed 4068 1700 unsuccessful (0.41 0.59) *
```

The output shows the split variable/value, along with how many samples were partitioned into the branch (223 for the second node in the output above). The majority class is also printed (successful for node 2) and the predicted class probabilities for samples that terminate in this node.

Prediction syntax is nearly the same as other models in R. The predict function, by default, produces probabilities for each class. Using predict(object, type = "class") generates a factor vector of the winning class.

The R implementation of C4.5 is in the RWeka package in a function called J48. The function also takes a model formula:

```
> library(RWeka)
> J48(Class ~ NumCI + Weekday, data = training[pre2008,])
J48 pruned tree
------------------

Weekday = Fri: unsuccessful (1422.0/542.0)
Weekday = Mon: successful (1089.0/455.0)
Weekday = Sat
|   NumCI <= 1: unsuccessful (1037.0/395.0)
|   NumCI > 1
|   |   NumCI <= 3: unsuccessful (378.0/185.0)
|   |   NumCI > 3: successful (61.0/26.0)
Weekday = Sun: successful (223.0)
Weekday = Thurs
|   NumCI <= 0: unsuccessful (47.0/21.0)
|   NumCI > 0: successful (520.0/220.0)
Weekday = Tues
|   NumCI <= 2
|   |   NumCI <= 0: unsuccessful (45.0/21.0)
|   |   NumCI > 0: successful (585.0/251.0)
```

---

[6] An example of this type of argument is shown in Sect. 16.9 where rpart is fit using with differential costs for different types of errors.

```
|   NumCI > 2: unsuccessful (56.0/22.0)
Weekday = Wed: unsuccessful (1170.0/521.0)

Number of Leaves  :     12

Size of the tree :  18
```

Recall that this implementation of C4.5 does not attempt to group the categories prior to pruning. The prediction function automatically produces the winning classes and the class probabilities can be obtained from predict(object, type = "prob").

When visualizing CART or J48 trees, the plot function from the partykit package can create detailed displays. The objects must be converted to the appropriate class with as.party, followed by the plot function.

A single C5.0 tree can be created from the C50 package:

```
> library(C50)
> C5tree <- C5.0(Class ~ NumCI + Weekday, data = training[pre2008,])
> C5tree

  Call:
  C5.0.formula(formula = Class ~ NumCI + Weekday, data
   = training[pre2008, ])

  Classification Tree
  Number of samples: 6633
  Number of predictors: 2

  Tree size: 2

  Non-standard options: attempt to group attributes
> summary(C5tree)

  Call:
  C5.0.formula(formula = Class ~ NumCI + Weekday, data
   = training[pre2008, ])


  C5.0 [Release 2.07 GPL Edition]      Thu Dec  6 13:53:14 2012
  -------------------------------

  Class specified by attribute `outcome'

  Read 6633 cases (3 attributes) from undefined.data

  Decision tree:

  Weekday in Tues,Mon,Thurs,Sun: successful (2565/1010)
  Weekday in Fri,Wed,Sat: unsuccessful (4068/1678)


  Evaluation on training data (6633 cases):

          Decision Tree
```

```
          ----------------
          Size      Errors

             2 2688(40.5%)    <<


          (a)   (b)     <-classified as
          ----  ----
          1555  1678    (a): class successful
          1010  2390    (b): class unsuccessful


     Attribute usage:

     100.00% Weekday

Time: 0.0 secs
```

Note that, unlike J48, this function is able to split the weekday values from groups of values. The control function for this model (C5.0Control) turns this feature off (subset = FALSE). Other options are available here, such as winnowing and the confidence factor for splitting. Like J48, the default prediction function produces classes and type = "prob" produces the probabilities.

There are wrappers for these models using the **caret** function train. For example, to fit the grouped category model for CART, we used:

```
> set.seed(476)
> rpartGrouped <- train(x = training[,factorPredictors],
+                       y = training$Class,
+                       method = "rpart",
+                       tuneLength = 30,
+                       metric = "ROC",
+                       trControl = ctrl)
```

Recall that the ctrl object specifies which data are in the holdout set and what performance measures should be calculated (e.g., sensitivity, specificity, and the area under the ROC curve). The model codes for J48 and C5.0 trees are J48 and C5.0Tree, respectively. The main differences here between train and the original model function are a unified interface to the models and the ability to tune the models with alternative metrics, such as the area under the ROC curve.

Note that rpart, C5.0, and J48 use the formula method differently than most other functions. Usually, the formula method automatically decomposes any categorical predictors to a set of binary dummy variables. These functions respect the categorical nature of the data and treat these predictors as grouped sets of categories (unless the data are already converted to dummy variables). The train function follows the more common convention in R, which is to create dummy variables prior to modeling. This is the main reason the code snippet above is written with the non-formula method when invoking train.

Rules

There are several rule-based models in the **RWeka** package. The PART function creates models based on Frank and Witten (1998). Its syntax is similar to J48:

```
> PART(Class ~ NumCI + Weekday, data = training[pre2008,])
  PART decision list
  ------------------

  Weekday = Fri: unsuccessful (1422.0/542.0)

  Weekday = Sat AND
  NumCI <= 1: unsuccessful (1037.0/395.0)

  Weekday = Mon: successful (1089.0/455.0)

  Weekday = Thurs AND
  NumCI > 0: successful (520.0/220.0)

  Weekday = Wed: unsuccessful (1170.0/521.0)

  Weekday = Tues AND
  NumCI <= 2 AND
  NumCI > 0: successful (585.0/251.0)

  Weekday = Sat AND
  NumCI <= 3: unsuccessful (378.0/185.0)

  Weekday = Sun: successful (223.0)

  Weekday = Tues: unsuccessful (101.0/43.0)

  Weekday = Sat: successful (61.0/26.0)

  : unsuccessful (47.0/21.0)

  Number of Rules  :  11
```

Other **RWeka** functions for rules can be found on the help page ?Weka_classifier_rules.

C5.0 rules are created using the C5.0 function in the same manner as trees, but with the rules = TRUE option:

```
> C5rules <- C5.0(Class ~ NumCI + Weekday, data = training[pre2008,],
+                 rules = TRUE)
> C5rules

  Call:
  C5.0.formula(formula = Class ~ NumCI + Weekday, data
   = training[pre2008, ], rules = TRUE)

  Rule-Based Model
  Number of samples: 6633
```

```
Number of predictors: 2

Number of Rules: 2

Non-standard options: attempt to group attributes
> summary(C5rules)
Call:
C5.0.formula(formula = Class ~ NumCI + Weekday, data
 = training[pre2008, ], rules = TRUE)


C5.0 [Release 2.07 GPL Edition]     Thu Dec  6 13:53:14 2012
-------------------------------

Class specified by attribute `outcome'

Read 6633 cases (3 attributes) from undefined.data

Rules:

Rule 1: (2565/1010, lift 1.2)
    Weekday in Tues, Mon, Thurs, Sun
    -> class successful   [0.606]

Rule 2: (4068/1678, lift 1.1)
    Weekday in Fri, Wed, Sat
    -> class unsuccessful  [0.587]

Default class: unsuccessful


Evaluation on training data (6633 cases):

          Rules
    ----------------
     No      Errors

      2 2688(40.5%)   <<


     (a)    (b)    <-classified as
    ----   ----
     1555   1678    (a): class successful
     1010   2390    (b): class unsuccessful


    Attribute usage:

    100.00% Weekday


Time: 0.0 secs
```

Prediction follows the same syntax as above. The variable importance scores for C5.0 trees and rules is calculated using the C5imp function or the varImp function in the caret package.

When working with the train function, model codes C5.0Rules and PART are available.

Other packages for single trees include party (conditional inference trees), tree (CART trees), oblique.tree (oblique trees), partDSA (for the model of Molinaro et al. (2010)), and evtree (trees developed using genetic algorithms). Another class of partitioning methods not discussed here called Logic Regression (Ruczinski et al. 2003) are implemented in several packages, including Logi-cReg.

Bagged Trees

The primary tree bagging package is ipred. The bagging function creates bagged versions of rpart trees using the formula method (another function, ipredbagg, uses the non-formula method). The syntax is familiar:

```
> bagging(Class ~ Weekday + NumCI, data = training[pre2008,])
```

The argument nbagg controls how many trees are in the ensemble (25 by default). The default for the standard predict method is to determine the winning class and type = "prob" will produce the probabilities.

Another function in the caret package, called bag, creates bag models more generally (i.e., models other than trees).

Random Forest

The R port of the original random forest program is contained in the randomForest package and its basic syntax is identical to the regression tree code shown on p. 215. The default value of $m_{try} \approx \sqrt{p}$ is different than in regression. One option, cutoff, is specific to classification and controls the voting cutoff(s) for determining the winning class from the ensemble of trees. This particular option is also available when using random forest's predict function.

The model takes the formula and non-formula syntax. In either case, any categorical predictors encoded as R factor variables are treated as a group. The predict syntax defaults to generating the winning class, but the type argument allows for predicting other quantities such as the class probabilities (type = "prob") or the actual vote counts type = "votes".

A basic example for the grant data, with output, is:

```
> library(randomForest)
> randomForest(Class ~ NumCI + Weekday, data = training[pre2008,])
  Call:
    randomForest(formula = Class ~ NumCI + Weekday, data = training[pre2008, ])
                    Type of random forest: classification
                          Number of trees: 500
  No. of variables tried at each split: 1

          OOB estimate of  error rate: 40.06%
  Confusion matrix:
                 successful unsuccessful class.error
  successful          1455         1778   0.5499536
  unsuccessful         879         2521   0.2585294
```

Since only two predictors are included, only a single predictor is randomly selected at each split.

The function prints the out-of-bag error estimate, as well as the analogous confusion matrix. Out-of-bag estimates of the sensitivity and the false positive rate (i.e., 1—specificity) are shown under the column class.error.

The model code for tuning a random forest model with train is "rf".

Other random forests functions are cforest (in the party package), obliqueRF (forests from oblique trees in the obliqueRF package), rFerns (for the random fern model of Ozuysal et al. (2010) in the rFerns package), and RRF (regularized random forest models in the RRF package).

Boosted Trees

The primary boosted tree package in R is gbm, which implements stochastic gradient boosting. The primary difference between boosting regression and classification trees is the choice of the distribution of the data. The gbm function can only accommodate two class problems and using distribution = "bernoulli" is an appropriate choice here. Another option is distribution = "adaboost" to replicate the loss function used by that methodology.

One complication when using gbm for classification is that it expects that the outcome is coded as 0/1. An example of a simple model for the grant data would be

```
> library(gbm)
> forGBM <- training
> forGBM$Class <- ifelse(forGBM$Class == "successful", 1, 0)
> gbmModel <- gbm(Class ~ NumCI + Weekday,
+                 data = forGBM[pre2008,],
+                 distribution = "bernoulli",
+                 interaction.depth = 9,
+                 n.trees = 1400,
+                 shrinkage = 0.01,
+                 ## The function produces copious amounts
```

```
+                        ## of output by default.
+                        verbose = FALSE)
```

The prediction function for this model does not predict the winning class. Using `predict(gbmModel, type = "response")` will calculate the class probability for the class encoded as a 1 (in our example, a successful grant was encoded as a 1). This can be converted to a factor variable with the winning class:

```
> gbmPred <- predict(gbmModel,
+                     newdata = head(training[-pre2008,]),
+                     type = "response",
+                     ## The number of trees must be
+                     ## explicitly set
+                     n.trees = 1400)
> gbmPred
  [1] 0.5697346 0.5688882 0.5688882 0.5688882 0.5697346 0.5688882
> gbmClass <- ifelse(gbmPred > .5, "successful", "unsuccessful")
> gbmClass <- factor(gbmClass, levels = levels(training$Class))
> gbmClass
  [1] successful successful successful successful successful successful
Levels: successful unsuccessful
```

Fitting this model with `train` simplifies the process considerably. For example, a factor variable can be used as the outcome format (`train` automatically does the conversion). When predicting the winning class, a factor is produced. If the class probabilities are required, then specify `predict(object, type = "prob")` (`train`'s prediction function automatically uses the number of trees that were found to be optimal during model tuning).

The original AdaBoost algorithm is available in the **ada** package. Another function for boosting trees is `blackboost` in the **mboost** package. This package also contains functions for boosting other types of models (such as logistic regression) as does the **bst** package.

To train boosted versions of **C5.0**, the `trials` argument is used (with values between 1 and 100).

```
> library(C50)
> C5Boost <- C5.0(Class ~ NumCI + Weekday, data = training[pre2008,],
+                  trials = 10)
> C5Boost

Call:
C5.0.formula(formula = Class ~ NumCI + Weekday, data
 = training[pre2008, ], trials = 10)

Classification Tree
Number of samples: 6633
Number of predictors: 2

Number of boosting iterations: 10 requested;  6 used due to early stopping
Average tree size: 2.5

Non-standard options: attempt to group attributes
```

By default, the algorithm has internal tests that assess whether the boosting is effective and will halt the model training when it diagnoses that it is no longer effective (note the message that ten iterations were requested but only six were used due to early stopping). This feature can be negated using C5.0Control(earlyStopping = FALSE).

These models can be tuned by train using method values of gbm, ada, or C5.0.

Exercises

14.1. Variable importance for the bagging, random forests, and boosting has been computed for both the independent categories and the factor model predictors. The top 16 important predictors for each method and predictor set are presented in Fig. 14.15.

(a) Within each modeling technique, which factors are in common between the independent category and factor models?

(b) How do these results compare with the most prolific predictors found in the PART model results discussed in Sect. 14.2?

14.2. For the churn data described in Exercise 12.3:

(a) Fit a few basic trees to the training set. Should the area code be encoded as independent dummy variables or as a grouped set of values?

(b) Does bagging improve the performance of the trees? What about boosting?

(c) Apply rule-based models to the data. How is the performance? Do the rules make any sense?

(d) Use lift charts to compare tree or rule models to the best techniques from previous chapters.

14.3. Exercise 12.1 gives a detailed description of the hepatic injury data set, where the primary scientific objective for these data is to construct a model to predict hepatic injury status. Recall that random forests can be performed with CART trees or conditional inference trees. Start R and use these commands to load the data:

```
> library(AppliedPredictiveModeling)
> data(hepatic)
```

(a) Fit a random forest model using both CART trees and conditional inference trees to the chemistry predictors, using the Kappa statistic as the metric as follows:

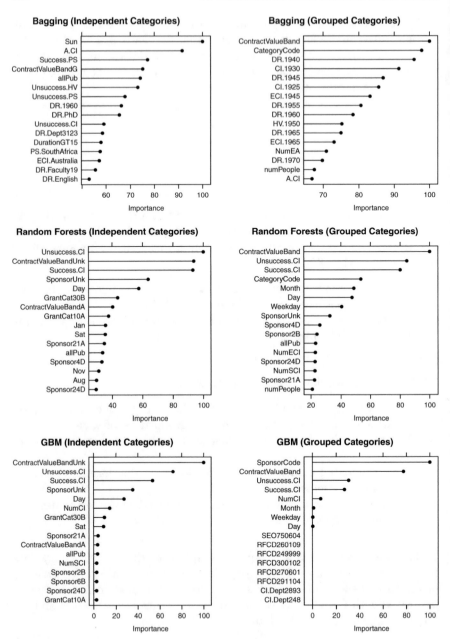

Fig. 14.15: A comparison of variable importance for the ensemble methods of bagging, random forests, and boosting for both the independent categories and grouped categories predictors

```
> library(caret)
> set.seed(714)
> indx <- createFolds(injury, returnTrain = TRUE)
> ctrl <- trainControl(method = "cv", index = indx)
> mtryValues <- c(5, 10, 25, 50, 75, 100)
> rfCART <- train(chem, injury,
+                  method = "rf",
+                  metric = "Kappa",
+                  ntree = 1000,
+                  tuneGrid = data.frame(.mtry = mtryValues))
> rfcForest <- train(chem, injury,
+                      method = "cforest",
+                      metric = "Kappa",
+                      tuneGrid = data.frame(.mtry = mtryValues))
```

Which model has better performance, and what are the corresponding tuning parameters?

(b) Use the following syntax to obtain the computation time for each model:

```
> rfCART$times$everything
> rfcForest$times$everything
```

Which model takes less computation time? Given the trade-off between performance and computation time, which model do you prefer?

(c) Use the following syntax to obtain the variable importance for the top ten predictors for each model:

```
> varImp(rfCART)
> varImp(rfcForest)
```

Are there noticeable differences in variable importance between the top ten predictors for each model? Explain possible reasons for the differences.

Chapter 15
A Summary of Grant Application Models

The previous three chapters used a variety of different philosophies and techniques to predict grant-funding success. In general, we believe that it is prudent to evaluate a number of different models for each data set since it is difficult to know which will do well *a priori* with any degree of certainty.

Before comparing models, recall that the data splitting process used the pre-2008 grants to tune the model, and, once final parameters were determined, the entire training set (which consisted of a fraction of the 2008 grants) was used to fit the model. The test set of 518, not yet used in our analyses, consisted completely of year 2008 grants. As discussed in Sect. 12.1, the performance on the test set is likely to be better than the results generated in the tuning process since the final model parameters were based on some 2008 information.

Figure 15.1 shows a visualization of the area under the ROC curve for the final models with the two data sets. Each point in the plot is for a particular model from the last three chapters. The correlation between the two estimates is high (0.96), although the tuning holdout set was more pessimistic than the test set. On average, the test set was 0.029 units larger. Again, this small but reproducible difference is likely due to the fact that the test set predictions were produced from a model built with some 2008 information, and these estimates are probably more relevant to predicting more recent grants. An important point is that, despite differences between the holdout and test set performance, model performance rankings are nearly the same regardless of the data splitting process (see Table 15.1).

Figure 15.2 shows the area under the ROC curves for each model, estimated using the test set grants. The bars represent 95 % confidence intervals that were derived using the bootstrap (Robin et al. 2011). These estimates of uncertainty help in two ways. First, the intervals give the consumers of the model an understanding about how good or bad the model may be. The interval quantifies the variation in the model but is also reflective of the data. For example, smaller test sets or noise (or mislabeling) in the response (see Sect. 20.2) can lead to wider intervals. In this way, the confidence

M. Kuhn and K. Johnson, *Applied Predictive Modeling*,
DOI 10.1007/978-1-4614-6849-3_15,
© Springer Science+Business Media New York 2013

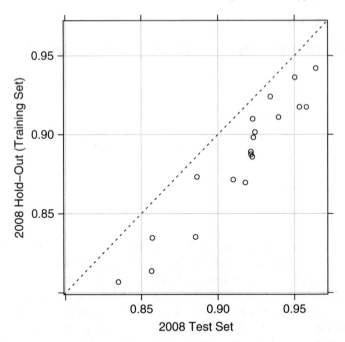

Fig. 15.1: A comparison of the year 2008 holdout areas under the ROC curve and the AUC values that result from evaluating the test set. Each point represents a model estimated in the last three chapters

interval helps gauge the weight of evidence available when comparing models. The second benefit of the confidence intervals is to facilitate trade-offs between models. If the confidence intervals for two models significantly overlap, this is an indication of (statistical) equivalence between the two and might provide a reason to favor the less complex or more interpretable model.

Finally, before comparing models, we echo the comment made in Sect. 14.7: the relative effectiveness of the models for these data cannot be used to extrapolate to other situations. A low-ranking model for these data may beat out others on a different data set. Any conclusions derived from these analyses should be considered "forward-looking statements" and should be taken with a grain of salt.

Across the models, which predictors had the largest effects?[1] In many of the models, the historical success and failure rates for the chief investigator played a large role in predicting grant outcomes ("nothing succeeds like

---

[1] As previously noted, more formal statistical methods are much better at making inferential statements on the importance of the predictors than variable importance measures.

Table 15.1: Ranked model performance across the 2008 holdout (training set) and the 2008 test set

Model	Holdout set	Test set
C5.0	1	1
Boosted tree	2	4
Bagged tree	4	3
Random forest	5	2
FDA	3	6
Neural networks	6	5
Sparse LDA	8	7
glmnet	7	9
SVM (polynomial)	9	8
CART	12	10
LDA	10	12
MDA	11	11
Logistic regression	14	14
Nearest shrunken centroids	13	15
PLS	15	13
J48	16	16
PART	17	17
Naive Bayes	18	18
KNN	19	19

The methods have similar ROC curve rankings between the two sets (rank correlation of the area under the curve: 0.96)

success"). Informative missingness seemed to occur in these data; unknown values of the contract value band and sponsor code were heavily used in many models. This itself is a likely surrogate or signal for some other piece of information. Similarly, why was there a strong seasonal effect such that grants in late December and early January (see Table 12.1 and Figs. 12.3 and 13.8) were likely to be more successful? In this case, it may be difficult to tell if increased success was due to the investigators that submit grants during this time or if the improvement was due to the grant reviewers. Finally, grants with category code 30B were associated with decreased success rates. Understanding this trend would help add another piece to the puzzle for those interested in improving success rates.

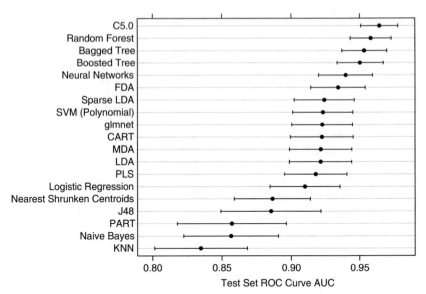

Fig. 15.2: A plot of the test set ROC curve AUCs and their associated 95 % confidence intervals

Chapter 16
Remedies for Severe Class Imbalance

When modeling discrete classes, the relative frequencies of the classes can have a significant impact on the effectiveness of the model. An imbalance occurs when one or more classes have very low proportions in the training data as compared to the other classes. Imbalance can be present in any data set or application, and hence, the practitioner should be aware of the implications of modeling this type of data.

Here are a few practical settings where class imbalance often occurs:

- Online advertising: An advertisement is presented to a viewer which creates an *impression*. The *click through rate* is the number of times an ad was clicked on divided by the total number of impressions and tends to be very low (Richardson et al. 2007 cite a rate less than 2.4%).
- Pharmaceutical research: High-throughput screening is an experimental technique where large numbers of molecules (10000s) are rapidly evaluated for biological activity. Usually only a few molecules show high activity; therefore, the frequency of interesting compounds is low.
- Insurance claims: Artis et al. (2002) investigated auto insurance damage claims in Spain between the years of 1993 and 1996. Of claims undergoing auditing, the rate of fraud was estimated to be approximately 22 %.

This chapter discusses the impact of class imbalance on performances measures, methodologies for post-processing model predictions, and predictive models that can mitigate the issue during training. However, before proceeding, we will describe another case study which we will use to illustrate the various approaches to addressing class imbalance.

16.1 Case Study: Predicting Caravan Policy Ownership

A data set generated by the computational intelligence and learning (CoIL) research network is used to illustrate methods for combatting class imbalances. The 2000 CoIL Challenge was to predict whether customers would purchase

M. Kuhn and K. Johnson, *Applied Predictive Modeling*,
DOI 10.1007/978-1-4614-6849-3_16,
© Springer Science+Business Media New York 2013

caravan insurance[1]; Van Der Putten and Van Someren (2004) discuss these data, the challenge, and some of the solutions to the problem. Our discussion of these data is limited to illustrating the effect of class imbalances.

The outcome, whether the costumer purchased caravan insurance, is highly unbalanced with only 6 % of customers having purchased policies. The predictors in the data set consisted of:

- Customer subtype designation, such as "Traditional Families" or "Affluent Young Families." There were 39 unique values, although many of the subtypes comprise less than 5 % of the customers.
- Demographic factors, such as religion, education level, social class, income, and 38 others. The values of the predictors were derived from data at the zip code level, so customers residing in the same zip code will have the same values for these attributes.[2]
- Product ownership information, such as the number of (or the contribution to) policies of various types.

In all there were 85 predictors. Many of the categorical predictors had 10 or more levels and the count-based predictors tended to be fairly sparse (i.e., few nonzero values).

To demonstrate different methodologies with these data, stratified random sampling (where the strata was the response variable) was used to create three different data sets:

- A training set of customers ($n = 6877$) that will be used to estimate model parameters, tuning models, etc.
- A small *evaluation* set of customers ($n = 983$) that will be used for developing post-processing techniques, such as alternative probability cutoffs
- A customer test set ($n = 1962$) that is solely used for final evaluations of the models

The rate of customers with caravan policies in each of these data sets was roughly the same across all three data sets (6 %, 5.9 %, and 6 %, respectively).

16.2 The Effect of Class Imbalance

To begin, three predictive models were used to model the data: random forest, a flexible discriminant analysis model (with MARS hinge functions), and logistic regression. To tune the models, 10-fold cross-validation was used; each holdout sample contained roughly 687 customers, which should provide

---

[1] We would like to thank Peter van der Putten for permission to use these data.

[2] Giving all customers within the same zip code the same values for the predictors implies that there is unseen noise within the predictors. The implications of predictor set noise are discussed in Sect. 20.3.

Table 16.1: Results for three predictive models using the evaluation set

Model	Accuracy	Kappa	Sensitivity	Specificity	ROC AUC
Random forest	93.5	0.091	6.78	99.0	0.757
FDA (MARS)	93.8	0.024	1.69	99.7	0.754
Logistic regression	93.9	0.027	1.69	99.8	0.727

reasonable estimates of uncertainty. To choose the optimal model, the area under the receiver operating characteristic (ROC) curve was optimized.[3]

The random forest model used 1500 trees in the forest and was tuned over 5 values of the m_{try} parameter (Sect. 8.5); the final model had an optimal m_{try} value of 126. The FDA model used first-degree features and was tuned over 25 values for the number of retained terms. The resampling process determined that 13 model terms was appropriate. Logistic regression utilized a simple additive model (i.e., no interactions or nonlinear terms) with a reduced predictor set (many near-zero variance predictors were removed so that the model resulted in a stable solution).

A number of different performance metrics were estimated including: overall accuracy, Kappa, area under the ROC curve, sensitivity, and specificity (where a purchased policy was defined as the "event" of interest). All models predicted the samples in the evaluation data set and yielded very similar results, as shown in Table 16.1. In each model, any patterns that were useful for predicting the outcome were overwhelmed by the large percentage of customers with no caravan insurance. In fact, none of the models predicted more than 13 customers on the evaluation set as having insurance, despite 59 customers with insurance in the evaluation set. The implication of these results is that the models achieve good specificity (since almost every customer is predicted no insurance) but have poor sensitivity.

The imbalance also had a severe effect on the predicted class probabilities. In the random forest model, for example, 82 % of the customers have a predicted probability of having insurance of 10 % or less. This highly left-skewed predicted probability distribution also occurs for the other two models.

Figure 16.1 shows the lift plots and ROC curves for the evaluation set. The lift curves are very similar and can be used to determine how many individuals would need to be contacted in order to capture a specific percent of those who might purchase the policy. For example, to find about 60 % of those with policies using the random forest model, around 30 % of the population would need to be sampled. The ROC curves show considerable overlap and does not differentiate the models.

---

[3] The results of the tuning process are summarized here. The full details of the process can be found in the Chapters directory of the AppliedPredictiveModeling package and in the Computing section of this chapter.

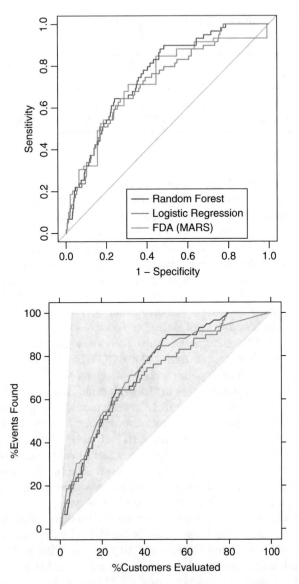

Fig. 16.1: *Top*: Evaluation set ROC curves for each of the three baseline models. *Bottom*: The corresponding lift plots

In this figure, there is a strong similarity between the lift and ROC curves. When classes are more balanced, lift plots and ROC curves are not this similar; rather, the similarity we see in Fig. 16.1 is due to class imbalance. In general, this is not the case but is an artifact of the severe class imbalance. When the classes are more balanced, the curves are unlikely to have similar patterns. For example, the maximum area on the lift curve is bounded by the event rate in the data (as shown with the grey background area in the loft plot) while the ROC curve has no such limitation.

The remaining sections discuss other strategies for overcoming class imbalances. The next section discusses how model tuning can be used to increase the sensitivity of the minority class while Sect. 16.4 demonstrates how alternative probability cutoffs can be derived from the data to improve the error rate on the minority class. This amounts to post-processing the model predictions to redefine the class predictions. Modifications of case weights and prior probabilities are also discussed. Another section examines how the training data can be altered to mitigate the class imbalance prior to model training. The last approach described in Sect. 16.6 demonstrates how, for some models, the model training process can be altered to emphasize the accuracy of the model for the less frequent class(es). In this case, the estimated model parameters are being modified instead of post-processing the model output.

16.3 Model Tuning

The simplest approach to counteracting the negative effects of class imbalance is to tune the model to maximize the accuracy of the minority class(es). For insurance prediction, tuning the model to maximize the sensitivity may help desensitize the training process to the high percentage of data without caravan policies in the training set. The random forest model that was tuned for these data did not show a meaningful trend in sensitivity across the tuning parameter. The FDA model did show a trend; as the number of model terms was increased, there was a rise in sensitivity from effectively 0 % for very simple models to 5.4 % when 16 terms were retained. This minor improvement in sensitivity comes at virtually no cost to specificity. Given that the increase in sensitivity is not high enough to be considered acceptable, this approach to solving the problem is not effective for this particular data set. The use of model tuning for this purpose is revisited in Sect. 16.8.

16.4 Alternate Cutoffs

When there are two possible outcome categories, another method for increasing the prediction accuracy of the minority class samples is to determine alternative cutoffs for the predicted probabilities which effectively changes the definition of a predicted event. The most straightforward approach is to use the ROC curve since it calculates the sensitivity and specificity across a continuum of cutoffs. Using this curve, an appropriate balance between sensitivity and specificity can be determined.

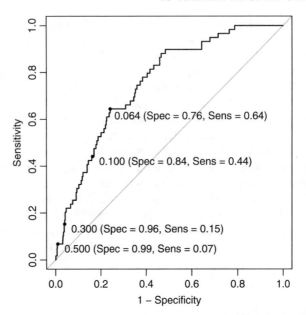

Fig. 16.2: The random forest ROC curve for predicting the classes using the evaluation set. The number on the left represents the probability cutoff, and the numbers in the parentheses are the specificity and sensitivity, respectively. Several possible probability cutoffs are used, including the threshold geometrically closest to the perfect model (0.064)

Figure 16.2 shows the ROC curve for the random forest model based on the evaluation set. Several cutoffs are shown on the curve and it is apparent that decreasing the cutoff for the probability of responding increases the sensitivity (at the expense of the specificity). There may be situations where the sensitivity/specificity trade-off can be accomplished without severely compromising the accuracy of the majority class (which, of course, depends on the context of the problem).

Several techniques exist for determining a new cutoff. First, if there is a particular target that must be met for the sensitivity or specificity, this point can be found on the ROC curve and the corresponding cutoff can be determined. Another approach is to find the point on the ROC curve that is closest (i.e., the shortest distance) to the perfect model (with 100 % sensitivity and 100 % specificity), which is associated with the upper left corner of the plot. In Fig. 16.2, a cutoff value of 0.064 would be the closest to the perfect model. Another approach for determining the cutoff uses Youden's J index (see Sect. 11.2), which measures the proportion of correctly predicted samples for both the event and nonevent groups. This index can be computed for each cutoff that is used to create the ROC curve. The cutoff associated with the largest value of the Youden index may also show superior performance relative

Table 16.2: Confusion matrices for the test set for random forests using the default and alternate cutoffs

| | 0.50 Cutoff | | 0.064 Cutoff | |
	Insurance	no insurance	Insurance	no insurance
Insurance	11	19	71	441
Noinsurance	105	1827	45	1,405

to the default 50 % value. For the random forest ROC curve, the cutoff that maximizes the Youden index (0.021) is similar to the point closest to the optimal model.

Using the evaluation set, the predicted sensitivity for the new cutoff of 0.064 is 64.4 %, which is a significant improvement over the value generated by the default cutoff. The consequence of the new cutoff is that the specificity is estimated to drop from 99 % to 75.9 %. This may or may not be acceptable based on the context of how the model will be used.

In our analysis, the alternate cutoff for the model was not derived from the training or test sets. It is important, especially for small samples sizes, to use an independent data set to derive the cutoff. If the training set predictions are used, there is likely a large optimistic bias in the class probabilities that will lead to inaccurate assessments of the sensitivity and specificity. If the test set is used, it is no longer an unbiased source to judge model performance. For example, Ewald (2006) found via simulation that *post hoc* derivation of cutoffs can exaggerate test set performance.

Table 16.2 contains confusion matrices derived from the test set for the default and alternate cutoffs. Predictions from the 50 % cutoff echo the same performances values shown by cross-validation (a sensitivity of 9.5 % and a specificity of 99 %). For the new cutoff, the test set sensitivity was found to be 61.2 % while the specificity was calculated to be 76.1 %. This estimated difference in sensitivity between the two data sets (64.4 % and 61.2 %) is likely due to the high uncertainty in the metric (which itself is a result of the low frequency of events). These two values may be equivalent given the experimental noise. To reiterate, this cutoff resulted from being as close as possible to the optimal model. This may not be applicable in the context of other problems in which case alternative trade-offs can be made.

It is worth noting that the core of the model has not changed. The same model parameters are being used. Changing the cutoff to increase the sensitivity does not increase the overall predictive effectiveness of the model. The main impact that an alternative cutoff has is to make trade-offs between particular types of errors. For example, in a confusion matrix, alternate cutoffs can only move samples up and down rows of the matrix (as opposed to moving them from the off-diagonals to the diagonals). In other words, using an alternative cutoff does not induce further separation between the classes.

Figure 16.2 and Table 16.2 demonstrate why, for many classification problems, comparing models on the basis of the default sensitivity and specificity may be misleading. Since a better cutoff may be possible, an analysis of the ROC curve can lead to improvements in these metrics. As shown in Fig. 16.2, a class imbalance can further exacerbate this issue. Consequently, performance metrics that are independent of probability cutoffs (such as the area under the ROC curve) are likely to produce more meaningful contrasts between models. However, some predictive models only produce discrete class predictions.

16.5 Adjusting Prior Probabilities

Some models use prior probabilities, such as naïve Bayes and discriminant analysis classifiers. Unless specified manually, these models typically derive the value of the priors from the training data. Weiss and Provost (2001a) suggest that priors that reflect the natural class imbalance will materially bias predictions to the majority class. Using more balanced priors or a balanced training set may help deal with a class imbalance.

For the insurance data, the priors are 6 % and 94 % for the insured and uninsured, respectively. The predicted probability of having insurance is extremely left-skewed for all three models and adjusting the priors can shift the probability distribution away from small values. For example, new priors of 60 % for the insured and 40 % for the uninsured in the FDA model increase the probability of having insurance significantly. With the default cutoff, predictions from the new model have a sensitivity of 71.2 % and a specificity of 66.9 % on the test set. However, the new class probabilities did not change the rankings of the customers in the test set and the model has the same area under the ROC curve as the previous FDA model. Like the previous tactics for an alternative cutoff, this strategy did not change the model but allows for different trade-offs between sensitivity and specificity.

16.6 Unequal Case Weights

Many of the predictive models for classification have the ability to use *case weights* where each individual data point can be given more emphasis in the model training phase. For example, previously discussed boosting approaches to classification and regression trees are able to create a sequence of models, each of which apply different case weights at each iteration.

One approach to rebalancing the training set would be to increase the weights for the samples in the minority classes (Ting 2002). For many models, this can be interpreted as having identical duplicate data points with the exact same predictor values. Logistic regression, for example, can utilize case weights in this way. This procedure for dealing with a class imbalance is related to the sampling methods discussed in next section.

16.7 Sampling Methods

When there is *a priori* knowledge of a class imbalance, one straightforward method to reduce its impact on model training is to select a training set sample to have roughly equal event rates during the initial data collection (see, e.g., Artis et al. 2002). Basically, instead of having the model deal with the imbalance, we can attempt to balance the class frequencies. Taking this approach eliminates the fundamental imbalance issue that plagues model training. However, if the training set is sampled to be balanced, the test set should be sampled to be more consistent with the state of nature and should reflect the imbalance so that honest estimates of future performance can be computed.

If an *a priori* sampling approach is not possible, then there are *post hoc* sampling approaches that can help attenuate the effects of the imbalance during model training. Two general *post hoc* approaches are *down-sampling* and *up-sampling* the data. Up-sampling is any technique that simulates or imputes additional data points to improve balance across classes, while down-sampling refers to any technique that reduces the number of samples to improve the balance across classes.

Ling and Li (1998) provide one approach to up-sampling in which cases from the minority classes are sampled with replacement until each class has approximately the same number. For the insurance data, the training set contained 6466 non-policy and 411 insured customers. If we keep the original minority class data, adding 6055 random samples (with replacement) would bring the minority class equal to the majority. In doing this, some minority class samples may show up in the training set with a fairly high frequency while each sample in the majority class has a single realization in the data. This is very similar to the case weight approach shown in an earlier section, with varying weights per case.

Down-sampling selects data points from the majority class so that the majority class is roughly the same size as the minority class(es). There are several approaches to down-sampling. First, a basic approach is to randomly sample the majority classes so that all classes have approximately the same size. Another approach would be to take a bootstrap sample across all cases such that the classes are balanced in the bootstrap set. The advantage of this approach is that the bootstrap selection can be run many times so that the estimate

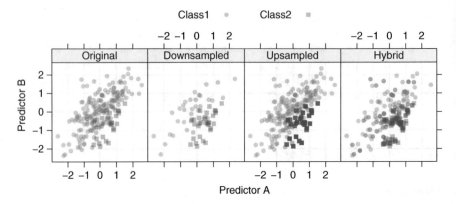

Fig. 16.3: *From left to right*: The original simulated data set and realizations of a down-sampled version, an up-sampled version, and sampling using SMOTE where the cases are sampled and/or imputed

of variation can be obtained about the down-sampling. One implementation of random forests can inherently down-sample by controlling the bootstrap sampling process within a *stratification variable*. If class is used as the stratification variable, then bootstrap samples will be created that are roughly the same size per class. These *internally down-sampled* versions of the training set are then used to construct trees in the ensemble.

The synthetic minority over-sampling technique (SMOTE), described by Chawla et al. (2002), is a data sampling procedure that uses both up-sampling and down-sampling, depending on the class, and has three operational parameters: the amount of up-sampling, the amount of down-sampling, and the number of neighbors that are used to impute new cases. To up-sample for the minority class, SMOTE synthesizes new cases. To do this, a data point is randomly selected from the minority class and its K-nearest neighbors (KNNs) are determined. Chawla et al. (2002) used five neighbors in their analyses, but different values can be used depending on the data. The new synthetic data point is a random combination of the predictors of the randomly selected data point and its neighbors. While the SMOTE algorithm adds new samples to the minority class via up-sampling, it also can down-sample cases from the majority class via random sampling in order to help balance the training set.

Figure 16.3 shows an example of sampling methods using a simulated data set. The original data contain 168 samples from the first class and 32 from the second (a 5.2:1 ratio). The down-sampled version of the data reduced the total sample size to 64 cases evenly split between the classes. The up-sampled data have 336 cases, now with 168 events. The SMOTE version of the data has a smaller imbalance (with a 1.3:1 ratio) resulting from having 128 samples from the first class and 96 from the second. For the most part, the new synthetic samples are very similar to other cases in the data set; the space encompassing the minority class is being filled in instead of expanding.

It should be noted that when using modified versions of the training set, resampled estimates of model performance can become biased. For example, if the data are up-sampled, resampling procedures are likely to have the same sample in the cases that are used to build the model as well as the holdout set, leading to optimistic results. Despite this, resampling methods can still be effective at tuning the models.

A substantial amount of research has been conducted on the effectiveness of using sampling procedures to combat skewed class distributions, most notably Weiss and Provost (2001b), Batista et al. (2004), Van Hulse et al. (2007), Burez and Van den Poel (2009), and Jeatrakul et al. (2010). These and other publications show that, in many cases, sampling can mitigate the issues caused by an imbalance, but there is no clear winner among the various approaches. Also, many modeling techniques react differently to sampling, further complicating the idea of a simple guideline for which procedure to use.

These sampling methods were applied to the random forest models for the insurance data using the same tuning process as the original model. The ROC and lift curves for the evaluation set for three of the random forest models are shown in Fig. 16.4. Numerical summaries of the models are contained in Table 16.3. In this table, the area under the ROC curve is calculated for the evaluation and test sets. Using the evaluation set, new cutoffs for each model were derived by choosing the point on the ROC curve closest to the optimal model. The sensitivity and specificity values in this table are the result of applying those cutoffs to the test set.

The results show that the up-sampling procedure had no real improvement on the area under the curve. SMOTE showed an improvement in the evaluation set, but the increase in the area under the ROC curve was not reproduced in the larger test set. Simple down-sampling of the data also had a limited effect on model performance. However, down-sampling inside the random forest model had robust areas under the ROC curve in both data sets. This may be due to using independent realizations of the majority class in each tree. In all, the results are mixed. While these improvements are modest, the sampling approaches have the benefit of enabling better trade-offs between sensitivity and specificity (unlike modifying cutoffs or prior probabilities).

16.8 Cost-Sensitive Training

Instead of optimizing the typical performance measure, such as accuracy or impurity, some models can alternatively optimize a cost or loss function that differentially weights specific types of errors. For example, it may be

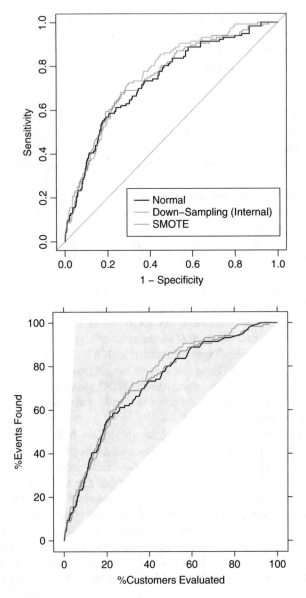

Fig. 16.4: *Top*: Test set ROC curves for three of the random forest models. *Bottom*: The corresponding lift plots

appropriate to believe that misclassifying true events (false negatives) is X times as costly as incorrectly predicting nonevents (false positives). Incorporation of specific costs during model training may bias the model towards less

Table 16.3: A summary of results for random forest models with different sampling mechanisms

Method	Evaluation	Test		
	ROC	ROC	Sensitivity	Specificity
Original	0.757	0.738	64.4	75.9
Down-sampling	0.794	0.730	81.4	70.3
Down-sampling (Internal)	0.792	0.764	78.0	68.3
Up-sampling	0.755	0.739	71.2	68.1
SMOTE	0.767	0.747	78.0	67.7

The test set sensitivity and specificity values were determined using the optimal cutoff derived from the evaluation set ROC curve

frequent classes. Unlike using alternative cutoffs, unequal costs can affect the model parameters and thus have the potential to make true improvements to the classifier.

For support vector machine (SVM) models, costs can be associated with specific classes (as opposed to specific types of errors). Recall that these models control the complexity using a cost function that increases the penalty if samples are on the incorrect side of the current class boundary. For class imbalances, unequal costs for each class can adjust the parameters to increase or decrease the sensitivity of the model to particular classes (Veropoulos et al. 1999). Note that this approach is different from one where specific types of errors can have differential costs. For support vector machines (SVMs), the entire class can be given increased importance. For two classes, these two approaches are similar.

One consequence of this approach is that class probabilities cannot be generated for the model, at least in the available implementation. Therefore we cannot calculate an ROC curve and must use a different performance metric. Instead we will now use the Kappa statistic, sensitivity, and specificity to evaluate the impact of weighted classes.

For the SVM model, we analyzed both weighted and unweighted models and compared the performance results. When tuning the models, the unweighted SVM required a fairly large value of the SVM cost parameter (256) to optimize the Kappa statistic. Applying the unweighted model to the test set, the Kappa statistic was 0.121 with a corresponding sensitivity of 15.5% and a specificity of 95.7%. The effects of weights ranging between 6 and 25 were assessed for the training set (using resampling) and the evaluation set. Across the range of weights selected, the model performance based on the Kappa statistic, sensitivity, and specificity was very similar for the two data sets (Fig. 16.5). Smaller weights optimize Kappa, while moderate to

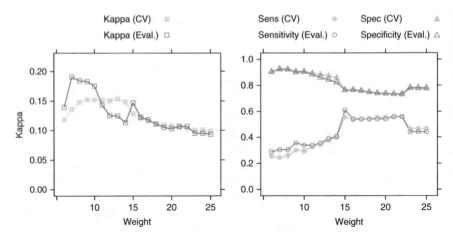

Fig. 16.5: Tuning results for class weighted support vector machine determined with cross-validation and the evaluation set

high weights optimize sensitivity. Using the plot, the modeler can decide the appropriate operating characteristics of the model for the problem at hand as described in Sect. 16.3.

Additionally, many classification tree models can incorporate differential costs, including CART and C5.0 trees. The potential cost of a prediction takes into account several factors (Johnson and Wichern 2001):

- The cost of the particular mistake
- The probability of making that mistake
- The prior probability of the classes

To illustrate how costs can be taken into account, let's return to the concepts and notation used in Sect. 13.6. Let π_i represent the prior probability of a sample being in class i, and let $Pr[j|i]$ be the probability of mistakenly predicting a class i sample as class j. For a two-class problem, the total probability of misclassifying a sample is then

$$Pr[2|1]\pi_1 + Pr[1|2]\pi_2$$

In practice we rarely know $Pr[j|i]$ and instead use the estimated probability of the ith class, p_i.

For two classes, the above equation can then be transformed into a rule for classifying a sample into class 1, if

$$\frac{p_1}{p_2} > \frac{\pi_2}{\pi_1}$$

This rule assumes that the costs of misclassifying a class 1 sample into class 2 or a class 2 sample into class 1 are equal. Conveniently, the equation can easily be extended to consider the scenario where the costs are not the same.

Let $C(j|i)$ be the cost of mistakenly predicting a class i sample as class j. Then the total expected cost of misclassification is

$$\text{Expected Cost} = C(2|1)Pr[2|1]\pi_1 + C(1|2)Pr[1|2]\pi_2$$

And the revised decision boundary for classifying a sample into class 1 is

$$\frac{p_1}{p_2} > \left(\frac{C(1|2)}{C(2|1)}\right)\left(\frac{\pi_2}{\pi_1}\right)$$

For equal priors, the first class is only predicted when the probability ratio is greater than the cost ratio. If $p_1 = 0.75$ and $p_2 = 0.25$, the second class would be predicted when the cost of erroneously predicting that class is greater than 3.0.

Once the cost of each type of error is specified, CART trees can incorporate them into the training process. Breiman et al. (1984) discuss the use of a generalized Gini criterion:

$$\begin{aligned}Gini^* &= C(1|2)p_1(1 - p_1) + C(2|1)p_2(1 - p_2)\\ &= [C(1|2) + C(2|1)]\, p_1 p_2\end{aligned}$$

where p_1 and p_2 are the observed class probabilities induced by the split. Note that, in this case, the two costs are lumped together when using the Gini index to determine splits. With more than two classes, this same issue arises. As such, using costs with the Gini matrix symmetrizes the costs, that is to say, that the costs $C(i|j)$ and $C(j|i)$ are averaged when determining the overall costs for the split. Breiman et al. (1984) also point out that, in some cases, using unequal costs becomes equivalent to using modified prior probabilities. In their examples, they note that the cost-sensitive trees tended to be smaller than the trees produced by the nominal procedure. The reasoning was that in the growing phase, the tree greedily splits to produce accurate predictions of the potentially costly errors but does not work as hard to be accurate on the remaining errors that have lower costs.

For trees (and rules), the predicted class probabilities (or confidence values) might not be consistent with the discrete class predictions when unequal costs are used. The final class prediction for a sample is a function of the class probability *and* the cost structure. As previously shown, the class probabilities in the terminal node may be appreciably favoring the one class but also have a large expected cost. For this reason, there is a disconnect between the confidence values and the predicted class. Therefore, simple class probabilities (or confidence values) should not be used under these circumstances.

To demonstrate cost-sensitive model training, single CART trees were fit to the data with equal costs as well as a wide range of cost values (2.5 to 30) similar to the previous weighted SVM model. Figure 16.6 shows the results for the training and evaluation sets. The trends shown in these plots are noisy (due to the instability of CART trees), especially for sensitivity, which has

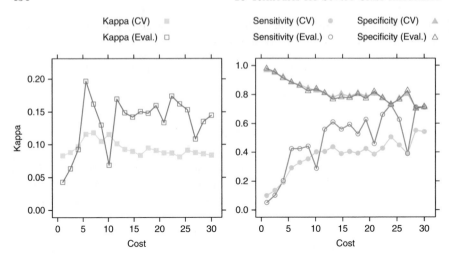

Fig. 16.6: Tuning results for cost-sensitive classification tree models determined with cross-validation and the evaluation set

the smaller sample size. The resampled estimate of the sensitivity was more pessimistic than the evaluation set. The results show that the sensitivity and specificity of the model start to converge at high cost values.

Recall that C5.0 does not use the Gini criterion for splitting. With costs, the previous formula is used and assumes equal prior probabilities[4]:

$$\text{Expected Cost} = C(2|1)p_1 + C(1|2)p_2$$

Again, new samples are predicted as the class associated with the lowest expected cost.

For C5.0, the models were tuned over the model type (i.e., trees or rules) and the number of boosting iterations. Figure 16.7 shows the patterns for cost-sensitive learning with false-negative costs ranging from 5 to 50. Like the SVM analysis, the curves are consistent between the training and evaluation sets. To optimize the concordance via the Kappa statistic, smaller costs values are required and to increase the sensitivity, moderate to large costs are needed. Here, there is a clear trade-off between sensitivity and specificity, but the sensitivity appears to plateau for costs values greater than 25 or 30.

---

[4] An alternative view of this criterion is that the priors are to be included into the appropriate cost value.

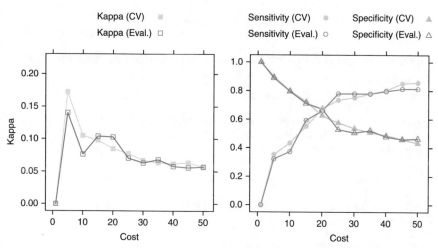

Fig. 16.7: Performance profiles for C5.0 models using cost-sensitive learning

16.9 Computing

This section uses the following packages: caret, C50, DMwR, DWD, kernlab, pROC, and rpart.

The insurance data are contained in the DWD package, and can be loaded as follows:

```
> library(DWD)
> data(ticdata)
```

There are several factor variables in the data set. Many of the factor levels have nonstandard characters, such as "%," commas, and other values. When these are converted to dummy variable columns, the values violate the rules for naming new variables. To bypass this issue, we re-encode the names to be more simplistic:

```
> recodeLevels <- function(x)
+   {
+     x <- as.numeric(x)
+     ## Add zeros to the text version:
+     x <- gsub(" ", "0",format(as.numeric(x)))
+     factor(x)
+   }
> ## Find which columns are regular factors or ordered factors
> isOrdered <- unlist(lapply(ticdata, is.ordered))
> isFactor <- unlist(lapply(ticdata, is.factor))
> convertCols <- names(isOrdered)[isOrdered | isFactor]

> for(i in convertCols) ticdata[,i] <- recodeLevels(ticdata[,i])
> ## Make the level 'insurance' the first factor level
```

```
> ticdata$CARAVAN <- factor(as.character(ticdata$CARAVAN),
+                           levels = rev(levels(ticdata$CARAVAN)))
```

The training and test sets were created using stratified random sampling:

```
> library(caret)
> ## First, split the training set off
> set.seed(156)
> split1 <- createDataPartition(ticdata$CARAVAN, p = .7)[[1]]
> other    <- ticdata[-split1,]
> training <- ticdata[ split1,]

> ## Now create the evaluation and test sets
> set.seed(934)
> split2 <- createDataPartition(other$CARAVAN, p = 1/3)[[1]]
> evaluation  <- other[ split2,]
> testing     <- other[-split2,]
> ## Determine the predictor names
> predictors <- names(training)[names(training) != "CARAVAN"]
```

Dummy variables are useful for several models being fit in this section. The `randomForest` function has a limitation that all factor predictors must not have more than 32 levels. The customer type predictor has 39 levels, so a predictor set of dummy variables is created for this and other models using the `model.matrix` function:

```
> ## The first column is the intercept, which is eliminated:
> trainingInd   <- data.frame(model.matrix(CARAVAN ~ .,
+                                           data = training))[,-1]
> evaluationInd <- data.frame(model.matrix(CARAVAN ~ .,
+                                           data = evaluation))[,-1]
> testingInd    <- data.frame(model.matrix(CARAVAN ~ .,
+                                           data = testing))[,-1]

> ## Add the outcome back into the data set
> trainingInd$CARAVAN   <- training$CARAVAN
> evaluationInd$CARAVAN <- evaluation$CARAVAN
> testingInd$CARAVAN    <- testing$CARAVAN

> ## Determine a predictor set without highly sparse and unbalanced
    distributions:
> isNZV <- nearZeroVar(trainingInd)
> noNZVSet <- names(trainingInd)[-isNZV]
```

To obtain different performance measures, two wrapper functions were created:

```
> ## For accuracy, Kappa, the area under the ROC curve,
> ## sensitivity and specificity:
> fiveStats <- function(...) c(twoClassSummary(...),
+                              defaultSummary(...))
> ## Everything but the area under the ROC curve:
> fourStats <- function (data, lev = levels(data$obs), model = NULL)
```

```
+ {
+
+    accKapp <- postResample(data[, "pred"], data[, "obs"])
+    out <- c(accKapp,
+                sensitivity(data[, "pred"], data[, "obs"], lev[1]),
+                specificity(data[, "pred"], data[, "obs"], lev[2]))
+    names(out)[3:4] <- c("Sens", "Spec")
+    out
+ }
```

Two control functions are developed for situations when class probabilities can be created and when they cannot:

```
> ctrl <- trainControl(method = "cv",
+                        classProbs = TRUE,
+                        summaryFunction = fiveStats,
+                        verboseIter = TRUE)
> ctrlNoProb <- ctrl
> ctrlNoProb$summaryFunction <- fourStats
> ctrlNoProb$classProbs <- FALSE
```

The three baseline models were fit with the syntax:

```
> set.seed(1410)
> rfFit <- train(CARAVAN ~ ., data = trainingInd,
+                method = "rf",
+                trControl = ctrl,
+                ntree = 1500,
+                tuneLength = 5,
+                metric = "ROC")

> set.seed(1410)
> lrFit <- train(CARAVAN ~ .,
+                data = trainingInd[, noNZVSet],
+                method = "glm",
+                trControl = ctrl,
+                metric = "ROC")

> set.seed(1401)
> fdaFit <- train(CARAVAN ~ ., data = training,
+                method = "fda",
+                tuneGrid = data.frame(.degree = 1, .nprune = 1:25),
+                metric = "ROC",
+                trControl = ctrl)
>
```

A data frame is used to house the predictions from different models:

```
> evalResults <- data.frame(CARAVAN = evaluation$CARAVAN)
> evalResults$RF <- predict(rfFit,
+                        newdata = evaluationInd,
+                        type = "prob")[,1]
```

```
> evalResults$FDA <- predict(fdaFit,
+                              newdata = evaluation[, predictors],
+                              type = "prob")[,1]
> evalResults$LogReg <- predict(lrFit,
+                                 newdata = valuationInd[, noNZVSet],
+                                 type = "prob")[,1]
```

The ROC and lift curves are created from these objects. For example:

```
> library(pROC)
> rfROC <- roc(evalResults$CARAVAN, evalResults$RF,
+              levels = rev(levels(evalResults$CARAVAN)))
> ## Create labels for the models:
> labs <- c(RF = "Random Forest", LogReg = "Logistic Regression",
+           FDA = "FDA (MARS)")
> lift1 <- lift(CARAVAN ~ RF + LogReg + FDA, data = evalResults,
+               labels = labs)

> rfROC

  Call:
  roc.default(response = evalResults$CARAVAN, predictor = evalResults$RF,
      levels = rev(levels(evalResults$CARAVAN)))

  Data: evalResults$RF in 924 controls (evalResults$CARAVAN noinsurance) <
        59 cases (evalResults$CARAVAN insurance).
  Area under the curve: 0.7569
> lift1

  Call:
  lift.formula(x = CARAVAN ~ RF + LogReg + FDA, data = evalResults,
               labels = labs)

  Models: Random Forest, Logistic Regression, FDA (MARS)
  Event: insurance (6%)
```

To plot the curves:

```
> plot(rfROC, legacy.axes = TRUE)
> xyplot(lift1,
+        ylab = "%Events Found", xlab =  "%Customers Evaluated",
+        lwd = 2, type = "l")
```

Alternate Cutoffs

After the ROC curve has been created, there are several functions in the pROC package that can be used to investigate possible cutoffs. The coords function returns the points on the ROC curve as well as deriving new cutoffs. The main arguments are x, which specifies what should be returned. A value of x = "all" will return the coordinates for the curve and their associated cutoffs. A value of "best" will derive a new cutoff. Using x = "best" in conjunction with the best.method (either "youden" or "closest.topleft") can be informative:

```
> rfThresh <- coords(rfROC, x = "best", best.method = "closest.topleft")
> rfThresh
    threshold specificity sensitivity
   0.06433333  0.75865801  0.64406780
```

For this, new predicted classes can be calculated:

```
> newValue <- factor(ifelse(evalResults$RF > rfThresh,
+                           "insurance", "noinsurance"),
+                    levels = levels(evalResults$CARAVAN))
```

Sampling Methods

The caret package has two functions, downSample and upSample, that readjust
the class frequencies. Each takes arguments for the predictors (called x) and
the outcome class (y). Both functions return a data frame with the sampled
version of the training set:

```
> set.seed(1103)
> upSampledTrain <- upSample(x = training[,predictors],
+                            y = training$CARAVAN,
+                            ## keep the class variable name the same:
+                            yname = "CARAVAN")
> dim(training)
  [1] 6877    86
> dim(upSampledTrain)
  [1] 12932    86
> table(upSampledTrain$CARAVAN)

   insurance noinsurance
        6466        6466
```

The down-sampling function has the same syntax. A function for SMOTE
can be found in the DMwR package. It takes a model formula as an input,
along with parameters (such as the amount of over- and under-sampling and
the number of neighbors). The basic syntax is

```
> library(DMwR)
> set.seed(1103)
> smoteTrain <- SMOTE(CARAVAN ~ ., data = training)
> dim(smoteTrain)
  [1] 2877    86
> table(smoteTrain$CARAVAN)

   insurance noinsurance
        1233        1644
```

These data sets can be used as inputs into the previous modeling code.

Cost-Sensitive Training

Class-weighted SVMs can be created using the kernlab package. The syntax for the ksvm function is the same as previous descriptions, but the class.weights argument is put to use. The train function has similar syntax:

```
> library(kernlab)
> ## We will train over a large cost range, so we precompute the sigma
> ## parameter and make a custom tuning grid:
> set.seed(1157)
> sigma <- sigest(CARAVAN ~ ., data = trainingInd[, noNZVSet], frac = .75)
> names(sigma) <- NULL
> svmGrid <- data.frame(.sigma = sigma[2],
+                       .C = 2^seq(-6, 1, length = 15))
> ## Class probabilities cannot be generated with class weights, so
> ## use the control object 'ctrlNoProb' to avoid estimating the
> ## ROC curve.
> set.seed(1401)
> SVMwts <- train(CARAVAN ~ .,
+                 data = trainingInd[, noNZVSet],
+                 method = "svmRadial",
+                 tuneGrid = svmGrid,
+                 preProc = c("center", "scale"),
+                 class.weights = c(insurance = 18, noinsurance = 1),
+                 metric = "Sens",
+                 trControl = ctrlNoProb)


> SVMwts

  6877 samples
   203 predictors
     2 classes: 'insurance', 'noinsurance'

Pre-processing: centered, scaled
Resampling: Cross-Validation (10-fold)

Summary of sample sizes: 6189, 6190, 6190, 6189, 6189, 6189, ...

Resampling results across tuning parameters:

  C        Accuracy  Kappa   Sens   Spec
  0.0156   0.557     0.0682  0.742  0.545
  0.0221   0.614     0.0806  0.691  0.609
  0.0312   0.637     0.0864  0.669  0.635
  0.0442   0.644     0.0883  0.662  0.643
  0.0625   0.658     0.0939  0.657  0.658
  0.0884   0.672     0.0958  0.633  0.674
  0.125    0.684     0.101   0.625  0.688
  0.177    0.7       0.106   0.611  0.705
  0.25     0.711     0.108   0.591  0.719
  0.354    0.724     0.111   0.572  0.734
  0.5      0.737     0.112   0.543  0.75
```

```
0.707    0.75      0.109   0.506  0.765
1        0.765     0.104   0.46   0.785
1.41     0.776     0.097   0.416  0.799
2        0.791     0.102   0.394  0.817
```

```
Tuning parameter 'sigma' was held constant at a value of 0.00245
Sens was used to select the optimal model using  the largest value.
The final values used for the model were C = 0.0156 and sigma = 0.00245.
```

(The standard deviation columns were not shown to save space) Prediction uses the same syntax as unweighted models.

For cost-sensitive CART models, the rpart package is used with the parms argument, which is a list of fitting options. One option, loss, can take a matrix of costs:

```
> costMatrix <- matrix(c(0, 1, 20, 0), ncol = 2)
> rownames(costMatrix) <- levels(training$CARAVAN)
> colnames(costMatrix) <- levels(training$CARAVAN)
> costMatrix
```

```
            insurance noinsurance
insurance          0          20
noinsurance        1           0
```

Here, there would be a 20-fold higher cost of a false negative than a false positive. To fit the model:

```
> library(rpart)
> set.seed(1401)
> cartCosts <- train(x = training[,predictors],
+                    y = training$CARAVAN,
+                    method = "rpart",
+                    trControl = ctrlNoProb,
+                    metric = "Kappa",
+                    tuneLength = 10,
+                    parms = list(loss = costMatrix))
```

Similar to the support vector machine model, the syntax for generating class predictions is the same as the nominal model. However, any class probabilities generated from this model may not match the predicted classes (which are a function of the cost and the probabilities).

C5.0 has similar syntax to rpart by taking a cost matrix, although this function uses the transpose of the cost matrix structure used by rpart:

```
> c5Matrix <- matrix(c(0, 20, 1, 0), ncol = 2)
> rownames(c5Matrix) <- levels(training$CARAVAN)
> colnames(c5Matrix) <- levels(training$CARAVAN)
> c5Matrix
```

```
            insurance noinsurance
insurance          0           1
noinsurance       20           0
```

```
> library(C50)
> set.seed(1401)
> C5Cost <- train(x = training[, predictors],
+                 y = training$CARAVAN,
+                 method = "C5.0",
+                 metric = "Kappa",
+                 cost = c5Matrix,
+                 trControl = ctrlNoProb)
```

When employing costs, the predict function for this model only produces the discrete classes (i.e. no probabilities).

Exercises

16.1. The "adult" data set at the UCI Machine Learning Repository is derived from census records.[5] In these data, the goal is to predict whether a person's income was large (defined in 1994 as more than $50K) or small. The predictors include educational level, type of job (e.g., never worked, and local government), capital gains/losses, work hours per week, native country, and so on.[6] After filtering out data where the outcome class is unknown, there were 48842 records remaining. The majority of the data were associated with a small income level (75.9 %).

The data are contained in the arules package and the appropriate version can be loaded using data(AdultUCI).

(a) Load the data and investigate the predictors in terms of their distributions and potential correlations.
(b) Determine an appropriate split of the data.
(c) Build several classification models for these data. Do the results favor the small income class?
(d) Is there a good trade-off that can be made between the sensitivity and specificity?
(e) Use sampling methods to improve the model fit.
(f) Do cost-sensitive models help performance?

16.2. The direct marketing data of Larose (2006, Chap. 7) discussed previously in Chap. 11 can be found at the author's web site.[7] The goal of the

---

[5] These data are first referenced in Kohavi (1996). A description of the data collection and a summary of the results of previous models can be found at the UCI Machine Learning Repository (http://archive.ics.uci.edu/ml/machine-learning-databases/adult/adult.names).

[6] Another attribute, "fnlwgt," only contains information about the data collection process and should not be used as a predictor.

[7] http://www.dataminingconsultant.com/data.

analysis was to predict which customers would respond to a promotional opportunity via mail.

Of the 65220 customers in the data set, 16.6 % responded to the promotion. The predictors in the data set include

- Spending habits, in aggregate and broken down by month and frequently visited store locations
- The types of products purchased
- Time between visits
- Historical promotion response rates
- Predefined customer cluster memberships

Larose (2006) discussed the class imbalance for this problem and demonstrates several techniques to achieve effective results.

(a) Read the data into R, conduct exploratory analyses, and determine the best method for encoding the predictors.
(b) Determine an appropriate split of the data and build several classification models for these data.
(c) Construct lift plots to understand a possible strategy regarding how many customers should be contacted to capture an estimated 60 % of responders.
(d) Use sampling methods with several models. Do these models have better lift charts, and can they be used to contact fewer customers to achieve a 60 % response rate (of those who were given the promotion)?

Chapter 17
Case Study: Job Scheduling

High-performance computing (HPC) environments are used by many technology and research organizations to facilitate large-scale computations. An HPC environment usually consists of numerous "compute nodes" networked to handle computations required by the users. These can be structured in different ways, such as a network of many computers each with fewer processors, or a network of fewer computers with many processors. The amount of memory on each may vary from environment to environment and often is built based on a balance between available funds and the nature of the types of computations required by an institution.

A specific unit of computations (generally called a *job* here) can be launched by users for execution in the HPC environment. The issue is that, in many cases, a large number of programs are executed simultaneously and the environment has to manage these jobs in a way that returns the job results in the most efficient manner. This may be a complicated task. For example:

- There are times where the existing jobs outnumber the capacity of the environment. In these cases, some jobs will be required to stay pending prior to launch until the appropriate resources are available.
- The frequency of submissions by users may vary. If one user submits a large number of jobs at once, it may be undesirable for the system to let a single user consume the majority of resources at the expense of the other users.
- All compute jobs may not be treated equally. Higher priority projects may require more privileged access to the hardware resources. For example, jobs at a pharmaceutical company needed to support a time-sensitive regulatory submission may need to have a higher priority than jobs related to research-oriented tasks.

A common solution to this problem is to use a *job scheduler*—a software that prioritizes jobs for submissions, manages the computational resources, and initiates submitted jobs to maximize efficiency. The scheduler can enact a queuing system based on several factors such as resource requirements for

M. Kuhn and K. Johnson, *Applied Predictive Modeling*,
DOI 10.1007/978-1-4614-6849-3_17,
© Springer Science+Business Media New York 2013

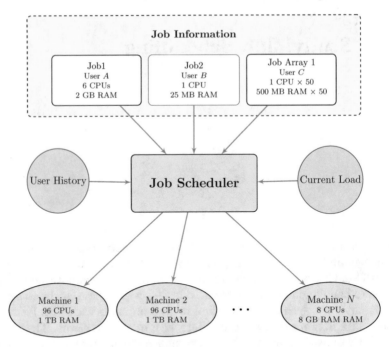

Fig. 17.1: A hypothetical example of a job scheduler in a high-performance computing environment

a job (e.g., number of processors required, memory requirements), project priority, and the current load of the environment. The scheduler may also consider the submission history of specific users when delegating jobs to computational resources.

Figure 17.1 shows a schematic of such a system. The top shows three hypothetical jobs that are submitted at the same time. The first two have a single set of computations each but have different requirements. For example, the first job could be a scientific computation that spreads the computations across multiple processors on the same physical machine. The second job may be a short database query that a scientist makes interactively from a web site. This job is expected to run quickly with low overhead. The third case represents a cohesive set of computations that are launched at once but correspond to a set of independent calculations (such as a simulation) that use the same program. This *job array* launches 50 independent calculations that can be run on different machines but should be managed and supervised as a single entity. Again the goal of the scheduler is to allocate these jobs to the system in a manner that maximizes efficiency.

The efficiency of the scheduler can be significantly affected by the amount and quality of job information that is known at the time of submission. This allows the scheduler to place the jobs on suitable machines at the appropriate time. For computations that are repeated a large number of times, it is straightforward to record information on existing jobs then make resource predictions on new jobs. For example, it may be helpful to predict the execution time or maximum memory requirements for a job at the time of submission. The requirements for such a prediction are that it be quick and accurate. However, the accuracy requirements should take into account the fact that prediction errors do not likely have the same impact on the environment's performance. For example, if the predicted amount of memory needed is severely underestimated, this could cause physical machine resources to be overburdened and may drastically affect all the jobs on that machine. The cost of this type of error should be high in order for the scheduler to avoid this problem. The converse problem is not true: overestimation of memory needs may cause abnormally low utilization of a hardware resource but will not critically affect existing jobs on the system. A cost should be assigned to this error, but likely not as high as the other type of error.

As an example, Pfizer runs a large number of jobs in its HPC environment. One class of jobs for characterizing compounds is run regularly, some of which can be computationally burdensome. Over a period of time, resource utilization information was logged about this class of jobs. Additionally, there are several task characteristics that can be collected at the time of job launch:

- Protocol: Several different analytical techniques, called *protocols*, can be used to calculate results for each compound. The protocols are coded as letters A through O; protocol J was used the most (22.8 % of all the jobs) while protocol K was rarely invoked (0.1 %).
- Number of compounds: The number of compounds processed by the job. This number varied wildly across the data.
- Number of input fields: Each task can process a number of different input fields in the data, depending on what the scientist would like to analyze. This predictor is also right skewed.
- Number of iterations: Each protocol can run for a pre-specified number of iterations. The default is 20 iterations, which occurs most frequently in these data.
- Pending job count: A count of how many jobs were pending at the time launch was recorded. This is meant to measure the workload of the environment at the time of the launch. All other things being equal, the number of pending jobs should not directly affect execution time of the jobs but may capture the amount of resources being used at the time. For these data, most jobs were launched at a time when there were available resources, so no jobs were pending. However, a minority of requests were made when the hardware was in high demand (thousands of jobs were already pending).
- Time of day: The time of day (Eastern Standard Time) that the job was launched (0 to 24). The distribution is multimodal, which reflects users coming online in three different time zones on two continents.
- Day of the week: The day of the week when the job was launched.

Execution time was recorded for each job. Time spent in pending or suspended states were not counted in these values. While the outcome is continuous in nature, the scheduler required a qualitative representation for this information. Jobs were required to be classified as either very fast (1 m or less), fast (1–5 m), moderate (5–30 m), or long (greater than 30 m). Most of the jobs fall into either the very fast category (51.1%) or the fast category (31.1%) while only 11.9% were classified as moderate and 6% were long.

The goal of this experiment is to predict the class of the jobs using the information given in Table 17.1. Clearly, the types of errors are not equal and there should be a greater penalty for classifying jobs as very short that are in fact long. Also, since the prediction equation will need to be implemented in software and quickly computed, models with simpler prediction equations are preferred.

Over the course of two years, changes were made to some of the hardware in the HPC environment. As a consequence, the same job run on two different vintages of hardware may produce different execution times. This has the effect of inflating the inherent variation in the execution times and can lead to potential mislabeling of the observed classes. While there is no way to handle this in the analysis, any model for classifying execution times should be revisited over time (on the assumption that new hardware will decrease execution time).

Before delving into model building, it is important to investigate the data. Prior to modeling, one would expect that the main drivers of the execution time would be the number of compounds, the number of tasks, and, which protocol is being executed. As an initial investigation, Fig. 17.2 shows the relationship between the protocols and the execution time classes using a *mosaic plot*. Here the widths of the boxes are indicative of the number of jobs run for the protocol (e.g., protocol J was run the most and K the least). To predict the slow jobs, one can see that only a few protocols produce long execution times. Others, such as protocol D, are more likely to be executed very quickly. Given these relationships, we might expect the protocol information to be potentially important to the model.

Figure 17.3 shows another visualization of the data using a *table plot*. Here, the data are ordered by the class then binned into 100 slices. Within each slice, the average value of the numeric predictors is determined. Similarly, the frequency distribution of the categorical predictors is determined. The results for each predictor are shown in columns so that the modeler can have a better understanding of how each predictor relates to the outcome. In the figure, we can see that:

- The jobs associated with a large number of compounds tend to be either large or moderate in execution time.
- Many of the jobs of moderate length were submitted when the number of pending jobs was very high. However, this trend does not reproduce itself in the very long jobs. Because of this, it would be important to

Table 17.1: Predictors for the job scheduler data

7 Variables   4331 Observations

Protocol
  n missing unique
4331   0   14

	A	C	D	E	F	G	H	I	J	K	L	M	N	O
Frequency	94	160	149	96	170	155	321	381	989	6	242	451	536	581
%	2	4	3	2	4	4	7	9	23	0	6	10	12	13

Compounds
  n missing unique Mean 0.05 0.10 0.25 0.50 0.75 0.90 0.95
4331   0   858 497.7 27   37   98 226 448 967 2512

lowest :   20   21   22   23   24
highest: 14087 14090 14091 14097 14103

InputFields
  n missing unique Mean 0.05 0.10 0.25 0.50 0.75 0.90 0.95
4331   0 1730 1537 26   48 134 426 991 4165 7594

lowest :   10   11   12   13   14
highest: 36021 45420 45628 55920 56671

Iterations
  n missing unique Mean 0.05 0.10 0.25 0.50 0.75 0.90 0.95
4331   0   11 29.24 10   20   20   20   20   50 100

	10	11	15	20	30	40	50	100	125	150	200
Frequency	272	9	2	3568	3	7	153	188	1	2	126
%	6	0	0	82	0	0	4	4	0	0	3

NumPending
  n missing unique Mean 0.05 0.10 0.25 0.50 0.75 0.90 0.95
4331   0   303 53.39 0.0 0.0 0.0 0.0 0.0 33.0 145.5

lowest :   0   1   2   3   4, highest: 3822 3870 3878 5547 5605

Hour
  n missing unique Mean 0.05 0.10   0.25   0.50   0.75   0.90   0.95
4331   0   924 13.73 7.025 9.333 10.900 14.017 16.600 18.250 19.658

lowest : 0.01667 0.03333 0.08333 0.10000 0.11667
highest: 23.20000 23.21667 23.35000 23.80000 23.98333

Day
  n missing unique
4331   0   7

	Mon	Tue	Wed	Thu	Fri	Sat	Sun
Frequency	692	900	903	720	923	32	161
%	16	21	21	17	21	1	4

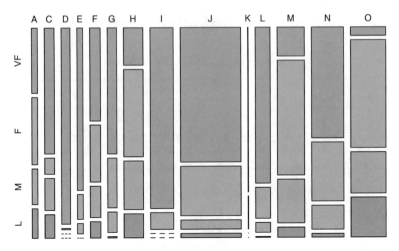

Fig. 17.2: A mosaic plot of the class frequencies for each protocol. The width of the boxes is determined by the number of jobs observed in the data set

prospectively validate this observation to make sure that it is not a fluke of this particular data set.

- When the number of iterations is large, the job tends to go long.

One shortcoming of this particular visualization is that it obscures the relationships between predictors. Correlation plots and scatter plot matrices are effective methods for finding these types of relationships.

Additionally, Fig. 17.4 shows scatter plots for the number of compounds versus the number of input fields by protocol. In these plots, the jobs are colored by class. For some cases, such as protocols A, C, D, H, I, and K, the number of compounds and fields appears to provide information to differentiate the classes. However, these relationships are class specific; the patterns for protocols I and K are different. Another interesting aspect of this analysis is that the correlation pattern between the number of compounds versus the number of input fields is protocol-specific. For example, there is very little correlation between the two predictors for some protocols (e.g., J, O) and a strong correlation in others (such as D, E, and H). These patterns might be important and are more likely to be discovered when the modeler looks at the actual data points.

17.1 Data Splitting and Model Strategy

There are 4331 samples available; 80% will be used for training the algorithms while the remainder will be used to evaluate the final candidate models. The data were split using stratified random sampling to preserve the class

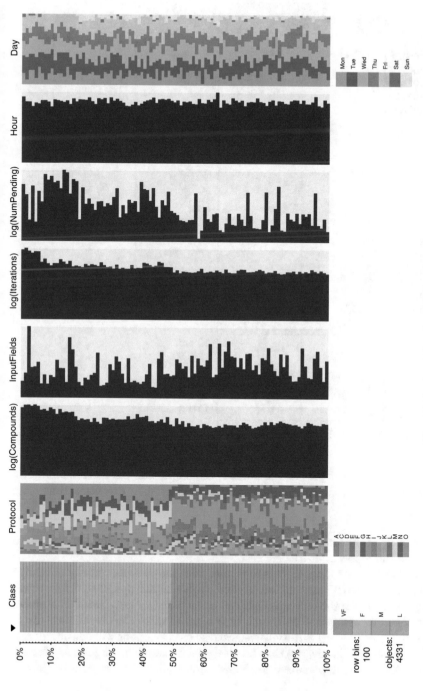

Fig. 17.3: A table plot of the data

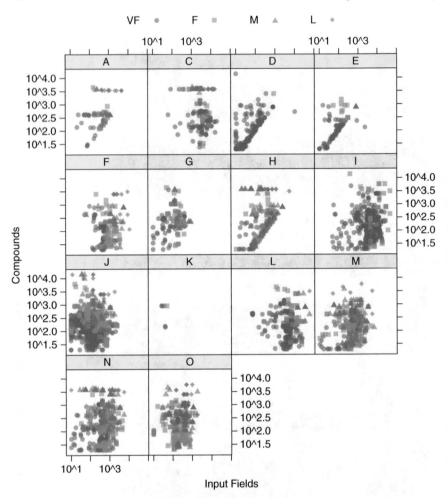

Fig. 17.4: A scatter plot of the number of compounds versus the number of fields for each protocol. The points are colored by their execution time class

distribution of the outcome. Five repeats of 10-fold cross–validation were used to tune the models.

Rather than creating models that maximize the overall accuracy or Kappa statistics, a custom cost function is used to give higher weight to errors where long and medium jobs are misclassified as fast or very fast. Table 17.2 shows how the costs associated with each type of error affect the overall measure of performance. The cost is heavily weighted so that long jobs will not be submitted to queues (or hardware) that are designed for small, quick jobs. Moderate-length jobs are also penalized for being misclassified as more efficient jobs.

Table 17.2: Cost structure used to optimize the model

	Observed Class			
	VF	F	M	L
VF	0	1	5	10
F	1	0	5	5
M	1	1	0	1
L	1	1	1	0

Longer jobs that are misclassified as fast are penalized more in this criterion

The best possible approach to model training is when this cost function is used to estimate the model parameters (see Sect. 16.8). A few tree-based models allow for this, but most of the models considered here do not.

A series of models were fit to the training set. The tuning parameter combination associated with the smallest average cost value was chosen for the final model and used in conjunction with the entire training set. The following models were investigated:

- Linear discriminant analysis: This model was created using the standard set of equations as well as with the penalized version that conducts feature selection during model training. Predictor subset sizes ranging from 2 to 112 were investigated in conjunction with several values of the ridge penalty: 0, 0.01, 0.1, 1 and 10.
- Partial least squares discriminant analysis: The PLS model was fit with the number of components ranging from 1 to 91.
- Neural networks: Models were fit with hidden units ranging from 1 to 19 and 5 weight decay values: 0, 0.001, 0.01, 0.1, and 0.5.
- Flexible discriminant analysis: First-degree MARS hinge functions were used and the number of retained terms was varied from 2 to 23.
- Support vector machines (SVMs): Two different models were fit with the radial basis function. One using equal weights per class and another where the moderate jobs were given a fivefold weight and long jobs were upweighted tenfold. In each case, the analytical calculations for estimating the RBF kernel function were used in conjunction with cost values ranging from 2^{-2} to 2^{12} in the log scale.
- Single CART trees: Similarly, the CART models were fit with equal costs per class and another where the costs mimic those in Table 17.2. In each case, the model was tuned over 20 values of the complexity parameter.
- Bagged CART trees: These models used 50 bagged CART trees with and without incorporating the cost structure.
- Random forests: The model used 2,000 trees in the forest and was tuned over 6 values of the tuning parameter.

- C5.0: This model was evaluated with tree- and rule-based models, with and without winnowing, with single models and with up to 100 iterations of boosting. An alternative version of this model was fit that utilized the cost structure shown in Table 17.2.

For this application, there is a bias towards models which are conducive to fast predictions. If the prediction equation(s) for the model can be easily encoded in software (such as a simple tree or neural network) or can be executed from a simple command-line interface (such as C5.0), the model is preferred over others.

17.2 Results

The model results are shown in Fig. 17.5 where box plots of the resampling estimates of the mean cost value are shown. The linear models, such as LDA and PLS, did not do well here. Feature selection did not help the linear discriminant model, but this may be due to that model's inability to handle nonlinear class boundaries. FDA also showed poor performance in terms of cost.

There is a cluster of models with average costs that are likely to be equivalent, mostly SVMs and the various tree ensemble methods. Using costs/weights had significant positive effects on the single CART tree and SVMs. Figure 17.6 shows the resampling profiles for these two models in

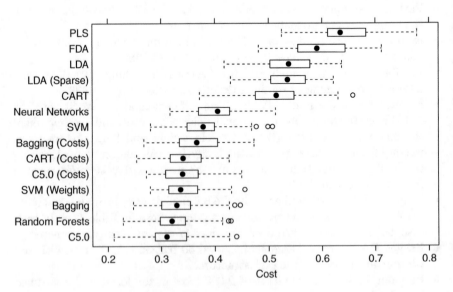

Fig. 17.5: Average cost resampling profiles for various models

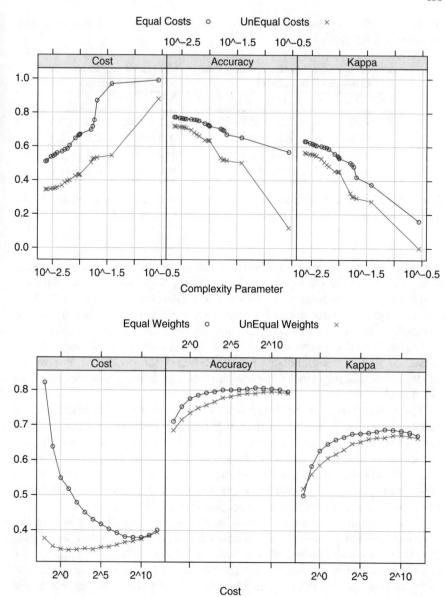

Fig. 17.6: The effect of incorporating the cost structure into the CART training process (*top*) and weights for support vector machines (*bottom*)

terms of their estimates of the cost, overall accuracy and Kappa statistic. The CART model results show that using the cost has a negative effect on accuracy and Kappa but naturally improved the cost estimates. No matter the metric, the tuning process would have picked the same CART model

Table 17.3: Resampled confusion matrices for the random forest and cost-sensitive CART models

	Cost-sensitive CART				Random forests			
	VF	F	M	L	VF	F	M	L
VF	157.0	24.6	2.0	0.2	164.7	18.0	1.3	0.2
F	10.3	43.2	3.1	0.2	11.9	83.7	11.5	1.8
M	9.6	38.3	34.5	5.8	0.2	5.5	27.4	1.8
L	0.0	1.7	1.6	14.6	0.0	0.6	0.9	17.0

Each value is the average number of jobs that occurred in that cell across the 50 holdout data sets. The columns are the true job classes

for final training. The support vector machine (SVM) results are somewhat different. Using class weights also had a slight negative effect on accuracy and Kappa, but the improvement in the estimated cost was significant. Also, the unweighted model would be optimized with a much higher SVM cost parameter (and thus more complex models) than the weighted version.

Oddly, the C5.0 model without costs did very well, but adding the cost structure to the tree-building process *increased* the estimated cost of the model. Also, bagging CART trees with costs had a small negative effect on the model

Trees clearly did well for these data, as did support vector machines and neural networks. Is there much of a difference between the top models? One approach to examining these results is to look at a confusion matrix generated across the resamples. Recall that for resampling, there were 50 hold–out sets that contained, on average, about 347 jobs. For each one of these hold–out sets, a confusion matrix was calculated and the average confusion matrix was calculated by averaging the cell frequencies.

Table 17.3 shows two such tables for the random forests model and the cost-sensitive CART model. For random forest, the average number of long jobs that were misclassified as very fast was 0.2 while the same value for the classification tree was 0.24. The CART tree shows very poor accuracy for the fast jobs compared to the random forest model. However, the opposite is true for moderately long jobs; random forest misclassified 72.56% of those jobs (on average), compared to 65.52% for the single tree. For long jobs, the single tree has a higher error rate than the ensemble method. How do these two models compare using the test set? The test set cost for random forest was 0.316 while the single classification trees had a average cost of 0.37. Table 17.4 shows the confusion matrices for the two models. The trends in the test set are very similar to the resampled estimates. The single tree does worse with fast and long jobs while random forests have issues predicting the moderately

Table 17.4: Test set confusion matrices for the random forest and cost-sensitive CART models

	Cost-sensitive CART				Random forests			
	VF	F	M	L	VF	F	M	L
VF	383	61	5	1	414	45	3	0
F	32	106	7	2	28	206	27	5
M	26	99	87	15	0	18	71	6
L	1	3	3	33	0	0	1	40

The columns are the true job classes

long jobs. In summary, the overall differences between the two models are not large.

17.3 Computing

The data are contained in the AppliedPredictiveModeling package. After loading the data, a training and test set were created:

```
> library(AppliedPredictiveModeling)
> data(schedulingData)
> set.seed(1104)
> inTrain <- createDataPartition(schedulingData$Class,
+                                p = .8,
+                                list = FALSE)
> schedulingData$NumPending <- schedulingData$NumPending + 1
> trainData <- schedulingData[ inTrain,]
> testData  <- schedulingData[-inTrain,]
```

Since the costs defined in Table 17.2 will be used to judge the models, functions were written to estimate this value from a set of observed and predicted classes:

```
> cost <- function(pred, obs)
+   {
+     isNA <- is.na(pred)
+     if(!all(isNA))
+       {
+         pred <- pred[!isNA]
+         obs <- obs[!isNA]
+         cost <- ifelse(pred == obs, 0, 1)
+         if(any(pred == "VF" & obs == "L"))
+           cost[pred == "L" & obs == "VF"] <- 10
+         if(any(pred == "F" & obs == "L"))
+           cost[pred == "F" & obs == "L"] <- 5
```

```
+           if(any(pred == "F" & obs == "M"))
+               cost[pred == "F" & obs == "M"] <- 5
+           if(any(pred == "VF" & obs == "M"))
+               cost[pred == "VF" & obs == "M"] <- 5
+           out <- mean(cost)
+         } else out <- NA
+       out
+     }
> costSummary <- function (data, lev = NULL, model = NULL)
+ {
+     if (is.character(data$obs))  data$obs <- factor(data$obs,
+         levels = lev)
+     c(postResample(data[, "pred"], data[, "obs"]),
+       Cost = cost(data[, "pred"], data[, "obs"]))
+ }
```

The latter function is used in the control object for future computations:

```
> ctrl <- trainControl(method = "repeatedcv", repeats = 5,
+                       summaryFunction = costSummary)
```

For the cost-sensitive tree models, a matrix representation of the costs was also created:

```
> costMatrix <- ifelse(diag(4) == 1, 0, 1)
> costMatrix[1,4] <- 10
> costMatrix[1,3] <- 5
> costMatrix[2,4] <- 5
> costMatrix[2,3] <- 5
> rownames(costMatrix) <- levels(trainData$Class)
> colnames(costMatrix) <- levels(trainData$Class)
> costMatrix
```

The tree-based methods did not use independent categories, but the other models require that the categorical predictors (e.g., protocol) are decomposed into dummy variables. A model formula was created that log transforms several of the predictors (given the skewness demonstrated in Table 17.1):

```
> modForm <- as.formula(Class ~ Protocol + log10(Compounds) +
+                       log10(InputFields)+ log10(Iterations) +
+                       log10(NumPending) + Hour + Day)
```

The specifics of the models fit to the data can be found in the Chapter directory of the AppliedPredictiveModeling package and follow similar syntax to the code shown in previous chapters. However, the cost-sensitive and weighted model function calls are

```
> ## Cost-Sensitive CART
> set.seed(857)
> rpFitCost <- train(x = trainData[, predictors],
+                     y = trainData$Class,
+                     method = "rpart",
+                     metric = "Cost",
+                     maximize = FALSE,
```

```
+                     tuneLength = 20,
+                     ## rpart structures the cost matrix so that
+                     ## the true classes are in rows, so we
+                     ## transpose the cost matrix
+                     parms =list(loss = t(costMatrix)),
+                     trControl = ctrl)

> ## Cost- Sensitive C5.0
> set.seed(857)
> c50Cost <- train(x = trainData[, predictors],
+                   y = trainData$Class,
+                   method = "C5.0",
+                   metric = "Cost",
+                   maximize = FALSE,
+                   costs = costMatrix,
+                   tuneGrid = expand.grid(.trials = c(1, (1:10)*10),
+                                          .model = "tree",
+                                          .winnow = c(TRUE, FALSE)),
+                   trControl = ctrl)

> ## Cost-Sensitive bagged trees
> rpCost <- function(x, y)
+   {
+     costMatrix <- ifelse(diag(4) == 1, 0, 1)
+     costMatrix[4, 1] <- 10
+     costMatrix[3, 1] <- 5
+     costMatrix[4, 2] <- 5
+     costMatrix[3, 2] <- 5
+     library(rpart)
+     tmp <- x
+     tmp$y <- y
+     rpart(y~.,
+           data = tmp,
+           control = rpart.control(cp = 0),
+           parms = list(loss = costMatrix))
+   }
> rpPredict <- function(object, x) predict(object, x)
> rpAgg <- function (x, type = "class")
+ {
+   pooled <- x[[1]] * NA
+   n <- nrow(pooled)
+   classes <- colnames(pooled)
+   for (i in 1:ncol(pooled))
+     {
+       tmp <- lapply(x, function(y, col) y[, col], col = i)
+       tmp <- do.call("rbind", tmp)
+       pooled[, i] <- apply(tmp, 2, median)
+     }
+   pooled <- apply(pooled, 1, function(x) x/sum(x))
+   if (n != nrow(pooled)) pooled <- t(pooled)
+   out <- factor(classes[apply(pooled, 1, which.max)],
+                 levels = classes)
```

```
+    out
+ }
> set.seed(857)
> rpCostBag <- train(trainData[, predictors],
+                    trainData$Class,
+                    "bag",
+                    B = 50,
+                    bagControl = bagControl(fit = rpCost,
+                                            predict = rpPredict,
+                                            aggregate = rpAgg,
+                                            downSample = FALSE),
+                    trControl = ctrl)
>


> ## Weighted SVM
> set.seed(857)
> svmRFitCost <- train(modForm, data = trainData,
+                      method = "svmRadial",
+                      metric = "Cost",
+                      maximize = FALSE,
+                      preProc = c("center", "scale"),
+                      class.weights = c(VF = 1, F = 1,
+                                        M = 5, L = 10),
+                      tuneLength = 15,
+                      trControl = ctrl)
```

The resampled versions of the confusion matrices were computed using the
confusionMatrix function on the objects produced by the train function, such
as

```
> confusionMatrix(rpFitCost, norm = "none")
  Cross-Validated (10-fold, repeated 5 times) Confusion Matrix

  (entries are un-normalized counts)

            Reference
  Prediction   VF     F     M     L
          VF 157.0  24.6   2.0   0.2
          F   10.3  43.2   3.1   0.2
          M    9.6  38.3  34.5   5.8
          L    0.0   1.7   1.6  14.6
```

The norm argument determines how the raw counts from each resample should
be normalized. A value of "none" results in the average counts in each cell
of the table. Using norm = "overall" first divides the cell entries by the total
number of data points in the table, then averages these percentages.

Part IV
Other Considerations

Chapter 18
Measuring Predictor Importance

Often, we desire to quantify the strength of the relationship between the predictors and the outcome. As the number of attributes becomes large, exploratory analysis of the all the predictors may be infeasible and concentrating on those with strong relationships with the outcome may be an effective triaging strategy. Ranking predictors in this manner can be very useful when sifting through large amounts of data.

One of the primary reasons to measure the strength or relevance of the predictors is to filter which should be used as inputs in a model. This *supervised feature selection* can be data driven based on the existing data. The results of the filtering process, along with subject matter expertise, can be a critical step in creating an effective predictive model. As will be seen in the next chapter, many feature selection algorithms rely on a quantitative relevance score for filtering.

Many predictive models have built-in or *intrinsic* measurements of predictor importance and have been discussed in previous chapters. For example, MARS and many tree-based models monitor the increase in performance that occurs when adding each predictor to the model. Others, such as linear regression or logistic regression can use quantifications based on the model coefficients or statistical measures (such as *t*-statistics). The methodologies discussed in this chapter are not specific to any predictive model. If an effective model has been created, the scores derived from that model are likely to be more reliable than the methodologies discussed in this chapter because they are directly connected to the model.

In this chapter, the notion of variable importance is taken to mean an overall quantification of the relationship between the predictor and outcome. Most of the methodologies discussed cannot inform the modeler as to the *nature* of the relationship, such as "increasing the predictor results in a decrease in the outcome." Such detailed characterizations can only result from models having precise parametric forms such as linear or logistic regression, multivariate adaptive regression splines, and a few others. For example, Sect. 8.5 discussed variable importance scores for random forest. In

M. Kuhn and K. Johnson, *Applied Predictive Modeling*,
DOI 10.1007/978-1-4614-6849-3_18,
© Springer Science+Business Media New York 2013

essence, this measurement of predictor relevance is derived by permuting each predictor individually and assessing the loss in performance when the effect of the predictor is negated. In this case, a substantial drop in performance is indicative of an important predictor. While this can be an effective approach, it does not enlighten the modeler as to the exact form of the relationship. Despite this, these measurements can be useful for guiding the user to focus more closely on specific predictors via visualizations and other means.

Many variable importance scores are specific to the type of data. For example, techniques for numeric outcomes may not be appropriate for categorical outcomes. This chapter is divided based on the nature of the outcome. Section 18.1 discusses techniques for numeric outcomes and Sect. 18.2 focuses on categorical outcomes. Finally, Sect. 18.3 discussed more general approaches to the problem. Several examples from previous chapters are used to illustrate the techniques.

18.1 Numeric Outcomes

For numeric predictors, the classic approach to quantifying each relationship with the outcome uses the sample correlation statistic. This quantity measures *linear* associations; if the relationship is nearly linear or curvilinear, then Spearman's correlation coefficient (Sect. 5.1) may be more effective. These metrics should be considered rough estimates of the relationship and may not be effective for more complex relationships.

For example, the QSAR data used in the previous regression chapters contained a number of numeric predictors. Figure 18.1 shows scatter plots of two predictors and the outcome. The relationship between solubility and number of carbon atoms is relatively linear and straightforward. The simple correlation was estimated to be -0.61 and the rank correlation was -0.67. For the surface area predictor, the situation is more complicated. There is a group of compounds with low surface area and, for these compounds, solubility is also low. The remainder of the compounds have higher solubility up to a point, after which there is a marginal trend. This could be a valuable piece of information to the modeler and would not be captured by the correlation statistic. For this predictor, simple correlation was estimated to be 0.27 and the rank correlation was 0.14. These values are relatively low and would rank accordingly low (17th out of 20 predictors).

An alternative is to use more flexible methods that may be capable of modeling general nonlinear relationships. One such technique is the locally weighted regression model (known more commonly as LOESS) of Cleveland and Devlin (1988). This technique is based on a series polynomial regressions that model the data in small neighborhoods (similar to computing a moving average). The approach can be effective at creating smooth regression trends that are extremely adaptive. The red lines in Fig. 18.1 are the LOESS

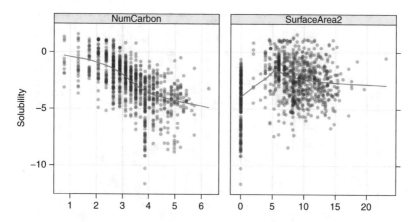

Fig. 18.1: Scatter plots for two numeric predictors (on transformed scales) for the solubility data. The *red lines* are smoother model fits

smoother fits. From the model fit, a pseudo-R^2 statistic can be calculated derived from the residuals. For the solubility data shown in Fig. 18.1, the LOESS pseudo-R^2 for the surface area was 0.22, which ranks higher (7th out of 20) than the correlation scores.

Figure 18.2 shows the relationship between importance scores for all of the continuous predictors. The third metric, the maximal information coefficient (MIC), is discussed in Sect. 18.3. The rank correlation and LOESS pseudo-R^2 tend to give the same results, with the exception of two surface area predictors. Both methods reflect three distinct clusters of predictors, based on their ranks: a set of four high scoring predictors (two significantly overlap in the plot), a set of moderately important predictors, and another set of very low importance. The only inconsistency between the methods is that the two surface area predictors score higher using LOESS than the other methods. These predictors are shown as red squares in the image.

Each of these techniques evaluates each predictor without considering the others. This can be potentially misleading in two ways. First, if two predictors are highly correlated with the response and with each other, then the univariate approach will identify both as important. As we have seen, some models will be negatively impacted by including this redundant information. Pre-processing approaches such as removing highly correlated predictors can alleviate this problem. Second, the univariate importance approach will fail to identify groups of predictors that together have a strong relationship with the response. For example, two predictors may not be highly correlated with the response; however, their interaction may be. Univariate correlations will not capture this predictive relationship. A sensible strategy would be to further explore these aspects of the predictors instead of using the rankings as the sole method for understanding the underlying trends. Knowing which relationship to explore often requires expert knowledge about the data.

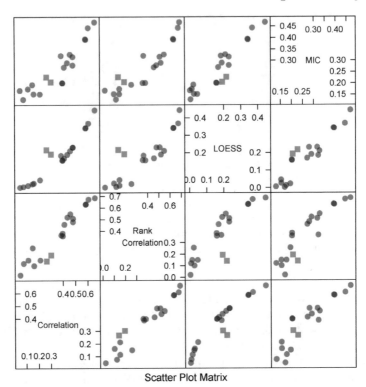

Scatter Plot Matrix

Fig. 18.2: A scatter plot matrix importance metrics for the 20 continuous predictors in the solubility data. The two surface area predictors are shown as *red squares*

When the predictors are categorical, different methodologies are required. In the solubility data, there were 208 fingerprint predictors, which are indicator variables representing particular atomic structures in the compound. The most straightforward method for determining the relevance of each binary predictor is to evaluate whether the average outcome in each category is different. Consider fingerprint FP175; the difference between the mean solubility value with and without the structure is −0.002. Given that solubility ranges from −11.6 to 1.6, this is likely to be negligible. On the other hand, fingerprint FP044 has a difference of −4.1 log units. This is larger but on its own may not be informative. The variability in the data should also be considered.

The most natural method for comparing the mean of two groups is the standard t-statistic, which is essentially a signal-to-noise ratio (the difference in means is divided by a function of the variabilities in the groups). A p-value can be produced by this procedure where the null hypothesis is that there is no difference between the groups. The assumption for the statistic

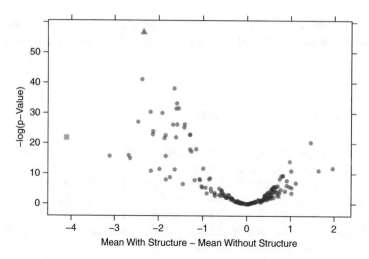

Fig. 18.3: A volcano plot of the t-test results applied to the fingerprint predictors. The *red square* is fingerprint FP044 (which has the largest difference in means) while the *blue triangle* is fingerprint FP076 and is the most statistically significant

is that the data are normally distributed. If this assumption is unlikely to be true, other methods (such as the Wilcoxon rank sum test) may be more appropriate.

For each of the 208 fingerprint predictors, a t-test was used. Instead of solely relying on the p-value, Fig. 18.3 shows a *volcano plot* where a transformed version of the p-value is shown on the y-axis and the difference in solubility means is shown on the x-axis. Higher values of the y-axis are indicative of strong statistical significance (i.e., low p-value). Most of the mean differences are negative, indicating that solubility tends to be higher without the structure. FP044 has the largest difference (and is shown as a red square). However, this difference is not the most statistically significant. Fingerprint FP076 is the most statistically significant (shown as a blue triangle) and has a difference in means of -2.3 log units. As previously mentioned, the t-statistic is a signal-to-noise ratio. While fingerprint FP044 has the largest signal, it also has appreciable variability which diminishes its significance. This is reflected in the 95 % confidence intervals for the mean differences: (3.6, 4.7) for FP044 and (2.1, 2.6) for fingerprint FP076. Which predictor is more important depends on the context and the particular data set. If the signal is large enough, the model may be able to overcome the noise. In other cases, smaller but more precise differences may generate better performance.

When the predictor has more than two values, an analysis of variance (ANOVA) model can be used to characterize the statistical significance of the predictors. However, if the means of the categories are found to be different, the natural next step is to discover which are different. For this reason, it may be helpful to decompose the categories into multiple binary dummy variables and apply the procedure outlined above to determine the relevance of each category.

18.2 Categorical Outcomes

With categorical outcomes and numeric predictors, there are several approaches to quantifying the importance of the predictor. The image segmentation data from Chap. 3 will be used to illustrate the techniques. Figure 18.4 shows histograms of two predictors (the fiber width for channel 1 and the spot fiber count for channel 4) for each class. Fiber width shows a shift in the average values between the classes while the spot fiber count distribution appears very similar between classes.

One approach when there are two classes is to use the area under the ROC curve to quantify predictor relevance. Sections 11.3 and 16.4 utilized the ROC curve with predicted class probabilities as inputs. Here, we use the predictor data as inputs into the ROC curve. If the predictor could perfectly separate the classes, there would be a cutoff for the predictor that would achieve a sensitivity and specificity of 1 and the area under the curve would be one. As before, a completely irrelevant predictor would have an area under the curve of approximately 0.5. Figure 18.5 shows the area under the curve for the fiber width and spot fiber count predictors. The area under the ROC

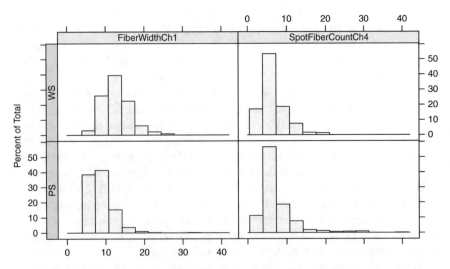

Fig. 18.4: Histograms for two predictors in the cell segmentation data, separated for each class

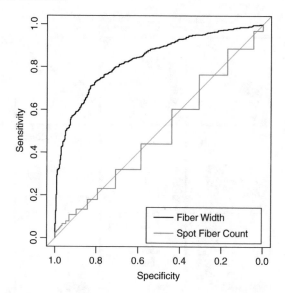

Fig. 18.5: ROC curves for two predictors in the cell segmentation data

curve for the fiber width data was 0.836 while the value for the spot fiber count was 0.538. This echoes the trends seen in Fig. 18.4 where the fiber width showed more separation between classes.

When there are multiple classes, the extensions of ROC curves described by Hanley and McNeil (1982), DeLong et al. (1988), Venkatraman (2000), and Pepe et al. (2009) can also be used. Alternatively, a set of "one versus all" ROC curves can be created by lumping all but one of the classes together. In this way, there would be a separate AUC for each class and the overall relevance can be quantified using the average or maximum AUC across the classes.

Another, more simplistic approach is to test if the mean values of predictors within each class are different. This is similar to the technique described in the previous section, but, in this context, the predictor is being treated as the outcome. Volcano plots cannot be used since the each of the differences may be on different scales. However, the t-statistics can be used to compare the predictors on different scales. For the fiber width, the t-statistic value was -19, indicating a clear signal above the noise. The signal was much weaker for the spot fiber count, with a value of 3.

For the segmentation data, the 58 continuous predictors were evaluated using each of these methods along with the random forest variable importance score and two methods that are described in Sect. 18.3 (MIC and Relief). The methods are roughly concordant (Fig. 18.6). The area under the ROC curve shows a tight, curvilinear relationship with the random forest score and a strong linear relationship with the t-statistic. The t-statistic and random

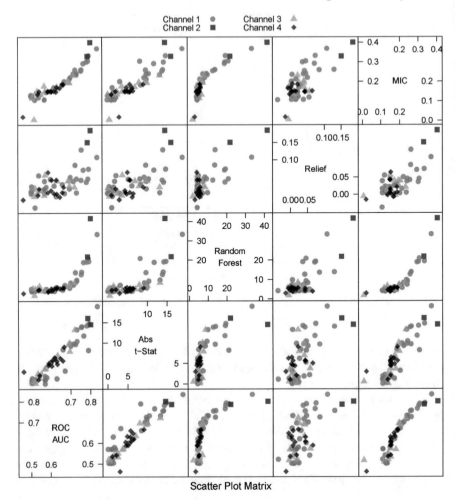

Fig. 18.6: A scatter plot matrix of several different metrics for ranking predictors with the image segmentation data set

forest appear to rank the same predictors as less important, but there are differences in the scores for those quantified as most important. Three predictors tend to be ranked very highly across the methods: average intensity (channel 2), fiber width (channel 1), and total intensity (channel 2).

When the predictor is categorical, there are several metrics that may be appropriate. For binary predictors and two classes, one effective method for measuring the relevance is the odds ratio. Recall that the odds of a probability are $p/(1-p)$. The probability of an event can be calculated for both levels of the predictor. If these are denoted as p_1 and p_2, the odds ratio (Bland and

Table 18.1: Statistics for three binary categorical predictors in the grant data

| | Grant success | | | | | |
	Yes	No	%	OR	p-value	Gain ratio
Sponsor						
62B	7	44	14			
Other	3226	3356	49	6.0	2.6e^{-07}	0.04726
CVB						
Band unknown	644	2075	24			
Band known	2589	1325	66	6.3	1.7e^{-263}	0.13408
RFCD code						
240302	13	15	46			
Other code	3220	3385	49	1.1	8.5e^{-01}	0.00017

Altman 2000; Agresti 2002) is

$$OR = \frac{p_1(1 - p_2)}{p_2(1 - p_1)}$$

and represents the increase in the odds of the event when going from the first level of the predictor to the other.

To illustrate this approach, the grant application data from previous chapters is used. For these data there are 226 binary predictors with at least 25 entries in each cell of the 2×2 table between the predictor and outcome. Table 18.1 shows cross tabulations for three predictors in the grant data. For contract value band, the probability of grant success is determined when the band is known ($p_1 = 0.661$) and unknown ($p_2 = 0.237$). The corresponding odds ratio is 6.3, meaning that there is more than a sixfold increase in the odds of success when the band is known. As with the discussion on the differences in means, the odds ratio only reflects the signal, not the noise. Although there are formulas for calculating the confidence interval for the odds ratio, a more common approach is to conduct a statistical hypothesis test that the odds ratio is equal to one (i.e., equal odds between the predictor levels). When there are two categories and two values for the predictor, Fisher's exact test (Agresti 2002) can be used to evaluate this hypothesis and can be summarized by the resulting p-value. For this predictor, the p-value was effectively zero, which indicates that levels of contract value band are related to grant success. Table 18.1 shows another predictor for Sponsor 62B that has a similar odds ratio (OR = 6), but the number of grants with this sponsor is very low. Here, the p-value was still small but would be ranked much lower using statistical significance. The left-hand panel of Fig. 18.7 shows a volcano

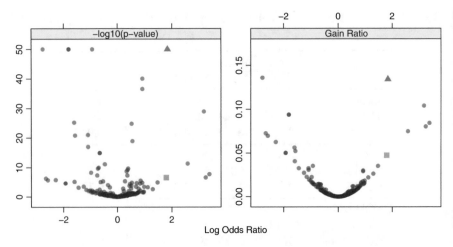

Fig. 18.7: The log odds ratio plotted against two other statistics. *Left*: a function of the *p*-values from Fisher's exact test is shown. The largest value in the data is 263; this image truncates at 50 to preserve the perspective. *Right*: The gain ratio for each predictor. The *red square* is the predictor for sponsor 62B and the *blue triangle* is for unknown contract value band

plot for the odds ratio and the corresponding *p*-value for 226 binary grant predictors.

When there are more than two classes or the predictors have more than two levels, other methods can be applied. Fisher's exact test can still be used to measure the association between the predictor and the classes. Alternatively, the gain ratio used for C4.5 can be applied to quantify relationship between two variables, where larger is better. Recall that the gain ratio adjusts for the number of levels in the predictor to remove the bias against attributes with few levels. For this reason, the information gain can be applied to all categorical predictors, irrespective of their characteristics. Table 18.1 shows the information gain for three of the grant predictors and Fig. 18.7 contrasts the gain statistics versus the odds ratio. Like the *p*-value for Fisher's exact test, the gain statistics favor the contract value band predictor over the one for Sponsor 62B, despite the similarities in their odds ratio.

18.3 Other Approaches

The Relief algorithm (Kira and Rendell 1992) is a generic method for quantifying predictor importance. It was originally developed for classification problems with two classes but has been extended to work across a

1	Initialize the predictor scores S_j to zero
2	**for** $i = 1 \ldots m$ *randomly selected training set samples* (R_i) **do**
3	Find the nearest miss and hit in the training set
4	**for** $j = 1 \ldots p$ *predictor variables* **do**
5	Adjust the score for each predictor based on the proximity of R_j to the nearest miss and hit:
6	$S_j = S_j - diff_j(R_j, Hit)^2/m + diff_j(R_j, Miss)^2/m$
7	**end**
8	**end**

Algorithm 18.1: The original Relief algorithm for ranking predictor variables in classification models with two classes

wider range of problems. It can accommodate continuous predictors as well as dummy variables and can recognize nonlinear relationships between the predictors and the outcome. It uses random selected points and their nearest neighbors to evaluate each predictor in isolation.

For a particular predictor, the score attempts to characterize the separation between the classes in isolated sections of the data. Algorithm 18.1 shows the procedure.

For a randomly selected training set sample, the algorithm finds the nearest samples from both classes (called the "hits" and "misses"). For each predictor, a measure of difference in the predictor's values is calculated between the random data point and the hits and misses. For continuous predictors, Kira and Rendell (1992) suggested the distance between the two points be divided by the overall range of the predictor:

$$\mathrm{diff}(x, y) = (x - y)/C$$

where C is a constant for the predictor that scales the difference to be between 0 and 1. For binary (i.e., 0/1) data, a simple indicator for equivalence can be used:

$$\mathrm{diff}(x, y) = |x - y|$$

so that these values are also between 0 and 1.

The overall score (S_j) is an accumulation of these differences such that the score is decreased if the hit is far away from the randomly selected value but is increased if the miss is far away. The idea is that a predictor that shows a separation between the classes should have hits nearby and missed far away. Given this, larger scores are indicative of important predictors.

For example, Fig. 18.8 presents a set of data for several predictors. The top panel shows a predictor that completely separates the classes. Suppose the sampling procedure selects the second to last sample on the left-hand side

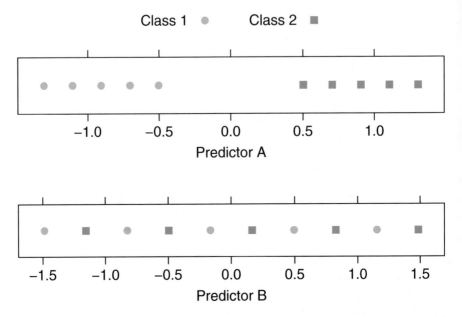

Fig. 18.8: Three data sets that illustrate the Relief algorithm. In the *top panel*, predictor A shows complete separation with a ReliefF score of 0.19. The *middle panel* shows a completely non-informative predictor with a corresponding ReliefF score of 0

(predictor $A = -1.1$). The nearest hit is on either side of this data point, with a difference of approximately 0.2 (we'll forgo the constant here). The nearest miss is far away ($A = 0.5$) with a corresponding difference of -1.61. If this were the first randomly selected training set point, the score would be

$$S_A = 0 - 0.2^2 + -1.61^2 = 2.55$$

This value would be divided by m and new values would be accumulated. As a counter example, predictor B in Fig. 18.8 is completely non-informative. Each hit and miss is adjacent to any randomly selected sample, so the differences will always offset each other and the score for this predictor is $S_B = 0$.

This procedure was subsequently improved by Kononenko (1994). The modified algorithm, called ReliefF, uses more than a single nearest neighbor, uses a modified difference metric, and allows for more than two classes as well as missing predictor values. Additionally, Robnik-Sikonja and Kononenko (1997) adapted the algorithm for regression (i.e., numeric outcomes).

The bottom panel of Fig. 18.9 illustrates an hypothetical data set with two classes and two correlated predictors (denoted as C and D). The class boundary was created using a simple logistic regression model equation with two strong main effects and a moderate interaction effect:

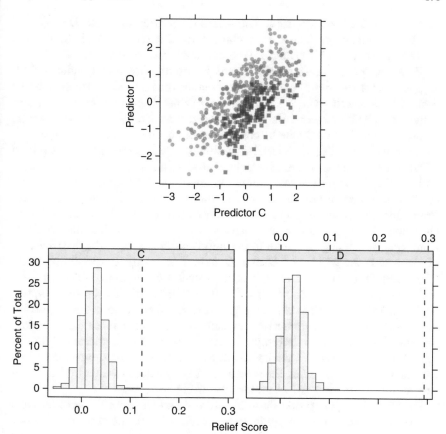

Fig. 18.9: *Top*: two predictors with distinct class boundary. In this example, the ReliefF scores for predictors C and D are 0.17 and 0.25, respectively. *Bottom*: the permutation distribution of the scores when there is no relationship between the predictors and the classes. The *dashed lines* indicate the observed ReliefF scores

$$\log \left(\frac{\pi}{1 - \pi} \right) = -4C - 4D + 2CD$$

The data shown in Fig. 18.9 were simulated with this class boundary. For these data, a logistic regression model was able to achieve a cross-validated accuracy rate of 90.6%. Knowing the true model equation, both predictors should be quantified as being important. Since there is an interaction effect in the model equation, one would expect the ReliefF algorithm to show a larger signal than other methods that only consider a single predictor at a time. For these data, the ReliefF algorithm was used with $m = 50$ random samples and $k = 10$-nearest neighbors. The two predictors were centered and scaled prior to running the algorithm. The scores for predictors C and D were 0.17 and 0.25, respectively. The areas under the ROC curves for predictors C and D were moderate, with values of 0.65 and 0.69, respectively.

What cutoff for these scores should be used? Kira and Rendell (1992) suggest that a threshold "can be much smaller than $1/\sqrt{\alpha m}$," where α is the desired false-positive rate (i.e., the percent of time that an irrelevant predictor is judged to be important). Using this yardstick with a 5 % false positive rate, values greater than 0.63 may be considered important. Another alternative is to use a well-established statistical method called a *permutation test* (Good 2000) to evaluate the scores. Here, the true class labels are randomly shuffled and the ReliefF scores are recalculated many times. This should provide some sense of the distribution of the scores when the predictor has no relevance. From this, the observed score can be contrasted against this distribution to characterize how extreme it is relative to the assumption that the predictor is not relevant. Using 500 random permutations of the data, the distributions of the scores for predictors C and D resembled normally distributed data (Fig. 18.9). For predictor C, the score values ranged from -0.05 to 0.11, while for predictor D, the range was -0.05 to 0.11. In this context, the two observed values for the data in Fig. 18.9 are indicative of very important predictors. Given the symmetric, normally distributed shapes of the random permutations, it can be determined that the scores for predictors C and D are 4.5 and 11.6 standard deviations away from what should be expected by chance. Given how extreme the scores are, the conclusion would be that both predictors are important factors for separating the classes.

For the cell segmentation data, Fig. 18.6 shows the ReliefF scores for each predictor. These values are moderately correlated with the other metrics but show larger variability in the relationships. For example, the area under the ROC curve shows less noise in the relationships with the other metrics. This may be due to the metrics measuring different aspects of the data or may be due to the random sampling used by ReliefF.

Reshef et al. (2011) describe a new metric to quantify the relationship between two variables called the MIC. Their method partitions the two-dimensional area defined by the predictor and outcome into sets of two-dimensional grids. For example, Fig. 18.10 shows the scatter plot of the solubility data where four random 4×3 grids are created for the number of carbon atoms predictor. Within each grid, the number of data points is calculated and used to compute the *mutual information* statistic (Brillinger 2004), which is related to the information criteria described in Chap. 14 for C4.5 and C5.0 decision trees. Many different configurations of the same grid size are evaluated and the largest mutual information value is determined. This process is repeated for many different grid sizes (e.g., 2×2, 10×3). The compendium of mutual information values across all the bins are normalized and the largest value across all the bin configurations is used as the strength of association between the predictor and the outcome.

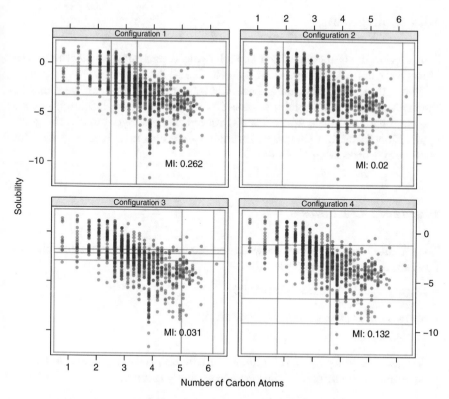

Fig. 18.10: Examples of how the maximal information criterion (MIC) is created. Each panel shows a random configuration of 4×3 grids for one of the solubility predictors with the corresponding the mutual information statistic

The authors demonstrate that this method can detect many types of relationships, such as sin waves, ellipses, and other highly nonlinear patterns. The metric has a similar scale to the simple correlation statistic where a value of zero indicates no relationship, whereas a value of one is indicative of an extremely strong relationship. One potential issue with such a general technique is that it may not do as well as others under some circumstances. For example, if the true relationship between the predictor and outcome were linear, the simple correlation statistic may perform better since it is specific to linear trends.

The MIC statistic was previously shown in Fig. 18.1 for the continuous solubility predictors. Here, the MIC values have a strong relationship with the other metrics. For the cell segmentation data shown in Fig. 18.6, the MIC statistic has a strong correlation with the absolute t-statistics, the area under the ROC curve, and random forest scores. There is smaller correlation with ReliefF.

18.4 Computing

This section uses functions from the following R packages: AppliedPredictive-
Modeling, caret, CORElearn, minerva, pROC, and randomForest.

The cell segmentation data from Chap. 3 are used and can be found in
the caret package. The solubility data from Chaps. 6 through 9 are also used
and can be found in the AppliedPredictiveModeling package. Finally, the grant
application data from Chaps. 12 through 15 are also used (see Sect. 12.7 for
reading and processing these data).

Numeric Outcomes

To estimate the correlations between the predictors and the outcome, the cor
function is used. For example,

```
> library(AppliedPredictiveModeling)
> data(solubility)
> cor(solTrainXtrans$NumCarbon, solTrainY)

  [1] -0.6067917
```

To get results for all of the numeric predictors, the apply function can be
used to make the same calculations across many columns

```
> ## Determine which columns have the string "FP" in the name and
> ## exclude these to get the numeric predictors
> fpCols<- grepl("FP", names(solTrainXtrans))
> ## Exclude these to get the numeric predictor names
> numericPreds <- names(solTrainXtrans)[!fpCols]

> corrValues <- apply(solTrainXtrans[, numericPreds],
+                     MARGIN = 2,
+                     FUN = function(x, y) cor(x, y),
+                     y = solTrainY)
> head(corrValues)

    MolWeight     NumAtoms NumNonHAtoms    NumBonds NumNonHBonds
   -0.6585284   -0.4358113   -0.5836236  -0.4590395   -0.5851968
  NumMultBonds
   -0.4804159
```

The obtain the rank correlation, the corr function has an option
method = "spearman".

The LOESS smoother can be accessed with the loess function in the stats
library. The formula method is used to specify the model:

```
> smoother <- loess(solTrainY ~ solTrainXtrans$NumCarbon)
> smoother
```

```
Call:
loess(formula = solTrainY ~ solTrainXtrans$NumCarbon)

Number of Observations: 951
Equivalent Number of Parameters: 5.3
Residual Standard Error: 1.548
```

The lattice function `xyplot` is convenient for displaying the LOESS fit:

```
> xyplot(solTrainY ~ solTrainXtrans$NumCarbon,
+         type = c("p", "smooth"),
+         xlab = "# Carbons",
+         ylab = "Solubility")
```

The caret function `filterVarImp` with the `nonpara = TRUE` option (for nonparametric regression) creates a LOESS model for each predictor and quantifies the relationship with the outcome:

```
> loessResults <- filterVarImp(x = solTrainXtrans[, numericPreds],
+                               y = solTrainY,
+                               nonpara = TRUE)
> head(loessResults)
                 Overall
  MolWeight     0.4443931
  NumAtoms      0.1899315
  NumNonHAtoms  0.3406166
  NumBonds      0.2107173
  NumNonHBonds  0.3424552
  NumMultBonds  0.2307995
```

The minerva package can be used to calculate the MIC statistics between the predictors and outcomes. The `mine` function computes several quantities including the MIC value:

```
> library(minerva)
> micValues <- mine(solTrainXtrans[, numericPreds], solTrainY)
> ## Several statistics are calculated
> names(micValues)

  [1] "MIC"    "MAS"    "MEV"    "MCN"    "MICR2"
> head(micValues$MIC)

                     Y
  MolWeight     0.4679277
  NumAtoms      0.2896815
  NumNonHAtoms  0.3947092
  NumBonds      0.3268683
  NumNonHBonds  0.3919627
  NumMultBonds  0.2792600
```

For categorical predictors, the simple `t.test` function computes the difference in means and the p-value. For one predictor:

```
> t.test(solTrainY ~ solTrainXtrans$FP044)

        Welch Two Sample t-test

data:  solTrainY by solTrainXtrans$FP044
t = 15.1984, df = 61.891, p-value < 2.2e-16
alternative hypothesis: true difference in means is not equal to 0
95 percent confidence interval:
 3.569300 4.650437
sample estimates:
mean in group 0 mean in group 1
     -2.472237       -6.582105
```

This approach can be extended to all predictors using `apply` in a manner
similar to the one shown above for correlations.

```
> getTstats <- function(x, y)
+   {
+     tTest <- t.test(y~x)
+     out <- c(tStat = tTest$statistic, p = tTest$p.value)
+     out
+   }
> tVals <- apply(solTrainXtrans[, fpCols],
+                MARGIN = 2,
+                FUN = getTstats,
+                y = solTrainY)
> ## switch the dimensions
> tVals <- t(tVals)
> head(tVals)

          tStat.t              p
FP001 -4.022040 6.287404e-05
FP002 10.286727 1.351580e-23
FP003 -2.036442 4.198619e-02
FP004 -4.948958 9.551772e-07
FP005 10.282475 1.576549e-23
FP006 -7.875838 9.287835e-15
```

Categorical Outcomes

The `filterVarImp` function also calculates the area under the ROC curve when
the outcome variable is an R factor variable:

```
> library(caret)
> data(segmentationData)
> cellData <- subset(segmentationData, Case == "Train")
> cellData$Case <- cellData$Cell <- NULL
> ## The class is in the first column
> head(names(cellData))

[1] "Class"       "AngleCh1"    "AreaCh1"    "AvgIntenCh1"
[5] "AvgIntenCh2" "AvgIntenCh3"
```

```
> rocValues <- filterVarImp(x = cellData[,-1],
+                           y = cellData$Class)
> ## Column is created for each class
> head(rocValues)
                   PS        WS
AngleCh1     0.5025967 0.5025967
AreaCh1      0.5709170 0.5709170
AvgIntenCh1  0.7662375 0.7662375
AvgIntenCh2  0.7866146 0.7866146
AvgIntenCh3  0.5214098 0.5214098
AvgIntenCh4  0.6473814 0.6473814
```

This is a simple wrapper for the functions roc and auc in the pROC package. When there are three or more classes, filterVarImp will compute ROC curves for each class versus the others and then returns the largest area under the curve.

The Relief statistics can be calculated using the CORElearn package. The function attrEval will calculate several versions of Relief (using the estimator option):

```
> library(CORElearn)
> reliefValues <- attrEval(Class ~ ., data = cellData,
+                          ## There are many Relief methods
+                          ## available. See ?attrEval
+                          estimator = "ReliefFequalK",
+                          ## The number of instances tested:
+                          ReliefIterations = 50)
> head(reliefValues)
    AngleCh1      AreaCh1 AvgIntenCh1 AvgIntenCh2 AvgIntenCh3 AvgIntenCh4
  0.01631332   0.02004060  0.09402596  0.17200400  0.09268398  0.02672168
```

This function can also be used to calculate the gain ratio, Gini index, and other scores. To use a permutation approach to investigate the observed values of the ReliefF statistic, the AppliedPredictiveModeling package has a function permuteRelief:

```
> perm <- permuteRelief(x = cellData[,-1],
+                       y = cellData$Class,
+                       nperm = 500,
+                       estimator = "ReliefFequalK",
+                       ReliefIterations = 50)
```

The permuted ReliefF scores are contained in a sub-object called permutations:

```
> head(perm$permutations)
    Predictor        value
1    AngleCh1  -0.009364024
2    AngleCh1   0.011170669
3    AngleCh1  -0.020425694
4    AngleCh1  -0.037133238
5    AngleCh1   0.005334315
6    AngleCh1   0.010394028
```

The permutation distributions for the ReliefF scores can be helpful. Histograms, such as those show in Fig. 18.9, can be created with the syntax:

```
> histogram(~ value|Predictor,
+             data = perm$permutations)
```

Also, the standardized versions of the scores are in the sub-object called standardized and represent the number of standard deviations that the observed ReliefF values (i.e., without permuting) are from the center of the permuted distribution:

```
> head(perm$standardized)
     AngleCh1      AreaCh1 AvgIntenCh1 AvgIntenCh2 AvgIntenCh3 AvgIntenCh4
    -1.232653     3.257958    3.765691    8.300906    4.054288    1.603847
```

The MIC statistic can be computed as before but with a binary dummy variable encoding of the classes:

```
> micValues <- mine(x = cellData[,-1],
+                    y = ifelse(cellData$Class == "PS", 1, 0))
>
```

```
> head(micValues$MIC)
                     Y
AngleCh1     0.1310570
AreaCh1      0.1080839
AvgIntenCh1  0.2920461
AvgIntenCh2  0.3294846
AvgIntenCh3  0.1354438
AvgIntenCh4  0.1665450
```

To compute the odds ratio and a statistical test of association, the fisher.test function in the stats library can be applied. For example, to calculate these statistics for the grant objects created in Sect. 12.7:

```
> Sp62BTable <- table(training[pre2008, "Sponsor62B"],
+                     training[pre2008, "Class"])
> Sp62BTable

    successful unsuccessful
  0       3226         3356
  1          7           44
> fisher.test(Sp62BTable)
        Fisher's Exact Test for Count Data

data:  Sp62BTable
p-value = 2.644e-07
alternative hypothesis: true odds ratio is not equal to 1
95 percent confidence interval:
  2.694138 15.917729
sample estimates:
odds ratio
  6.040826
```

When the predictor has more than two classes, a single odds ratio cannot be computed, but the p-value for association can still be utilized:

```
> ciTable <- table(training[pre2008, "CI.1950"],
+                  training[pre2008, "Class"])
> ciTable

    successful unsuccessful
  0       2704         2899
  1        476          455
  2         45           39
  3          7            7
  4          1            0
> fisher.test(ciTable)
        Fisher's Exact Test for Count Data

data:  ciTable
p-value = 0.3143
alternative hypothesis: two.sided
```

In some cases, Fisher's exact test may be computationally prohibitive. In these cases, the χ^2 test for association can be computed:

```
> DayTable <- table(training[pre2008, "Weekday"],
+                   training[pre2008, "Class"])
> DayTable

      successful unsuccessful
  Fri        542          880
  Mon        634          455
  Sat        615          861
  Sun        223            0
  Thurs      321          246
  Tues       377          309
  Wed        521          649
> chisq.test(DayTable)
        Pearson's Chi-squared test

data:  DayTable
X-squared = 400.4766, df = 6, p-value < 2.2e-16
```

Model-Based Importance Scores

As described in the previous chapters, many models have built-in approaches for measuring the aggregate effect of the predictors on the model. The caret package contains a general class for calculating or returning these values. As of this writing, there are methods for 27 R classes, including: C5.0, JRip, PART, RRF, RandomForest, bagEarth, classbagg, cubist, dsa, earth, fda, gam, gbm, glm, glmnet, lm, multinom, mvr, nnet, pamrtrained, plsda, randomForest, regbagg, rfe, rpart, sbf, and train.

To illustrate, a random forest model was fit to the cell segmentation data:

```
> library(randomForest)
> set.seed(791)
> rfImp <- randomForest(Class ~ ., data = segTrain,
+                        ntree = 2000,
+                        importance = TRUE)
```

The randomForest package contains a function called importance that returns the relevant metric. The varImp function standardizes across models:

```
> head(varImp(rfImp))
                  PS        WS
AngleCh1    -1.002852 -1.002852
AreaCh1      8.769884  8.769884
AvgIntenCh1 21.460666 21.460666
AvgIntenCh2 22.377451 22.377451
AvgIntenCh3  7.690371  7.690371
AvgIntenCh4  9.108741  9.108741
```

Note that some models return a separate score for each class while others do not.

When using the train function, the varImp function executes the appropriate code based on the value of the method argument. When the model does not have a built-in function for measuring importances, train employs a more general approach (as described above).

Exercises

18.1. For the churn data described in Exercise 12.3:

(a) Calculate the correlations between predictors. Are there strong relationships between these variables? How does this compare to what one would expect with these attributes?
(b) Assess the importance of the categorical predictors (i.e., area code, voice mail plan, etc) individually using the training set.
(c) Also estimate the importance scores of the continuous predictors individually.
(d) Now use ReliefF to jointly estimate the importance of the predictors. Is there a difference in rankings? Why or why not?

18.2. For the oil type data described in Exercise 4.4, estimate variable importance scores. Does the large number of classes affect the process of quantifying the importances?

18.3. The UCI Abalone data (http://archive.ics.uci.edu/ml/datasets/Abalone) consist of data from 4,177 abalones. The data contain measurements of the type (male, female, and infant), the longest shell measurement, the diameter,

height, and several weights (whole, shucked, viscera, and shell). The outcome
is the number of rings. The age of the abalone is the number of rings plus 1.5.
The data are contained in the AppliedPredictiveModeling package:

```
> library(AppliedPredictiveModeling)
> data(abalone)
> str(abalone)
'data.frame':      4177 obs. of  9 variables:
  $ Type        : Factor w/ 3 levels "F","I","M": 3 3 1 3 2 2 1 1 3 1 ...
  $ LongestShell : num  0.455 0.35 0.53 0.44 0.33 0.425 0.53 0.545 ...
  $ Diameter    : num  0.365 0.265 0.42 0.365 0.255 0.3 0.415 0.425 ...
  $ Height      : num  0.095 0.09 0.135 0.125 0.08 0.095 0.15 0.125  ...
  $ WholeWeight : num  0.514 0.226 0.677 0.516 0.205 ...
  $ ShuckedWeight: num  0.2245 0.0995 0.2565 0.2155 0.0895 ...
  $ VisceraWeight: num  0.101 0.0485 0.1415 0.114 0.0395 ...
  $ ShellWeight : num  0.15 0.07 0.21 0.155 0.055 0.12 0.33 0.26 ...
  $ Rings       : int  15 7 9 10 7 8 20 16 9 19 ...
> head(abalone)
```

	Type	LongestShell	Diameter	Height	WholeWeight	ShuckedWeight
1	M	0.455	0.365	0.095	0.5140	0.2245
2	M	0.350	0.265	0.090	0.2255	0.0995
3	F	0.530	0.420	0.135	0.6770	0.2565
4	M	0.440	0.365	0.125	0.5160	0.2155
5	I	0.330	0.255	0.080	0.2050	0.0895
6	I	0.425	0.300	0.095	0.3515	0.1410

	VisceraWeight	ShellWeight	Rings
1	0.1010	0.150	15
2	0.0485	0.070	7
3	0.1415	0.210	9
4	0.1140	0.155	10
5	0.0395	0.055	7
6	0.0775	0.120	8

(a) Plot the data to assess the functional relationships between the predictors
and the outcome.

(b) Use scatter plots and correlation plots to understand how the predictors
relate to one another.

(c) Estimate variable importance scores for each predictor. Develop an
approach to determining a reduced set of nonredundant predictors.

(d) Apply principal component analysis to the continuous predictors to
determine how many distinct underlying pieces of information are in the
data. Would feature extraction help these data?

Chapter 19
An Introduction to Feature Selection

Determining which predictors should be included in a model is becoming one of the most critical questions as data are becoming increasingly high-dimensional. For example:

- In business, companies are now more proficient at storing and accessing large amounts of information on their customers and products. Large databases are often mined to discover crucial relationships (Lo 2002).
- In pharmaceutical research, chemists can calculate thousands of predictors using quantitative structure-activity relationship (QSAR) methodology described in the regression chapters for numerically describing various aspects of molecules. As an example, one popular software suite calculates 17 flavors of a compound's surface area. These predictors can be categorical or continuous and can easily number in the tens of thousands.
- In biology, a vast array of biological predictors can be measured at one time on a sample of biological material such as blood. RNA expression profiling microarrays can measure thousands of RNA sequences at once. Also, DNA microarrays and sequencing technologies can comprehensively determine the genetic makeup of a sample, producing a wealth of numeric predictors. These technologies have rapidly advanced over time, offering ever larger quantities of information.

From a practical point of view, a model with less predictors may be more interpretable and less costly especially if there is a cost to measuring the predictors. Statistically, it is often more attractive to estimate fewer parameters. Also, as we will soon see, some models may be negatively affected by non-informative predictors.

Some models are naturally resistant to non-informative predictors. Tree- and rule-based models, MARS and the lasso, for example, intrinsically conduct feature selection. For example, if a predictor is not used in any split during the construction of a tree, the prediction equation is functionally independent of the predictor.

M. Kuhn and K. Johnson, *Applied Predictive Modeling*,
DOI 10.1007/978-1-4614-6849-3_19,
© Springer Science+Business Media New York 2013

An important distinction to be made in feature selection is that of *supervised* and *unsupervised* methods. When the outcome is ignored during the elimination of predictors, the technique is *unsupervised*. Examples of these filters were described in Chap. 3 and included removing predictors that have high correlations with other predictors or that have very sparse and unbalanced distributions (i.e., near-zero variance predictors). In each case, the outcome is independent of the filtering calculations. For *supervised methods*, predictors are specifically selected for the purpose of increasing accuracy or to find a subset of predictors to reduce the complexity of the model. Here, the outcome is typically used to quantify the importance of the predictors (as illustrated s in Chap. 18).

The issues related to each type of feature selection are very different, and the literature for this topic is large. Subsequent sections highlight several critical topics including the need for feature selection, typical approaches, and common pitfalls.

19.1 Consequences of Using Non-informative Predictors

Feature selection is primarily focused on removing non-informative or redundant predictors from the model. As with many issues discussed in this text, the importance of feature selection depends on which model is being used. Many models, especially those based on regression slopes and intercepts, will estimate parameters for every term in the model. Because of this, the presence of non-informative variables can add uncertainty to the predictions and reduce the overall effectiveness of the model.

The solubility QSAR data which were analyzed in Chaps. 6–9 and 20 will again be used to demonstrate the effect of non-informative predictors on various models. The data most likely contain non-informative predictors already. Despite this, we will tune and rebuild several models after adding more irrelevant predictors. To do this, the original predictor data are altered by randomly shuffling their rows (independently for each column). As a result, there should be no connection between the new predictors and the solubility values. This procedure preserves the nature of the individual predictors (i.e., fingerprints with the same frequency distribution) but has the side effect of eliminating the between-predictor correlations. If the inclusion of correlated predictors would add additional injury to a particular model, that impact will not be reflected in this exercise.

To quantify the effect of additional predictors, models were created that used the original 228 predictors in the data and then supplemented with either 10, 50, 100, 200, 300, 400, or 500 additional, non-informative predictors. The models were tuned and finalized, and the test set RMSE values were calculated. The models assessed in this manner were linear regression, partial

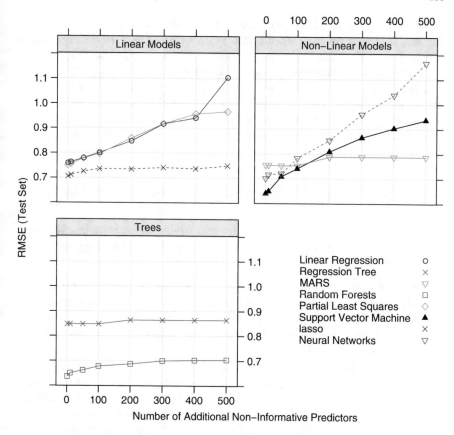

Fig. 19.1: Test set RMSE profiles for solubility models when non-informative predictors are added

least squares, single regression trees, multivariate adaptive regression splines, random forests, neural networks, and radial basis function support vector machines.

Figure 19.1 shows the test set results. As expected, regression trees and MARS models were not affected due to the built-in feature selection. Random forests showed a moderate degradation in performance. The issue here is that the random selection of predictors for splitting can coerce the model into including some unimportant predictors. However, their inclusion does not seriously impact the overall model. The parametrically structured models, such as linear regression, partial least squares, and neural networks, were most affected. Neural networks appear to have the most extensive issues, perhaps due to the excess number of parameters added to the model. For example, a network with 5 hidden units would originally have estimated 961 regression parameters. Adding 500 irrelevant predictors increases the number of parameters to 3,461. Given that there are 951 data points in the training set, this may be too difficult of a problem to solve without over-fitting. Support vector machines also saw a substantial increase in the RMSE, which is consistent with comments made by Hastie et al. (2008, Chap. 12).

Given the potential negative impact, there is the need to find a smaller subset of predictors. Our basic goal is to reduce their number in a way that maximizes performance. This is similar to the previous discussions: how can we reduce complexity without negatively affecting model effectiveness?

19.2 Approaches for Reducing the Number of Predictors

Apart from models with built-in feature selection, most approaches for reducing the number of predictors can be placed into two main categories (John et al. 1994):

- *Wrapper* methods evaluate multiple models using procedures that add and/or remove predictors to find the optimal combination that maximizes model performance. In essence, wrapper methods are search algorithms that treat the predictors as the inputs and utilize model performance as the output to be optimized.
- *Filter methods* evaluate the relevance of the predictors outside of the predictive models and subsequently model only the predictors that pass some criterion. For example, for classification problems, each predictor could be individually evaluated to check if there is a plausible relationship between it and the observed classes. Only predictors with important relationships would then be included in a classification model. Saeys et al. (2007) survey filter methods.

Both approaches have advantages and drawbacks. Filter methods are usually more computationally efficient than wrapper methods, but the selection criterion is not directly related to the effectiveness of the model. Also, most filter methods evaluate each predictor separately, and, consequently, redundant (i.e., highly-correlated) predictors may be selected and important interactions between variables will not be able to be quantified. The downside of the wrapper method is that many models are evaluated (which may also require parameter tuning) and thus an increase in computation time. There is also an increased risk of over-fitting with wrappers.

The following two sections describe these methods in more detail, and a case study is used to illustrate their application.

19.3 Wrapper Methods

As previously stated, wrapper methods conduct a search of the predictors to determine which, when entered into the model, produce the best results. A simple example is classical forward selection for linear regression (Algorithm 19.1). Here, the predictors are evaluated (one at a time) in the current linear regression model. A statistical hypothesis test can be conducted to see if each of the newly added predictors is statistically significant (at some predefined threshold). If at least one predictor has a p-value below the threshold, the predictor associated with the smallest value is added to the model and the process starts again. The algorithm stops when none of the p-values for the remaining predictors are statistically significant. In this scheme, linear regression is the *base learner* and forward selection is the *search procedure*. The *objective function* is the quantity being optimized which, in this case, is statistical significance as represented by the p-value.

There are a few issues with this approach:

1. The forward search procedure is *greedy*, meaning that it does not reevaluate past solutions.
2. The use of repeated hypothesis tests in this manner invalidates many of their statistical properties since the same data are being evaluated numerous times. See Fig. 19.2 for a nontechnical illustration of this issue.
3. Maximizing statistical significance may not be the same as maximizing more relevant accuracy-based quantities.

1	Create an initial model containing only an intercept term.
2	**repeat**
3	**for** *each predictor not in the current model* **do**
4	Create a candidate model by adding the predictor to the current model
5	Use a hypothesis test to estimate the statistical significance of the new model term
6	**end**
7	**if** *the smallest p-value is less than the inclusion threshold* **then**
8	Update the current model to include a term corresponding to the most statistically significant predictor
9	**else**
10	Stop
11	**end**
12	**until** *no statistically significant predictors remain outside the model*

Algorithm 19.1: Classical forward selection for linear regression models

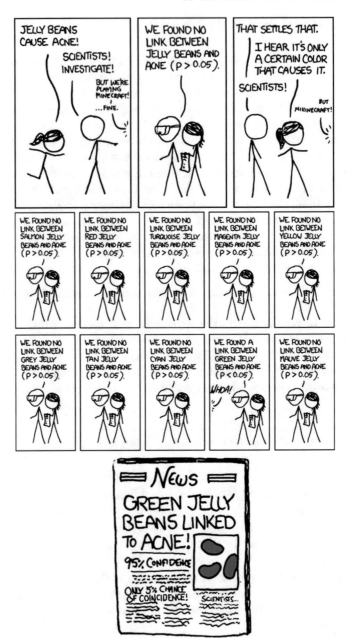

Fig. 19.2: The perils of repeated testing of the same data (Randall Munroe, http://xkcd.com/882, modified for space)

For the first issue, more complex search procedures may be more effective. Several such algorithms are discussed below. The second issue has been extensively studied (Derksen and Keselman 1992; Olden and Jackson 2000; Harrell 2001; Whittingham et al. 2006).[1] Harrell (2001) summarizes the use of p-values during automated model selection:

> ... if this procedure had just been proposed as a statistical method, it would most likely be rejected because it violates every principal of statistical estimation and hypothesis testing.

The second and third issues can be mitigated by using some measure of predictive performance such as RMSE, classification accuracy, or the area under the ROC curve.

Suppose that the RMSE was the objective function instead of statistical significance. Here, the algorithm would be the same but would add predictors to the model that results in the smallest model RMSE. The process would continue until some predefined number of predictors has been reached or the full model is used. From this process, the RMSE can be monitored to determine a point where the error began to increase. The subset size associated with the smallest RMSE would be chosen. As one would suspect, the main pitfall here is obtaining good estimates of the error rate that are not subject to over-fitting caused by the model or the feature selection process (see Sect. 19.5 below).

There are several other criteria that can penalize performance based on how many predictors are in the model. For example, when choosing between two models with the same RMSE, the simpler model with fewer predictors is preferable. For linear regression, a commonly used statistic is the *Akaike Information Criterion*, a penalized version of the sums of squares error:

$$\text{AIC} = n \log \left(\sum_{i=1}^{n} (y_i - \widehat{y}_i)^2 \right) + 2P$$

where P is the number of terms in the model. Here, no inferential statements are being made about this quantity, and, all other things being equal, simplicity is favored over complexity. Similar *AIC* statistics are also available for other models, such as logistic regression. Searching the predictor space for the model with the smallest *AIC* may help avoid over-fitting.[2]

Another approach is correlation-based feature selection (Hall and Smith 1997), which attempts to find the best subset of predictors that have strong

---

[1] The majority of the scholarship on this problem has revolved around *stepwise* model selection, a variant of forward selection. However, the results apply to any search procedure using hypothesis testing in this manner.

[2] It should be noted that the *AIC* statistic is designed for preplanned comparisons between models (as opposed to comparisons of many models during automated searches).

correlations with the outcome but weak between-predictor correlations. To do this, one possible metric is

$$G = \frac{P\,R_y}{\sqrt{P + P(P-1)\bar{R}_x}}$$

where R_y is a measure of correlation between the candidate predictor and the outcome, and $\bar{R}_x$ is the average correlation between the current predictor and the P predictors already included in the subset. At each stage of the search, this metric can rank predictors as a function of effectiveness and redundancy.

For models built *to predict*, rather than explain, there are two important overall points:

- Many of the criticisms of wrapper methods listed above[3] focus on the use of statistical hypothesis tests.
- As in many other cases presented in this text, methodologies based on dubious statistical principals may still lead to very accurate models. The key protection in these instances is a thorough, methodical validation process with independent data.

The following subsections describe different search methods to use with wrapper methods.

Forward, Backward, and Stepwise Selection

Classical forward selection was previously described in Algorithm 19.1. *Stepwise selection* is a popular modification where, after each candidate variable is added to the model, each term is reevaluated for removal from the model. In some cases, the p-value threshold for adding and removing predictors can be quite different (Derksen and Keselman 1992). Although this makes the search procedure less greedy, it exacerbates the problem of repeated hypothesis testing. In *backward selection*, the initial model contains all P predictors which are then iteratively removed to determine which are not significantly contributing to the model. These procedures can be improved using non-inferential criteria, such as the *AIC* statistic, to add or remove predictors from the model.

Guyon et al. (2002) described a backward selection algorithm (called *recursive feature elimination*) that avoids refitting many models at each step of the search. When the full model is created, a measure of variable importance is computed that ranks the predictors from most important to least. The importance calculations can be model based (e.g., the random forest importance criterion) or using a more general approach that is independent of the full model. At each stage of the search, the least important predictors are

---

[3] However, Derksen and Keselman (1992) and Henderson and Velleman (1981) make arguments against automated feature selection in general.

1	Tune/train the model on the training set using all P predictors
2	Calculate model performance
3	Calculate variable importance or rankings
4	**for** *each subset size S_i, $i = 1 \ldots S$* **do**
5	Keep the S_i most important variables
6	[Optional] Pre-process the data
7	Tune/train the model on the training set using S_i predictors
8	Calculate model performance
9	[Optional] Recalculate the rankings for each predictor
10	**end**
11	Calculate the performance profile over the S_i
12	Determine the appropriate number of predictors (i.e. the S_i associated with the best performance)
13	Fit the final model based on the optimal S_i

Algorithm 19.2: Backward selection via the recursive feature elimination algorithm of Guyon et al. (2002)

iteratively eliminated prior to rebuilding the model. As before, once a new model is created, the objective function is estimated for that model. The process continues for some predefined sequence, and the subset size corresponding to the best value of the objective function is used as the final model. This process is outlined in more detail in Algorithm 19.2 and is illustrated in Sect. 19.6.

While it is easy to treat the RFE algorithm as a black box, there are some considerations that should be made. For example, when the outcome has more than two classes, some classes may have a large degree of separation from the rest of the training set. As such, it may be easier to achieve smaller error rates for these classes than the others. When the predictors are ranked for selection, the predictors associated with the "easy" classes may saturate the positions for the highest ranks. As a result, the difficult classes are neglected and maintain high error rates. In this case, class-specific importance scores can aid in selecting a more balanced set of predictors in an effort to balance the error rates across all the classes.

Simulated Annealing

A multitude of modern search procedures exist that can be applied to the feature selection problem. *Simulated annealing* (Bohachevsky et al. 1986) mimics the process of metal cooling. Algorithm 19.3 describes this process in detail. An initial subset of predictors is selected and is used to estimate

---

1 Generate an initial random subset of predictors
2 for *iterations* $i = 1 \ldots t$ **do**
3   Randomly perturb the current best predictor set
4   [Optional] Pre-process the data
5   Tune/train the model using this predictor set
6   Calculate model performance (E_i)
7   **if** $E_i < E_{best}$ **then**
8   Accept current predictor set as best
9   Set $E_{best} = E_i$
10   **else**
11   Calculate the probability of accepting the current predictor set

$$p_i^a = \exp\left[(E_{best} - E_i)/T\right]$$

12   Generate a random number U between $[0, 1]$
13   **if** $p_i^a \leq U$ **then**
14   Accept current predictor set as best
15   Set $E_{best} = E_i$
16   **else**
17   Keep current best predictor set
18   **end**
19   **end**
20 end
21 Determine the predictor set associated with the smallest E_i across all iterations
22 Finalize the model with this predictor set

Algorithm 19.3: Simulated annealing for feature selection. E is a measure of performance where small values are best and T is a temperature value that changes over iterations

performance of the model (denoted here as E_1, for the initial error rate). The current predictor subset is slightly changed, and another model is created with an estimated error rate of E_2. If the new model is an improvement over the previous one (i.e., $E_2 < E_1$), the new feature set is accepted. However, if it is worse, it may still be accepted based on some probability p_i^a, where i is the iteration of the process. This probability is configured to decrease over time so that, as i becomes large, it becomes very unlikely that a suboptimal configuration will be accepted. The process continues for some pre-specified number of iterations and the best variable subset across all the iterations,

Parents   Reproduction   Children

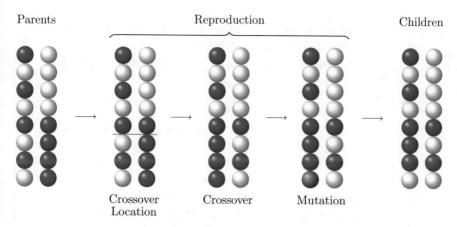

Crossover   Crossover   Mutation
Location

Fig. 19.3: A schematic of the reproduction phase of a genetic algorithm

is used. The idea is to avoid a local optimum (a solution that is currently best but is not best overall). By accepting "bad" solutions, the algorithm is able to continue the search in other spaces and therefore is less greedy.

Genetic Algorithms

A distant kin to simulated annealing are *genetic algorithms* (GAs) (Holland 1975; Goldberg 1989). This optimization tool is based on evolutionary principles of population biology and has been shown to be effective at finding optimal solutions of complex, multivariate functions. Specifically, GAs are constructed to imitate the evolutionary process by allowing the current population of solutions to reproduce, generating children which compete to survive. The most fit survivors are then allowed to reproduce, creating the next generation of children. Over time, generations converge to a fitness plateau (Holland 1992) and an optimal solution can be selected.

As we have seen thus far, the problem of feature selection is inherently a complex optimization problem, where we seek the combination of features that provides an optimal prediction of the response. To employ GAs towards this end, we must frame the feature selection problem in terms of the GA machinery. The subjects of this machinery are chromosomes, which consist of genes and are evaluated based on their fitness. To create the next generation of offspring, two chromosomes reproduce through the process of crossover and mutation, which is illustrated in Fig. 19.3. GAs have been shown to be effective feature selection tools in the fields of chemometrics (Lavine et al. 2002), image analysis (Bhanu and Lin 2003), and finance (Min et al. 2006; Huang et al. 2012).

1	Define the stopping criteria, number of children for each generation ($GenSize$), and probability of mutation (p_m)
2	Generate an initial random set of m binary chromosomes, each of length p
3	**repeat**
4	**for** *each chromosome* **do**
5	Tune and train a model and compute each chromosome's fitness
6	**end**
7	**for** *reproduction* $k = 1 \ldots GenSize/2$ **do**
8	Select two chromosomes based on the fitness criterion
9	Crossover: Randomly select a loci and exchange each chromosome's genes beyond the loci
10	Mutation: Randomly change binary values of each gene in each new child chromosome with probability, p_m
11	**end**
12	**until** *stopping criteria is met*

Algorithm 19.4: A genetic algorithm for feature selection

In the context of feature selection, the chromosome is a binary vector that has the same length as the number of predictors in the data set. Each binary entry of the chromosome, or gene, represents the presence or absence of each predictor in the data. The fitness of the chromosome is determined by the model using the predictors indicated by the binary vector. GAs are therefore tasked with finding optimal solutions from the 2^n possible combinations of predictor sets.

To begin the search process, GAs are often initiated with a random selection of chromosomes from the population of all possible chromosomes. Each chromosome's fitness is computed, which determines the likelihood of the chromosome's selection for the process of reproduction. Two chromosomes from the current population are then selected based on the fitness criterion and are allowed to reproduce. In the reproduction phase, the two parent chromosomes are split at a random position (also called *loci*), and the head of one chromosome is combined with the tail of the other chromosome and vice versa. After crossover, the individual entries of the new chromosomes can be randomly selected for mutation in which the current binary value is changed to the other value. Algorithm 19.4 lists these steps.

The crossover phase drives subsequent generations towards optimums in subspaces of similar genetic material. In other words, the search subspace will be narrowed to the space defined by the most fit chromosomes. This means that the algorithm could become trapped in a local optimum. In the context of feature selection, this means that the selected features may produce an optimal model, but other more optimal feature subsets may exist. The mutation phase enables the algorithm to escape local optimums by randomly perturbing the genetic material. Usually the probability of mutation is kept low (say, $p_m < 0.05$). However, if the practitioner is concerned about local optimums, then the mutation probability can be raised. The effect of raising the mutation probability is a slowing of the convergence to an optimal solution.

19.4 Filter Methods

As previously stated, filter methods evaluate the predictors prior to training the model, and, based on this evaluation, a subset of predictors are entered into the model. Since the scoring of predictors is disconnected from the model, many of the variable importance metrics discussed in Chap. 18 would be appropriate for filtering the variables. Most of these techniques are univariate, meaning that they evaluate each predictor in isolation. In this case, the existence of correlated predictors makes it possible to select important, but redundant, predictors. The obvious consequences of this issue are that too many predictors are chosen and, as a result, collinearity problems arise. Guyon and Elisseeff (2003) discuss several aspects of predictor redundancy during filtering.

Also, if hypothesis tests are used to determine which predictors have statistically significant relationships with the outcome (such as the t-test), the problem of *multiplicity* can occur (see Westfall and Young (1993) and Fig. 19.2). For example, if a confidence level of $\alpha = 0.05$ is used as a p-value threshold for significance, each individual test has a theoretical false-positive rate of 5 %. However, when a large number of simultaneous statistical tests are conducted, the overall false-positive probability increases exponentially. To account for this, p-value adjustment procedures can control the false positive rate. The *Bonferroni correction* (Bland and Altman 1995) is one such procedure. If a p-value cutoff of α is used to define statistical significance for each of M tests, using an alternative cutoff of α/M increases the stringency and will help control the probability of a false-positive results. However, this procedure can be very conservative and limit the number of true-positive results. Other approaches to dealing with multiplicity can be found in Westfall and Young (1993). Also, Ahdesmaki and Strimmer (2010) propose a modified t-test that accounts for the large number of tests being conducted as well as between-predictor correlations.

While filter methods tend to be simple and fast, there is a subjective nature to the procedure. Most scoring methods have no obvious cut point to declare which predictors are important enough to go into the model. Even in the case of statistical hypothesis tests, the user must still select the confidence level to apply to the results. In practice, finding an appropriate value for the confidence value α may require several evaluations until acceptable performance is achieved.

19.5 Selection Bias

While some filtering methods or search procedures are more effective than others, the more important question is related to how model performance is calculated (especially when the sample size is small). Over-fitting the predictors to the training data can occur and, without a proper validation, may go unnoticed. For example, Guyon et al. (2002) demonstrated recursive feature elimination with support vector machine classification models for a well-known colon cancer microarray data set. In these data, measurements on 2,000 unique RNA sequences were used as predictors of disease status (cancer or normal) in a set of 62 patients. No test set was used to verify the results. To monitor performance, leave-one-out cross-validation was used for each model (at Line 8 in Algorithm 19.2). Their analysis showed that the SVM model can achieve accuracy over 95 % using only 4 predictors and 100 % accuracy with models using 8–256 predictors.

The leave-one-out error rates were based on the SVM model *after* the features had been selected. One could imagine that if the feature selection were repeated with a slightly different data set, the results might change. It turns out that, in some cases, the uncertainty induced by feature selection can be much larger than the uncertainty of the model (once the features have been selected). To demonstrate this, Ambroise and McLachlan (2002) conducted the same RFE procedure with the same data set but scrambled the class labels (to coerce all the predictors into being non-informative). They showed that the leave-one-out cross-validation strategy used by Guyon et al. (2002) would achieve zero errors even when the predictors are completely non-informative.

The logical error in the original approach is clear. A model was created from the training set and, using these data, the predictors were evaluated and ranked. If the model is refit using only the important predictors, performance almost certainly improves on the same data set. In addition, the P to n ratio is extreme (2000:62) which appreciably increases the odds that a completely irrelevant predictor will be declared important by chance.

The methodological error occurred because the feature selection was not considered as part of the model-building process. As such, it should be included within the resampling procedure so that the variation of feature selection is captured in the results. The leave-one-out cross-validation procedure on Line 8 in Algorithm 19.2 is ignorant of the steps outside of the model training process that it measures. For example, even if the feature selection process arrives at the true model after evaluating a large number of candidate models, the performance estimates should reflect the process that led to the result.

To properly resample the feature selection process, an "outer" resampling loop is needed that encompasses the entire process. Algorithm 19.5 shows such an resampling scheme for recursive feature elimination. At Line 1, resampling is applied such that the entire feature selection process is within. For example, if 10-fold cross-validation were in this initial loop, 90 % of the data would be used to conduct the feature selection and the heldout 10 % would be used to evaluate performance (e.g., Line 10) for each subset of predictors. The entire feature selection process would be conducted nine additional times with a different set of heldout samples. In the end, these ten holdout sets determine the optimal number of predictors in the final model (Line 14). Given this result, the entire training set is used to rank the predictors and train the final model (Lines 16 and 17, respectively). Note that an additional "inner" layer of resampling may be needed to optimize any tuning parameters in the model (Lines 3 and 9).

Ambroise and McLachlan (2002) also showed that when the bootstrap, 10-fold cross-validation or repeated test set resampling methods were used properly, the model results were correctly determined to be around the value of the no-information rate.

The additional resampling layer can have a significant negative impact on the computational efficiency of the feature selection process. However, especially with small training sets, this process will drastically reduce the chances of over-fitting the predictors.

The critical point is that it is sometimes easy to commit errors in validating the results of feature selection procedures. For example, Castaldi et al. (2011) conducted a survey of articles that used classification techniques with biological data (e.g., RNA microarrays, proteins) and found that 64 % of the analyses did not appropriately validate the feature selection process. They also showed that these analyses had a significant difference between the re-sampled performance estimates and those calculated from an independent test set (the test set results were more pessimistic).

The risk of over-fitting in this way is not confined to recursive feature selection or wrappers in general. When using other search procedures or filters for reducing the number of predictors, there is still a risk.

The following situations increase the likelihood of selection bias:

- The data set is small.
- The number of predictors is large (since the probability of a non-informative predictor being falsely declared to be important increases).
- The predictive model is powerful (e.g., black-box models), which is more likely to over-fit the data.
- No independent test set is available.

When the data set is large, we recommend separate data sets for selecting features, tuning models, and validating the final model (and feature set). For small training sets, proper resampling is critical. If the amount of data is not too small, we also recommend setting aside a small test set to double check that no gross errors have been committed.

---

1 for *each resampling iteration* **do**

  2 | Partition data into training and test/hold-back set via resampling

  3 | Tune/train the model on the training set using all P predictors

  4 | Calculate model performance

  5 | Calculate variable importance or rankings

  6 | **for** *Each subset size S_i, $i = 1 \ldots S$* **do**

    7 | | Keep the S_i most important variables

    8 | | [Optional] Pre-process the data

    9 | | Tune/train the model on the training set using S_i predictors

    10 | | Calculate model performance using the held-back samples

    11 | | [Optional] Recalculate the rankings for each predictor

  12 | **end**

13 end

14 Calculate the performance profile over the S_i using the held-back samples

15 Determine the appropriate number of predictors

16 Determine the final ranks of each predictor

17 Fit the final model based on the optimal S_i using the original training set

---

Algorithm 19.5: Recursive feature elimination with proper resampling

19.6 Case Study: Predicting Cognitive Impairment

Alzheimer's disease (AD) is a cognitive impairment disorder characterized by memory loss and a decrease in functional abilities above and beyond what is typical for a given age. It is the most common cause of dementia in the elderly. Biologically, Alzheimer's disease is associated with amyloid-β ($A\beta$) brain plaques as well as brain tangles associated with a form of the Tau protein.

Diagnosis of AD focuses on clinical indicators that, once manifested, indicate that the progression of the disease is severe and difficult to reverse. Early diagnosis of Alzheimer's disease could lead to a significant improvement in patient care. As such, there is an interest in identifying *biomarkers*, which are measurable quantities that do not involve a clinical evaluation.[4]

---

[4] There are different types of biomarkers. For example, blood cholesterol levels are believed to indicate cardiovascular fitness. As such, they can be monitored to understand patient health but are also used to characterize the effect of treatments. In the

de Leon and Klunk (2006) and Hampel et al. (2010) contain broad discussion of biomarkers for Alzheimer's disease.

Although medical imaging may be helpful in predicting the onset of the disease there is also an interest in potential low-cost fluid biomarkers that could be obtained from plasma or cerebrospinal fluid (CSF). There are currently several accepted non-imaging biomarkers: protein levels of particular forms of the $A\beta$ and Tau proteins and the Apolipoprotein E genotype. For the latter, there are three main variants: E2, E3 and E4. E4 is the allele most associated with AD (Kim et al. 2009; Bu 2009). Prognostic accuracy may be improved by adding other biomarkers to this list.

Craig-Schapiro et al. (2011) describe a clinical study of 333 patients, including some with mild (but well characterized) cognitive impairment as well as healthy individuals. CSF samples were taken from all subjects. The goal of the study was to determine if subjects in the early states of impairment could be differentiated from cognitively healthy individuals. Data collected on each subject included:

- Demographic characteristics such as age and gender
- Apolipoprotein E genotype
- Protein measurements of $A\beta$, Tau, and a phosphorylated version of Tau (called pTau)
- Protein measurements of 124 exploratory biomarkers, and
- Clinical dementia scores

For these analyses, we have converted the scores to two classes: impaired and healthy. The goal of this analysis is to create classification models using the demographic and assay data to predict which patients have early stages of disease.

Given the relatively small sample size, one could argue that the best strategy for data splitting is to include all the subjects in the training set to maximize the amount of information for estimating parameters and selecting predictors. However, with the ratio of predictors to data points in these data, the possibility of selection bias is relatively high. For this reason, a small set of subjects will be held back as a test set to verify that no gross methodological errors were committed. The test set contained 18 impaired subjects and 48 cognitively healthy. Any measures of performance calculated from these data will have high uncertainty but will be adequate to detect over-fitting due to feature selection.

For the 267 subjects in the training set, five repeats of 10-fold cross-validation will be used to evaluate the feature selection routines (e.g., the "outer" resampling procedure). If models have additional tuning parameters, simple 10-fold cross-validation is used. Tuning these models will occur at every stage of the feature selection routine. During feature selection and model

---

latter case, the cholesterol information is treated as surrogate end points for the truly important attributes (e.g., mortality or morbidity).

Table 19.1: Training set frequencies for two encodings of the genotype data

	E2/E2	E2/E3	E2/E4	E3/E3	E3/E4	E4/E4	E2	E3	E4
Impaired	0	6	1	27	32	7	7	65	40
Control	2	24	6	107	51	4	32	182	61

tuning, the area under the ROC curve (for the predicted class probabilities) was optimized.

Figure 19.4 shows the 124×124 correlation matrix of the predictors. There are many strong between-predictor correlations, as indicated by the dark red and blue areas. The average pairwise correlation was 0.27. The minimum and maximum correlations were -0.93 and 0.99, respectively. Many of the correlations are contained within a large group of predictors (as shown by the large red block on the diagonal). This may have a negative effect on the modeling and feature selection process. The analysis shown below uses all the predictors to model the data. Applying an unsupervised filter to reduce the feature set prior to analysis may help improve the results (see Exercise 19.1).

Almost all of the predictors in the data are continuous. However, the Apolipoprotein E genotype is not. For the three genetic variants (E2, E3, and E4), there are six possible values as one copy of the gene is inherited from each parent. The breakdown of these values in the training set is shown in Table 19.1. When broken down into the maternal/paternal genetic combinations, some variants have very small frequencies (e.g., E2/E2). Some predictive models may have issues estimating some parameters, especially if the frequencies are reduced during resampling. An alternate encoding for these data is to create three binary indicators for each allele (e.g., E2, E3 and E4). This version of the information is shown in the three most right-hand columns in Table 19.1. Since these frequencies are not as sparse as the genotype pairs, this encoding is used for all the predictive models shown here.

To illustrate feature selection, recursive feature elimination was used for several models and 66 subset sizes ranging from 1 to 131. Models that require parameter tuning were tuned at each iteration of feature elimination. The following models were evaluated:

- Random forests: The default value of $m_{\text{try}} = \sqrt{p}$ was used at each iteration, and 1,000 trees were used in the forest.
- Linear discriminant analysis: The standard approach was used (i.e., no penalties or internal feature selection).
- Unregularized logistic regression: A model with only main effects was considered.
- K-nearest neighbors: The model was tuned over odd number of neighbors ranging from 5 to 43.

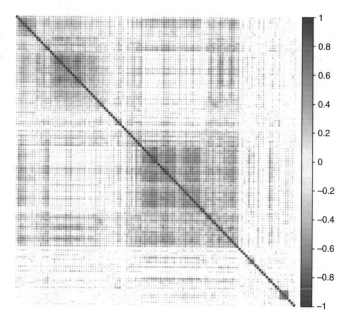

Fig. 19.4: Between predictor correlations for the AD data. Each *row* and *column* represents one of the predictors. The row and column orders have been sorted using clustering methods

- Naïve Bayes: Nonparametric kernel estimates were used for the continuous predictors
- Support Vector Machines: A radial basis function kernel was used. The analytical estimate of σ was used along with cost values ranging from 2^{-2} to 2^9.

The random forest variable importance scores (based on the initial first model) ranked predictors for that model, whereas logistic regression used the absolute value of the Z-statistic for each model parameter. The other models ranked predictors with the area under the ROC curve for each individual predictor.

Figure 19.5 shows the resampling profiles of the feature selection process for each model. Random forest showed very little change until important predictors were eventually removed from the model. This is somewhat expected since, even though random forests do minimal embedded filtering of predictors, non-informative predictors tend to have very little impact on the model predictions. The optimal number of predictors estimated for the model was 7, although there is considerable leeway in this number. LDA showed a large improvement and peaked at 35 predictors and the area under the ROC curve was estimated to be slightly better than the random forest model. Logistic regression showed very little change in performance until about 50 predic-

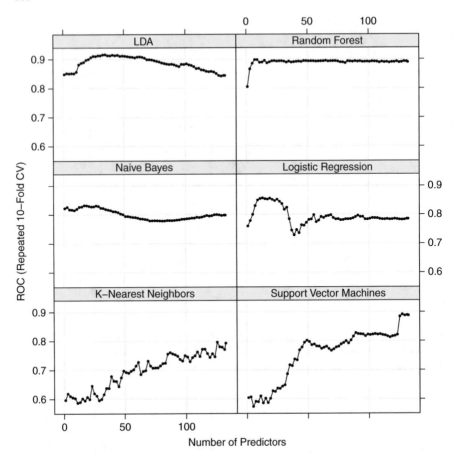

Fig. 19.5: The resampling profiles for the RFE procedure for several models

tors when, after an initial dip, performance improved considerably. The best subset size for this model was 13. However, there is a significant drop in performance for the model once important predictors are removed. Naïve Bayes showed a slight improvement as predictors were removed, culminating at approximately 17 predictors. Unlike the others, this model did not show a sharp downturn in performance when a small number of predictors were left. Both support vector machines and K-nearest neighbors suffered considerably when predictors were removed and were at their best with the full predictor set. In the case of support vector machines, the poor performance may be unrelated to selection bias. A closer examination of the SVM results indicates that the models have high specificity and low sensitivity (see the results in the computing section below). In other words, the poor results are likely a result of the class imbalance in the data.

Table 19.2: Cross-validation results for recursive feature selection

	Full set		Reduced set			
	ROC	C.I.	Size	ROC	C.I.	p-value
LDA	0.844	$(0.82 - 0.87)$	35	0.916	$(0.90 - 0.94)$	0
RF	0.891	$(0.87 - 0.91)$	7	0.898	$(0.88 - 0.92)$	0.1255
SVM	0.889	$(0.87 - 0.91)$	127	0.891	$(0.87 - 0.91)$	0.0192
Logistic reg.	0.785	$(0.76 - 0.81)$	13	0.857	$(0.83 - 0.88)$	0
N. Bayes	0.798	$(0.77 - 0.83)$	17	0.832	$(0.81 - 0.86)$	0.0002
K-NN	0.849	$(0.83 - 0.87)$	125	0.796	$(0.77 - 0.82)$	1.0000

The "C.I." column corresponds to 95 % confidence intervals while the
p-value column corresponds to a statistical test that evaluates whether the
ROC value for the reduced model was a larger than the curve associated
with all of the predictors

Table 19.2 contains a summary of the resampling results for each model.
The area under the ROC curve is shown for the full model (i.e., all of the
predictors) versus the models resulting from the recursive feature elimination process. In Table 19.2, 95 % confidence intervals are also shown. These
were calculated from the 50 resampled estimates produced by repeated cross-
validation. Of the models evaluated, LDA has the best estimate of performance. However, based on the confidence intervals, this value is similar in
performance to other models (at least within the experimental error reflected
in the intervals), including random forest (post feature selection) and support vector machines (before or after feature selection). The p-value column
is associated with a statistical test where the null hypothesis is that the reduced predictor set has a larger ROC value than the full set. This value was
computed using the paired resampling result process described in Sect. 4.8.
Although the support vector machine and K-nearest neighbors models were
not substantially enhanced, there was considerable evidence that the other
models were improved by recursive feature elimination.

Did the test set show the same trends as the resampling results? Figure 19.6
shows the estimates of the area under the ROC curve for the reduced models.
The y-axis corresponds to the resampled ROC values (and confidence intervals) shown previously in Table 19.2. The x-axis has similar values across
models, but these were calculated from ROC curves using predictions on the
test set of 66 subjects. There was much more uncertainty in the test set results; the widths of the test set confidence intervals tended to be more than
3 times the width of the corresponding intervals from resampling. There is a
moderate correlation between the ROC values calculated using the test set
and resampling. The test set results were more optimistic than the resampling results for the naïve Bayes, logistic regression, and K-nearest neighbors

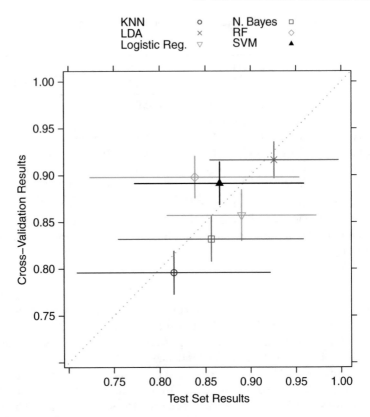

Fig. 19.6: Estimates of the area under the ROC curve for the reduced model using the test set and repeated cross-validation. The horizontal and vertical bars are the 95 % confidence intervals using each method

models. Also, the support vector machine model was ranked higher by cross-validation than the test set. Despite these inconsistencies, the test set results generally reinforce the results seen in Table 19.2; the feature selection process tended to show benefits for several models and did not result in severe selection bias.

The two leading models, LDA and random forests, are quite different. Did these models select the same predictors? This is a somewhat subjective question since, as shown in Fig. 19.5, neither of the profiles for these models had a single peak. Because of this, the optimal subset size is not clear. However, using the numerically optimal result, random forests used 7 and LDA selected 35. All of the random forest predictors are included in the LDA model, but 28 of the LDA predictors are not in the random forest model. Figure 19.7 shows the variable importance estimates for both models (recall that the area under the ROC curve was used for LDA). In this plot, the importance values are the averages of those found during the resampling process for the final subset size. For example, there are points on the plot for predictors only contained in the LDA model. These predictors have random forest values since that predictor was selected in at least one of the 50 resamples with a subset size of 7 predictors. The rug plot on the y-axis corresponds to the area under the ROC curve for predictors that were not selected in any of the random forest models. There is a fair amount of concordance between the two models; the rank correlation between the common predictors is 0.44. The discordant predictors tend to have low importance scores for both models. Both models contained two predictors, the Aβ and Tau protein assays, with a large influence on the models. The third most important predictor for both models was the modified Tau assay. After this, the importance scores begin to disagree with LDA/ROC using MMP10 and random forest using VEGF.

This underscores the idea that feature selection is a poor method for determining the most significant variables in the *data*, as opposed to which predictors most influenced the *model*. Different models will score the predictors differently. To assess which predictors have individual associations with the outcome, common classical statistical methods are far more appropriate. For example, Craig-Schapiro et al. (2011) also used analysis of covariance and other inferential models to evaluate possible associations. These techniques are designed to yield higher-quality, probabilistic statements about the potential biomarkers than any variable importance method. Finally, the biological aspects of the analysis potentially trump all of the empirical evaluations. While the study is aimed at finding novel biomarkers, a certain degree of scientific legitimacy is needed, as well as prospective experimentation to further validate the results found in these data.

The use of filters with linear discriminant analysis was also explored. For the continuous predictors, a simple t-test was used to generate a p-value for the difference in means of the predictor between the two classes. For the categorical predictors (e.g., gender, Apolipoprotein E genotype), Fisher's exact test was used to calculate a p-value that tests the association between the predictor and the class. Once the p-values were calculated, two approaches were used for filtering:

1. Retain the predictors with raw p-values less than 0.05, i.e., accept a 5 % false-positive rate for each individual comparison.
2. Apply a Bonferroni correction so that predictors are retained when their p-values are less than 0.000379 or 0.05/132.

For the first approach, the process retained 47 predictors out of 132. This process was also resampled using the same repeated cross-validation process used for the wrapper analysis. Across the 50 resamples, the filter selected 46.06 predictors on average, although this number ranged from 38 to 57. Using the predictor subset, an LDA model was fit. The resulting test set area under the ROC curve for this model was 0.918. When the filtering and modeling activities were resampled, a similar area under the curve resulted (AUC: 0.917). The filtered set of variables consisted of members with relatively small

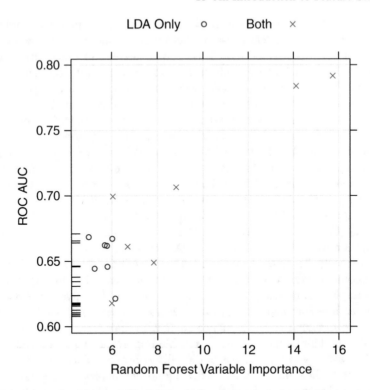

Fig. 19.7: A comparison of two methods for determining variable importance. The random forest values correspond to models with 7 predictors while the ROC values are based on the top 35 predictors (i.e., the best subset for LDA). The values are averaged across the 50 resamples. The "LDA Only" values are predictors that were in the final LDA model but not the random forest model. The hash marks, not the y-axis, are for LDA predictors that were not selected in any of the 50 resampled random forest models

between-correlations with one exception. The Tau and pTau predictors are strongly related (correlation: 0.91). Repeating this process without the pTau predictor resulted in no effective change in the area under the ROC curve.

When the p-value filter is modified to reduce the number of false-positive results, only 17 predictors were selected (13.46 were selected, on average, during cross-validation). Here, the impact on the model is not as clear. The test set area under the ROC curve was a slight improvement (AUC: 0.926), but the resampled estimate was considerably worse, with an area under the curve of 0.856. Given the sample size, there is considerable variability in the test set; the 95 % confidence interval for the area under the curve is (0.841, 1). While the cross-validation process only held out 27 patients on average, this process was repeated 50 times. For this reason, there may be more credence in the more pessimistic resampling estimates.

19.7 Computing

This section discusses data and/or functions from the following packages: AppliedPredictiveModeling, caret, klaR, leaps, MASS, pROC, rms, and stats.

The data are contained in the AppliedPredictiveModeling package. The data objects consist of a data frame of predictors called `predictors` and a factor vector of class values called `diagnosis` (with levels impaired and control). The following code was used to prepare the data for analysis:

```
> library(AppliedPredictiveModeling)
> data(AlzheimerDisease)
> ## Manually create new dummy variables
> predictors$E2 <- predictors$E3 <- predictors$E4 <- 0
> predictors$E2[grepl("2", predictors$Genotype)] <- 1
> predictors$E3[grepl("3", predictors$Genotype)] <- 1
> predictors$E4[grepl("4", predictors$Genotype)] <- 1
>

> ## Split the data using stratified sampling
> set.seed(730)
> split <- createDataPartition(diagnosis, p = .8, list = FALSE)
> ## Combine into one data frame
> adData <- predictors
> adData$Class <- diagnosis
> training <- adData[ split, ]
> testing  <- adData[-split, ]
> ## Save a vector of predictor variable names
> predVars <- names(adData)[!(names(adData) %in% c("Class",  "Genotype"))]

> ## Compute the area under the ROC curve, sensitivity, specificity,
> ## accuracy and Kappa
>
> fiveStats <- function(...) c(twoClassSummary(...),
+                              defaultSummary(...))
> ## Create resampling data sets to use for all models
> set.seed(104)
> index <- createMultiFolds(training$Class, times = 5)
> ## Create a vector of subset sizes to evaluate
> varSeq <- seq(1, length(predVars)-1, by = 2)
```

The code to reproduce the computations in this chapter is extensive and can be found in the AppliedPredictiveModeling package. This section demonstrates how feature selection can be conducted in R for a subset of the analyses.

Forward, Backward, and Stepwise Selection

There are several R functions for this class of wrappers:

- `step` in the stats package can be used to search for appropriate subsets for linear regression and generalized linear models (from the `lm` and `glm` functions, respectively). The `direction` argument controls the search method (e.g. "both," "backward," or "forward"). A more general function is the stepAIC function in the MASS package, which can handle additional model types. In either case, the AIC statistic (or its variants) is used as the objective function.

- The fastbw function in the rms package conducts similar searches but has the optional but unrecommended choice of using p-values as the objective function.
- The regsubsets function in the leaps package has similar functionality.
- The klaR package contains the stepclass function than searches the predictor space for models that maximize cross-validated accuracy rates. The function has built-in methods for several models, such as lda, but can be more broadly generalized.

The caret package function train has wrappers for leaps, stepAIC, and stepclass, so that the entire feature selection process can be resampled and the risk of selection bias is reduced.

For example, to use stepAIC with logistic regression, the function takes an initial model as input. To illustrate the function, a small model is used:

```
> initial <- glm(Class ~ tau + VEGF + E4 + IL_3, data = training,
+                    family = binomial)
> library(MASS)
> stepAIC(initial, direction = "both")

  Start:  AIC=189.46
  Class ~ tau + VEGF + E4 + IL_3

          Df Deviance    AIC
  - IL_3   1   179.69 187.69
  - E4     1   179.72 187.72
  <none>       179.46 189.46
  - VEGF   1   242.77 250.77
  - tau    1   288.61 296.61

  Step:  AIC=187.69
  Class ~ tau + VEGF + E4

          Df Deviance    AIC
  - E4     1   179.84 185.84
  <none>       179.69 187.69
  + IL_3   1   179.46 189.46
  - VEGF   1   248.30 254.30
  - tau    1   290.05 296.05

  Step:  AIC=185.84
  Class ~ tau + VEGF

          Df Deviance    AIC
  <none>       179.84 185.84
  + E4     1   179.69 187.69
  + IL_3   1   179.72 187.72
  - VEGF   1   255.07 259.07
```

```
- tau    1    300.69 304.69

Call: glm(formula = Class ~ tau + VEGF, family = binomial, data = training)

Coefficients:
(Intercept)           tau            VEGF
     9.8075       -4.2779          0.9761

Degrees of Freedom: 266 Total (i.e. Null);   264 Residual
Null Deviance:              313.3
Residual Deviance: 179.8              AIC: 185.8
```

The function returns a `glm` object with the final predictor set. The other functions listed above use similar strategies.

Recursive Feature Elimination

The caret and varSelRF packages contain functions for recursive feature elimination. While the `varSelRF` function in the **varSelRF** is specific to random forests, the `rfe` function in caret is a general framework for any predictive model. For the latter, there are predefined functions for random forests, linear discriminant analysis, bagged trees, naïve Bayes, generalized linear models, linear regression models, and logistic regression. The random forest functions are in a list called `rfFuncs`:

```
> library(caret)
> ## The built-in random forest functions are in rfFuncs.
> str(rfFuncs)
  List of 6
   $ summary    :function (data, lev = NULL, model = NULL)
   $ fit        :function (x, y, first, last, ...)
   $ pred       :function (object, x)
   $ rank       :function (object, x, y)
   $ selectSize:function (x, metric, maximize)
   $ selectVar :function (y, size)
```

Each of these function defines a step in Algorithm 19.2:

- The summary function defines how the predictions will be evaluated (Line 10 in Algorithm 19.2).
- The fit function allows the user to specify the model and conduct parameter tuning (Lines 19.2, 6, and 12).
- The pred function generates predictions for new samples.
- The rank function generates variable importance measures (Line 2).
- The selectSize function chooses the appropriate predictor subset size (Line 11).
- The selectVar function picks which variables are used in the final model.

These options can be changed. For example, to compute the expanded set of performance measures shown above,

```
> newRF <- rfFuncs
> newRF$summary <- fiveStats
```

To run the RFE procedure for random forests, the syntax is

```
> ## The control function is similar to trainControl():
> ctrl <- rfeControl(method = "repeatedcv",
+                    repeats = 5,
+                    verbose = TRUE,
+                    functions = newRF,
+                    index = index)

> set.seed(721)
> rfRFE <- rfe(x = training[, predVars],
+              y = training$Class,
+              sizes = varSeq,
+              metric = "ROC",
+              rfeControl = ctrl,
+              ## now pass options to randomForest()
+              ntree = 1000)
> rfRFE


Recursive feature selection

Outer resampling method: Cross-Validation (10-fold, repeated 5 times)

Resampling performance over subset size:

 Variables   ROC   Sens    Spec  Accuracy  Kappa Selected
         1 0.8051 0.5375 0.8806    0.7869 0.4316
         3 0.8661 0.6407 0.9167    0.8415 0.5801
         5 0.8854 0.6736 0.9365    0.8645 0.6386
         7 0.8980 0.6571 0.9414    0.8637 0.6300        *
         9 0.8978 0.6850 0.9506    0.8779 0.6679
        11 0.8886 0.6750 0.9609    0.8825 0.6756
        13 0.8895 0.6604 0.9609    0.8786 0.6636
        15 0.8950 0.6586 0.9629    0.8794 0.6628
        17 0.8867 0.6554 0.9621    0.8780 0.6576
        19 0.8900 0.6418 0.9642    0.8758 0.6514

         :      :      :       :         :      :        :

       129 0.8923 0.4439 0.9826    0.8351 0.4947
       131 0.8918 0.4439 0.9836    0.8360 0.4976
       132 0.8895 0.4439 0.9815    0.8345 0.4963

The top 5 variables (out of 7):
   Ab_42, tau, p_tau, VEGF, FAS
```

(This output has been truncated, and the columns for the standard deviations were removed to fit on the page.)

The process for predicting new samples is straightforward:

```
> predict(rfRFE, head(testing))
       pred Impaired Control
2   Control    0.291   0.709
6  Impaired    0.695   0.305
15  Control    0.189   0.811
16 Impaired    0.794   0.206
33  Control    0.302   0.698
38 Impaired    0.930   0.070
```

The built-in functions predict the classes and probabilities for classification.

There are also built-in functions to do recursive feature selection for models that require retuning at each iteration. For example, to fit support vector machines:

```
> svmFuncs <- caretFuncs
> svmFuncs$summary <- fivestats

> ctrl <- rfeControl(method = "repeatedcv",
+                    repeats = 5,
+                    verbose = TRUE,
+                    functions = svmFuncs,
+                    index = index)

> set.seed(721)
> svmRFE <- rfe(x = training[, predVars],
+               y = training$Class,
+               sizes = varSeq,
+               metric = "ROC",
+               rfeControl = ctrl,
+               ## Now options to train()
+               method = "svmRadial",
+               tuneLength = 12,
+               preProc = c("center", "scale"),
+               ## Below specifies the inner resampling process
+               trControl = trainControl(method = "cv",
+                                        verboseIter = FALSE,
+                                        classProbs = TRUE))
> svmRFE


Recursive feature selection

Outer resampling method: Cross-Validation (10-fold, repeated 5 times)

Resampling performance over subset size:

 Variables    ROC      Sens    Spec Accuracy     Kappa Selected
         1 0.6043 0.000000 0.9959   0.7237 -0.005400
         3 0.6071 0.005714 0.9858   0.7178 -0.010508
         5 0.5737 0.000000 0.9979   0.7252 -0.002718
         7 0.5912 0.005357 0.9969   0.7259  0.002849
         9 0.5899 0.000000 0.9979   0.7252 -0.002799
        11 0.6104 0.000000 0.9959   0.7237 -0.005625
        13 0.5858 0.000000 0.9979   0.7252 -0.002829
```

```
      :    :       :       :         :       :          :
    121 0.8172 0.513571 0.9241    0.8116  0.473426
    123 0.8210 0.514286 0.9199    0.8087  0.469536
    125 0.8844 0.608571 0.9559    0.8610  0.613538
    127 0.8914 0.671786 0.9548    0.8775  0.666157        *
    129 0.8877 0.647500 0.9445    0.8632  0.629154
    131 0.8891 0.644643 0.9487    0.8655  0.631925
    132 0.8879 0.647143 0.9455    0.8639  0.630313

  The top 5 variables (out of 127):
     Ab_42, tau, p_tau, MMP10, MIF
```

Here we can see that the poor performance is related to the class imbalance; the model is biased towards high specificity since most samples are controls.

The caret web page[5] contains more details and examples related to rfe.

Filter Methods

caret has a function called sbf (for Selection By Filter) that can be used to screen predictors for models and to estimate performance using resampling. Any function can be written to screen the predictors.

For example, to compute a p-value for each predictor, depending on the data type, the following approach could be used:

```
> pScore <- function(x, y)
+   {
+     numX <- length(unique(x))
+     if(numX > 2)
+       {
+         ## With many values in x, compute a t-test
+         out <- t.test(x ~ y)$p.value
+       } else {
+         ## For binary predictors, test the odds ratio == 1 via
+         ## Fisher's Exact Test
+         out <- fisher.test(factor(x), y)$p.value
+       }
+     out
+   }

> ## Apply the scores to each of the predictor columns
> scores <- apply(X = training[, predVars],
+                 MARGIN = 2,
+                 FUN = pScore,
+                 y = training$Class)
> tail(scores)
         p_tau         Ab_42         male            E4           E3
  1.699064e-07 8.952405e-13 1.535628e-02 6.396309e-04 1.978571e-01
            E2
  1.774673e-01
```

[5] http://caret.r-forge.r-project.org/.

A function can also be designed to apply a p-value correction, such as the Bonferroni procedure:

```
> pCorrection <- function (score, x, y)
+ {
+   ## The options x and y are required by the caret package
+   ## but are not used here
+   score <- p.adjust(score,  "bonferroni")
+   ## Return a logical vector to decide which predictors
+   ## to retain after the filter
+   keepers <- (score <= 0.05)
+   keepers
+ }
> tail(pCorrection(scores))
   p_tau Ab_42  male    E4    E3    E2
   TRUE   TRUE FALSE FALSE FALSE FALSE
```

As before, **caret** contains a number of built-in functions for filter methods: linear regression, random forests, bagged trees, linear discriminant analysis, and naïve Bayes (see ?rfSBF for more details). For example, ldaSBF has the following functions:

```
> str(ldaSBF)
List of 5
 $ summary:function (data, lev = NULL, model = NULL)
 $ fit    :function (x, y, ...)
 $ pred   :function (object, x)
 $ score  :function (x, y)
 $ filter :function (score, x, y)
```

These functions are similar to those shown for rfe. The score function computes some quantitative measure of importance (e.g., the p-values produced by the previous pScore function). The function filter takes these values (and the raw training set data) and determines which predictors pass the filter.

For the biomarker data, the filtered LDA model was fit using

```
> ldaWithPvalues <- ldaSBF
> ldaWithPvalues$score <- pScore
> ldaWithPvalues$summary <- fiveStats
> ldaWithPvalues$filter <- pCorrection
> sbfCtrl <- sbfControl(method = "repeatedcv",
+                       repeats = 5,
+                       verbose = TRUE,
+                       functions = ldaWithPvalues,
+                       index = index)
> ldaFilter <- sbf(training[, predVars],
+                   training$Class,
+                   tol = 1.0e-12,
+                   sbfControl = sbfCtrl)

> ldaFilter
```

```
Selection By Filter

Outer resampling method: Cross-Validation (10-fold, repeated 5 times)

Resampling performance:

   ROC   Sens   Spec Accuracy  Kappa  ROCSD SensSD  SpecSD AccuracySD
0.9168 0.7439 0.9136    0.867 0.6588 0.06458 0.1778 0.05973     0.0567
KappaSD
 0.1512

Using the training set, 47 variables were selected:
   Alpha_1_Antitrypsin, Apolipoprotein_D, B_Lymphocyte_Chemoattractant_BL,
   Complement_3, Cortisol...

During resampling, the top 5 selected variables (out of a possible 66):
   Ab_42 (100%), Cortisol (100%), Creatine_Kinase_MB (100%),
   Cystatin_C (100%), E4 (100%)

On average, 46.1 variables were selected (min = 38, max = 57)
```

Again, the caret package web site has additional detail regarding the rfe and sbf functions, including features not shown here.

Exercises

19.1. For the biomarker data, determine if the between-predictor correlations shown in Fig. 19.4 have an effect on the feature selection process. Specifically:

(a) Create an initial filter of the predictors that removes predictors to minimize the amount of multicollinearity in the data prior to modeling.
(b) Refit the recursive feature selection models.
(c) Did the RFE profiles shown in Fig. 19.4 change considerably? Which models would have been mostly likely affected by multicollinearity?

19.2. Use the same resampling process to evaluate a penalized LDA model. How does performance compare? Is the same variable selection pattern observed in both models?

19.3. Apply different combinations of filters and predictive models to the biomarker data. Are the same predictors retained across different filters? Do models react differently to the same predictor set?

19.4. Recall Exercise 7.2 where a simulation tool from Friedman (1991) utilized a nonlinear function of predictors:

$$y = 10\sin(\pi x_1 x_2) + 20(x_3 - 0.5)^2 + 10x_4 + 5x_5 + e$$

where the predictors x_1 through x_5 have uniform distributions and the error e is normally distributed with zero mean and a standard deviation that can be specified:

(a) Simulate a training and test set with $n = 500$ samples per data set. Plot the predictors against the outcome in the training set using scatter plots, correlation plots, table plots, and other visualizations.

(b) Use forward, backward, and stepwise algorithms for feature selection. Did the final models select the full set of predictors? Why or why not? If cross-validation was used with these search tools, was the performance similar to the test set?

(c) Use recursive feature selection with several different models? How did these methods perform? Were the informative predictors selected?

(d) Apply filter methods to the data using filters where each predictor is evaluated separately and others are evaluated simultaneously (e.g., the ReliefF algorithm). Were the two interacting predictors (x_1 and x_2) selected? Was one favored more than the other?

(e) Reduce the sample size of the training set and add a larger number of non-informative predictors. How do these search procedures perform under more extreme circumstances?

19.5. For the cell segmentation data:

(a) Use filter and wrapper methods to determine an optimal set of predictors.

(b) For linear discriminant analysis and logistic regression, use the alternative versions of these models with built-in feature selection (e.g., the glmnet and sparse LDA). How do the different approaches compare in terms of performance, the number of predictors required, and training time?

Chapter 20
Factors That Can Affect Model Performance

Several of the preceding chapters have focused on technical pitfalls of predictive models, such as over-fitting and class imbalances. Often, true success may depend on aspects of the problem that are not directly related to the model itself. For example, there may be limitations to what the data can support or perhaps there may be subtle obstacles related to the goal of the modeling effort. One issue not discussed here is related to the acceptance of modeling, especially in areas where these techniques are viewed as novel or disruptive. Ayres (2007) offers a broad discussion of this issue. Another important aspect of modeling not discussed in this chapter is *feature engineering*; that is, methods to encode one or more predictors for the model.

This chapter discusses several important aspects of creating and maintaining predictive models. The first section looks at "Type III" errors: developing a model that answers the wrong question. An illustrative example is used to show that, due to sampling issues with the training set, the model gives predictions that answer a different question than the one of interest.

Noise, or error, has varying degrees of impact on models' predictive performance and occurs in three general forms in most data sets:

- Since many predictors are measured, they contain some level of systematic noise associated with the measurement system. Any extraneous noise in the predictors is likely to be propagated directly through the model prediction equation and results in poor performance.
- A second way noise can be introduced into the data is by the inclusion of non-informative predictors (e.g., predictors that have no relationship with the response). Some models have the ability to filter out irrelevant information, and hence their predictive performance is relatively unaffected.
- A third way noise enters the modeling process is through the response variable. As with predictors, some outcomes can be measured with a degree of systematic, unwanted noise. This type of error gives rise to an upper bound on model performance for which no pre-processing, model complexity, or tuning can overcome. For example, if a measured categorical outcome is mislabeled in the training data 10 % of the time, it is unlikely

M. Kuhn and K. Johnson, *Applied Predictive Modeling*,
DOI 10.1007/978-1-4614-6849-3_20,
© Springer Science+Business Media New York 2013

that any model could truly achieve more than a 90 % accuracy rate. Of course, the modeler will not be aware of this and may expend considerable time chasing noise.

These aspects of modeling are explored in Sects. 20.2 and 20.3. Section 20.4 discusses the effect of discretizing outcomes on predictive performance while Sect. 20.5 examines the consequences of model *extrapolation*. We wrap up this chapter with an overview of how large data can impact model performance.

20.1 Type III Errors

One of the most common mistakes in modeling is to develop a model that answers the wrong question, otherwise known as a "Type III" error (Kimball 1957). Often, there can be a tendency to focus on the technical details and inadvertently overlook true nature of the problem. In other words, it is very important to focus on the overall strategy of the problem at hand and not just the technical tactics of the potential solution. For example, in business applications, the goal is almost always to maximize profit. When the observed outcome is categorical (e.g., purchase/no-purchase or churn/retention), it is key to tie the model performance and class predictions back to the expected profit.

A more subtle example of a problematic modeling strategy is related to *response modeling* in marketing. Recall the direct marketing example discussed in Chap. 11 where a group of customers for a clothing store were contacted with a promotion. For each customer, the *response* was recorded (i.e., whether a purchase was made).

The true goal of the clothing store is to increase profits, but this particular campaign did not sample from all of the appropriate populations. It only utilized customers who had been contacted and made the assumption that *all customers* would mimic the behavior demonstrated in this population.[1] Any model built from these data is limited to predicting the probability of a purchase *only if the customer was contacted*. This conditional statement is contrary to the goal of increasing overall profit. In fact, offering a promotion to customers who would always respond reduces profit.

For example, there is a subpopulation of customers who would make a purchase regardless of a promotional offer. These responders are likely to be in the observed data and the model would be unable to distinguish the reasons for the response. The goal of the model building exercise is to increase profits by making promotional offers to only those customers who would not have response without one.

---

[1] In marketing, Rzepakowski and Jaroszewicz (2012) defined the following classes of marketing models: "In the propensity models, historical information about purchases (or other success measures like visits) is used, while in the *response* models, all customers have been subject to a pilot campaign."

Siegel (2011) outlines four possible cases:

		No contact	
		Response	Non response
Contact	Response	A	B
	Non response	C	D

The cells in the table are:

- A: customers who would respond regardless of contact
- B: customers who would respond solely because of the promotion
- C: customers who have a negative response to the promotion and would have responded if they would not have been contacted
- D: customers who have absolutely no interest in responding

To increase profits, a model that accurately predicts which customers are in cell B is the most useful as this is the population associated with *new profit*. The potential negative consequences for the simple response model are:

- The response rate is overestimated since it contains customers who always respond. The overall estimated profit is not net profit since the baseline profit is embedded. For example, a lift curve generated from a response model might indicate that by contacting 30 % of the customers, a response rate of 70 % could be achieved. There is a good chance that the customers who always respond would be scored confidently by the model and consume some percentage of the 30 % designated for contact.
- Costs are increased by sending promotions to customers in cells C or D. For the cost structure described by Larose (2006, Chap. 7), the cost of the promotion was relatively low. However, in some situations, the costs can be much higher. For example, exposing customers to unwanted promotions can have a detrimental effect on their sentiment towards the business. Also, where response models are used for customer retention, there is the possibility that the contact will *trigger* churn since it is a reminder that they might find a better deal with another company.

These issues cannot be observed until the promotion is put into action.

Techniques that attempt to understand the impacts of customer response are called *uplift modeling* (Siegel 2011; Radcliffe and Surry 2011; Rzepakowski and Jaroszewicz 2012), *true lift models* (Lo 2002), *net lift modes*, *incremental lift models*, or *true response modeling*. Lo (2002) suggests that a control group of customers who are not contacted can be used to develop a separate response model to differentiate customers in cells A and C from those in cells B and D (although B and D cannot be differentiated by the model). In conjunction with a traditional response model that is created using customers who were contacted, a scoring strategy would be to find customers with large values of

$$Pr[\text{response}|\text{contact}] - Pr[\text{response}|\text{no contact}].$$

By subtracting off the probability of those customers who respond without contact, a more refined instrument is being used to find the appropriate customer set. The drawback with this approach is that it is indirect. Also, there is a likelihood that the model predictions would be highly correlated since they are modeling very similar events. If this is the case, there may be very few customers for which the two probabilities are not similar. Radcliffe and Surry (2011) describe tree-based models where the uplift is modeled directly with a control group of customers who have not been contacted.

Another approach could be to use more sophisticated sampling techniques to create an appropriate training set. For the table above, it is impossible to contact and to not contact the same customer. However, in medical research, this problem is often faced when evaluating a new treatment against an existing therapy. Here, clinical trials sometimes use *matched samples*. Two subjects are found that are nearly identical and are randomized into treatment groups. The idea is that the only differentiating factor is the treatment, and the patient response can be estimated more accurately than without matching. The important idea here is that the subjects are no longer the experimental unit. The matched pair itself becomes the primary data point in the analysis.

The same strategy can be applied to this situation. Suppose an initial sample of customers can be matched with others who have the same attributes such as demographic factors and income levels. Within each matched pair, a promotion could be randomly assigned to one customer in the pair. Now, for each matched pair, the above 2×2 table could be created. If the results are aggregated across all matched pairs, a classification model for the four different outcomes (A though D) can be created and customers can be scored on their probability of being in class B, which is the group of interest. This approach directly models the population of interest in a single model.

20.2 Measurement Error in the Outcome

What is the minimum error rate that a model could achieve? Recall the linear regression model shown in Eq. 6.1:

$$y_i = b_0 + b_1 x_{i1} + b_2 x_{i2} + \cdots + b_p x_{ip} + e_i.$$

The residuals e_i were assume, to have some variance denoted as σ^2. If we knew the true model structure (i.e., the exact predictors and their relationship with the outcome), then σ^2 would represent the lowest possible error achievable or the *irreducible error*. However, we do not usually know the true model structure, so this value becomes inflated to include *model error* (i.e., error

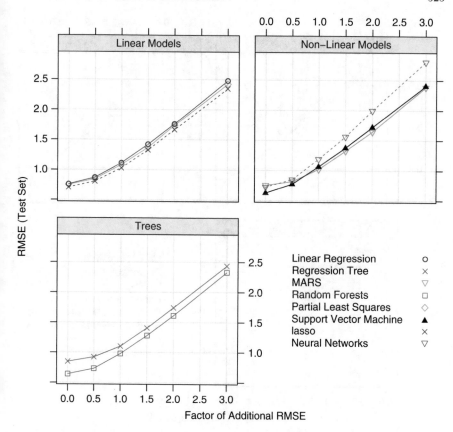

Fig. 20.1: Test set RMSE profiles for solubility models when measurement system noise increases

related to lack of fit). During the modeling process, the goal is to eliminate the model error.

However, there is another component that contributes to σ^2 that cannot be eliminated through the modeling process. If the outcome contains significant *measurement noise*, the irreducible error is increased in magnitude. The root mean squared error and R^2 then have respective lower and upper bounds due to this error. Therefore, the error term, in addition to containing the variation in the response that is not explained by the model, collects measurement system error. The better we understand the measurement system and its limits as well as the relationship between predictors and the response, the better we can foresee the limits of model performance. As mentioned in the introduction to this chapter, a similar problem occurs in classification.

To illustrate the impact of the degree of error in the response on model performance we will revisit the solubility QSAR data (Chaps. 6 through 9). The response for these data is the log of the solubility measurement (Fig. 6.2),

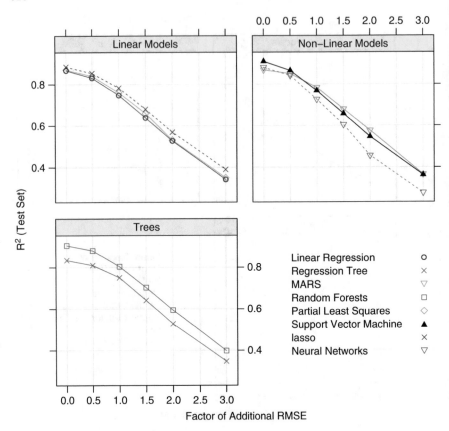

Fig. 20.2: Test set R^2 profiles for solubility models when measurement system noise increases

and the predictors were either continuous or binary (Sect. 6.1). The best linear regression model for these data had an RMSE of 0.7, which comprises the measurement system error, lack of fit error, and errors due to relevant predictors that are not included in the model. For our illustration, we will use this value as a base level for error and increase the error in the response proportionally. To do this, we have added noise to each compound's log solubility value that comes from a normal distribution with a mean of zero and a standard deviation of the linear regression model RMSE multiplied by a factor ranging from 0 to 3. For each level of additional noise, we trained and tuned the following models: linear regression, partial least squares, single regression trees, multivariate adaptive regression splines, random forests, neural networks, and radial basis function support vector machines. Performance for each of these models is evaluated based on RMSE and R^2 for the test set and the results are shown in Figs. 20.1 and 20.2. Clearly performance gets worse regardless of model type (linear models, nonlinear models, or trees) and worsens proportionally to the degree of additional error incorporated into the response.

There are two important take-aways from this simple illustration. First, this type of noise is, noise that no model can predict—we're simply stuck with it and we cannot break through the RMSE floor or R^2 ceiling. Thus, the more the modeler knows about the measurement system, the better one can understand expectations about model performance. Second, as noise increases, the models become virtually indistinguishable in terms of their predictive performance. This means that the advantages that some of the more complex models, like ensembles, bring are only advantageous when the measurement system error is relatively low. This makes sense because the complex underlying structure that a model (such as an ensemble) can find will become more fuzzy as the noise increases. Therefore, we will likely be able to perform just as well with a simple, computationally efficient model when measurement system noise is high.

20.3 Measurement Error in the Predictors

As shown in several of the data sets, many of the predictors are calculated. For example, the solubility data contained fingerprints that indicated the presence or absence of a particular chemical structure. In text mining, predictors may be the frequency of certain important words or phrases contained in the text. In other cases, the predictors are observed or may be the product of some external process. For example:

- The cell segmentation data measured different aspects of cells, such as the area of the nucleus.
- The grant data collected information about the number of successful and unsuccessful grants.

Traditional statistical models typically assume that the predictors are measured without error, but this is not always the case. The effect of randomness in the predictors can be drastic, depending on several factors: the amount of randomness, the importances of the predictors, the type of model being used, as well as others. In some cases, if the initial data that are in the training set are generated in very controlled conditions, then the randomness can be hidden. For example, suppose data are generated by a person manually measuring an object (such as a rating). There may be differences in how people perceive the object, resulting in rater-to-rater noise. If a single rater is used for the training set data but another rate is used for new data, the bias between raters is likely to cause issues.

As another example, consider the concrete mixture data discussed previously. Even though the exact proportions and amounts of each mixture ingredient are known, there is some deviation in these values when the mixtures are created. If the process of creating the concrete is complicated, the actual amount used may be different from the formula (although this difference is not measured or observed).

To illustrate the effect of random predictor noise on models, a simple *sin* wave was simulated with random error. Figure 20.3 shows the original data in the panel labeled "SD = 0". Here, the data on the x-axis are evenly spaced values between 2 and 10. The outcome was created by adding a small amount of normally distributed noise to the data. In each panel, the true relationship between the predictor and the response is shown as a solid black line. Two different regression models were used to fit the data. The left-hand column of panels shows an ordinary linear regression model where the true model form (i.e., $sin(x)$) is fit to the data. The right-hand column of panels corresponds to fits from a CART regression tree. The fitted curves from these models are shown as thick red lines.

The rows in Fig. 20.3 are the same data with no noise (in the top row) and when random error is incrementally added to the predictor values. Specifically, random normal values are added to the true values with different standard deviations. The small blue bell-shaped curves in this figure show the probability distribution of a data point with a mean of six and the corresponding standard deviation. The y-axis values are the same across all panels.

Linear regression is able to effectively model the true relationship with no additional noise. As noise is added to the predictors, the linear regression model begins to become poor at the apex and nadir points of the curve. The effect becomes very pronounced with a standard deviation of 0.75. However, the illustration is a somewhat optimistic assessment since it assumes that the modeler already knows the true relationship between x and y and has specified the model with this knowledge.

With no additional noise, the regression tree also approximates the pattern within the range of the observed data fairly well. The regression tree results are more problematic since the algorithm is having to determine the pattern in the data empirically. Additionally, this particular model is unstable (i.e., low bias but high variance). In this case, the difference between the predicted and true relationship begins to become more pronounced with smaller amounts of random error.

Measurement errors in the predictors can cause considerable issues when building models, especially in terms of reproducibility of the results on future data sets (similar in effect to over-fitting). In this case, future results may be poor because the underlying predictor data are different than the values used in the training set.

Case Study: Predicting Unwanted Side Effects

Pharmaceutical companies have departments for *derisking* compounds, that is, trying to detect if the candidate drug will have harmful side-effects or

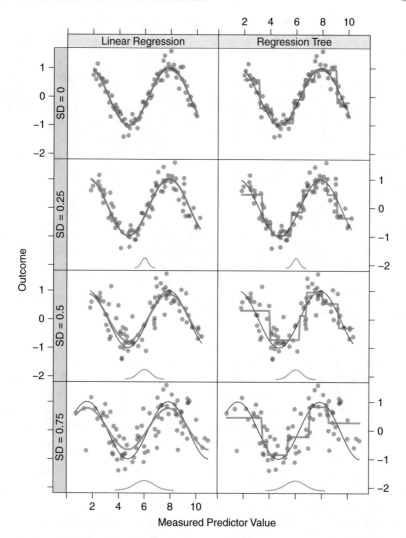

Fig. 20.3: A simulated *sin* wave and two model fits when different amounts of noise are added to the predictor values

toxicities in humans. One technique for detecting these issues is to create cell-based assays that signal if the compound is potentially dangerous. In conjunction with these lab results, a set of compounds with known issues are identified as well as a set of "clean" compounds with no known issues. Biological assays are created and used as inputs to predictive models. Much like the earlier example where solubility was predicted from chemical structures, these models use measurements of how cell lines react to the compounds to predict potential safety issues.

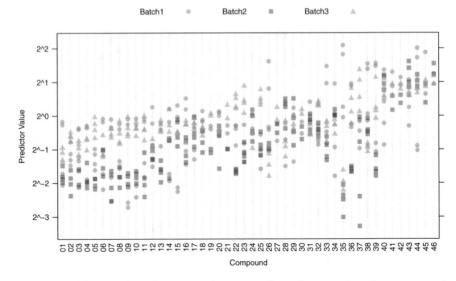

Fig. 20.4: The results of an experiment used to characterize the sources of unwanted noise in a set of biological assays

In the example presented here, the goal was to develop a predictive model for a specific toxicity. A set of about ten assays were created that measured the amount of RNA transcription (otherwise known as gene expression) in a specific type of cell. Around 250 compounds (either toxic or clean) were assayed and these results were used to train a set of models. The models resulted in sensitivities and specificities around 80 %.

However, when a new set of compounds was tested (along with several controls from the original training set), the results were no better than a random guessing. After reviewing the model building process for methodological errors, the quality of the assays was investigated.

An experiment was run where subset of 46 compounds were measured in three distinct batches (run over non-consecutive days). Within each batch, there were several replicates of each compound. A visualization of the individual data points for one of the assays is shown in Fig. 20.4, where the compounds are ordered by their average value. Clearly, there are batch-to-batch effects in the data, especially for some compounds. The trends are not uniform; in many cases, batch three had the largest values but not for every compound. Additionally, within a batch, the predictor values can range dramatically—sometimes across two logs. For example, compound 35 spans the entire range of the predictor data.

Statistical methods called variance component models (sometimes called *gauge reproducibility and repeatability* methods (Montgomery and Runger 1993)) quantify the source of the noise in the data. In this experimental design, the best possible case would be that the compound-to-compound variation in the data would account for 100 % of the noise (i.e., there would be no batch-to-batch or within-batch noise). Using a variance component analysis, the compounds accounted for about 38 % of the noise in the data. The batch-to-batch variation was 13 % of the total, and the within-batch variation was 49 %. Clearly, this is not an optimal situation since a large majority of the variation in the data is unwanted noise.[2] Since some of these compounds are toxic and others are not, it is unlikely that these measurements will help differentiate toxic and clean compounds. The other assays had similar results. It should be noted that these assays were chosen based on the data from other experiments that produced a sound biological rational for using them in this context. Therefore, we believe that there is some signal in these predictors, but it is being drowned out by the noise of the measurement system.

20.4 Discretizing Continuous Outcomes

In many fields, it may be desirable to work with a categorical response even if the original response is on a continuous scale.[3] This could be due to the fact that the underlying distribution of the response is truly bimodal. Consider Fig. 20.5 which illustrates two histograms of numeric outcomes from different data sets. The top histogram is the solubility data discussed thus far in the chapter while the histogram in the bottom of the figure represents the distribution of a measurement for another data set. While the solubility distribution is symmetric, the bottom distribution is clearly bimodal where most of the data are found at either end of the response, with relatively few in the midrange. Trying to categorize the data in the top distribution will be difficult, since there is no natural categorical distinction. Categorizing data in the bottom distribution, however, is more natural.

In other situations, the desire to work with the response on a categorical scale may be due to practical reasons. For the data that we have been examining thus far, solubility may be one of many characteristics that scientists evaluate in order to move forward in the drug discovery process. To simplify this multidimensional optimization problem, decision makers may prefer to know whether or not a compound is predicted to be *soluble enough* rather than the compound's predicted log solubility value. The selection of an optimal set of compounds can then be simplified into a checklist across the conditions of interest where the preferred compounds are the ones that satisfy the most properties of interest. While this process can grossly identify the most promising compounds for further research, more nuanced distinc-

---

[2] Note that, in this case, the noise in the predictors is *systematic* and random. In other words, we can attribute the source of variation to a specific cause.

[3] An example of this is the job scheduling data where the execution time of a job was binned into four groups. In this case, the queuing system cannot utilize estimates of job length but can use binned versions of this outcome.

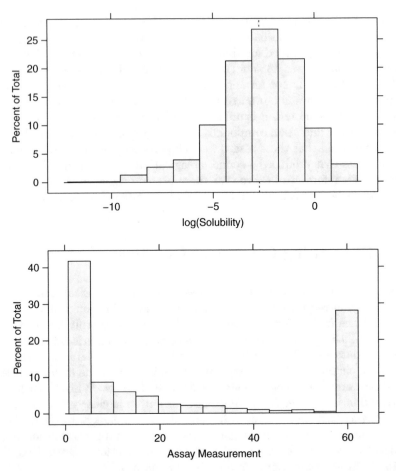

Fig. 20.5: Comparison of distributions between two data sets. *Top*: Solubility measurements on compounds previously discussed throughout this chapter. The dotted vertical line is the mean log solubility value which will be used to categorize these data. *Bottom*: Outcome values for another data set. This distribution is clearly bimodal and a categorization of data into two categories would be more natural

tions among compounds are lost because information in the outcome is being discarded.

When the response is bimodal (or multimodal), categorizing the response is appropriate. However, if the response follows a continuous distribution, as the solubility data do, then categorizing the response prior to modeling induces a loss of information, which weakens the overall utility of the model.

To illustrate this loss of information, we will continue to work with the solubility data. For this illustration, we have categorized the response as being above or below the mean (-2.72 log units) and tuned each classification model with a couple of necessary modifications. Linear regression has been replaced with logistic regression, MARS has been replaced with FDA, and the LASSO has been replaced with glmnet, where each replacement is the parallel classification technique. After training each model, we predict the probability of each compound in the test set in addition to the Kappa value for the test set. For each test set compound we also have the predicted continuous response which we can align with the predicted probability of a compound being soluble. We can then compare the scatter plots of the continuous prediction with the probability prediction across compounds.

Figure 20.6 illustrates the test set results for the regression and classification approaches for PLS, SVM, and random forests (results from other models are similar and are presented in Exercise 20.1). For each of the regression models, the observed and predicted log(solubility) values follow a line of agreement with predicted values falling within approximately four log(solubility) units of the actual values across the range of response. Looking at the center of the distribution, a predicted log(solubility) value of -4 traces back to observed values ranging between approximately -6 and -2 log units across the models. On the other hand, a predicted probability of 0.5 for the classification models traces back to actual values ranging between approximately -6 and 0 for PLS and -4 and 0 for SVM and random forests. The range of predictions at the extremes of the classification models is even wider. For example, a predicted probability near zero for SVM corresponds to actual log(solubility) values in the range of -10 to -2, and predicted probabilities near one correspond to actual values between -3.5 and 2 (similarly for random forests). In this example, working with the data in on the original scale provides more accurate predictions across the range of response for all models. Further comparisons of model results for these data are presented in Exercise 20.1.

A second common reason for wanting to categorize a continuous response is that the scientist may believe that the continuous response contains a high degree of error, so much so that only the response values in either extreme of the distribution are likely to be correctly categorized. If this is the case, then the data can be partitioned into three categories, where data in either extreme are classified generically as positive and negative, while the data in the midrange are classified as unknown or indeterminate. The middle category can be included as such in a model (or specifically excluded from the model tuning process) to help the model more easily discriminant between the two categories.

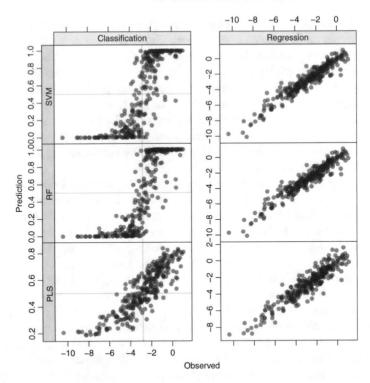

Fig. 20.6: Test set performance comparison of solubility models when response is modeled as a continuous and categorical value

20.5 When Should You Trust Your Model's Prediction?

We could view this section as "when should you *not* trust your model's prediction?" The predictive modeling process assumes that the underlying mechanism that generated the current, existing data for both the predictors and the response will continue to generate data from the same mechanism. For a simple example of a data-generating mechanism, consider the commercial food manufacturing business. Commercial food companies strive to create the same product over time so that customers can consistently have the same food tasting experience. Therefore companies keep the recipe, ingredients, and preparation process the same over time. If we were modeling moisture content of chocolate chip cookies from a commercial bakery, then we would expect that the predictors measured on a new batch of cookies would likely fall in the range as the predictors of the training set (collected at some past points in time). This means that new data will have similar characteristics and will occupy similar parts of the predictor space as the data on which the model was built.

For the examples used throughout this book, we have taken appropriate steps to create test sets that had similar properties across the predictor space as the training set. Principles underlying this process were described in Sect. 4.3. If new data are generated by the same data-generating mechanism as the training set, then we can have the confidence that the model will make sensible predictions for the new data. However, if the new data are not generated by the same mechanism, or if the training set was too small or sparse to adequately cover the range of space typically covered by the data-generating mechanism, then predictions from the model may not be trustworthy. *Extrapolation* is commonly defined as using a model to predict samples that are outside the range of the training data (Armitage and Berry 1994). It is important to recognize for high-dimensional data, however, that there may be regions within the predictors' range where no training data exist. Therefore, we need to extend our notion of extrapolation to include these vacuous interior regions of predictor space. Extrapolated predictions, whether outside the range of the predictors or within vacant regions of space, may not be trustworthy and can lead to poor decision making.

Understanding when a model is producing an extrapolated prediction can be difficult to diagnose, and the practitioner's first defense is a deep understanding of the mechanism used to generate both the training set and the new set of samples for which a prediction will be generated. Consider again the commercial chocolate chip cookie manufacturing process, and suppose that the manufacturer had changed the recipe, ingredients, and baking process. Using a previously developed model to predict moisture content for cookies from the current process may yield inaccurate predictions since the predictors for the new data are likely in a different part of space as those in the training data. If the practitioner knows this information about the data at hand, then she can use appropriate caution in applying the model and interpreting the resulting predictions.

Many times though, the practitioner does not know if the underlying data-generating mechanism is the same for the new data as the training data. Data sets with few predictors are much easier to understand and relationships between predictors in the training set and new set of samples can be examined via simple scatter plots and a comparison of distributions of each predictor. But as the dimension of the space increases, examining scatter plots and distributions is very inefficient and may not lead to a correct understanding of the predictor space between the training data and new data. In these circumstances there are a few tools that can be employed to better understand the similarity of the new data to the training data.

The *applicability domain* of a model is the region of predictor space where "the model makes predictions with a given reliability" (Netzeva et al. 2005). Different variations of this definition exist, but the most simplistic is to define the domain in terms of similarity to the training set data. If the new data being predicted are similar enough to the training set, the assumption would be that these points would, on average, have reliability that is characterized

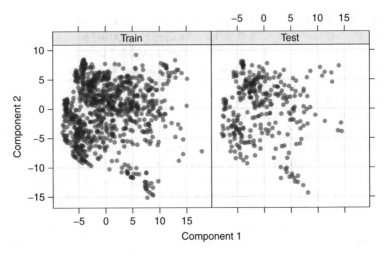

Fig. 20.7: PCA plots for the solubility data

by the model performance estimates (e.g., the accuracy rate derived from a test set).

A gross comparison of the space covered by the predictors from the training set and the new set can be made using routine dimension reduction techniques such as principal components analysis (Sect. 3.3) or multidimensional scaling (Davison 1983). If the training data and new data are generated from the same mechanism, then the projection of these data will overlap in the scatter plot. However, if the training data and new data occupy different parts of the scatter plot, then the data may not be generated by the same mechanism and predictions for the new data should be used with caution. Figure 20.7 displays the projection of the training and testing sets for the solubility data onto the first two principal components of the training data. In this case, the training and testing data appear to occupy the same space as determined by these components. Of course, this result is expected since the training set and test set were randomly partitioned from the original data set. But a further examination of similarity between training and test set samples is developed in Sect. 20.7 and Exercise 20.3.

When projecting many predictors into two dimensions, intricate predictor relationships as well as sparse and dense pockets of space can be masked. This means that while the training data and new data may appear to overlap in the projection plot, there may be regions within the predictor space where the model will inadequately predict new samples.

To address this problem, Hastie et al. (2008) describe an approach for quantifying the likelihood that a new sample is a member of the training data. In this approach, the training predictors are selected. Then a random multivariate uniform sample based on the ranges of the training predictors is

---

1 Compute the variable importance for the original model and identify the top 20 predictors

2 Randomly permute these predictors from the training set

3 Row-wise concatenate the original training set's top predictors and the randomly permuted version of these predictors

4 Create a classification vector that identifies the rows of the original training set and the rows of the permuted training set

5 Train a classification model on the newly created data

6 Use the classification model to predict the probability of new data being in the class of the training set.

Algorithm 20.1: Algorithm for determining similarity to the training set

generated such that it has the same number of samples as the training data. The response vector is categorical with the original training data identified as the training set and the random uniform sample identified as the random set. Any classification model can then be built on this set, and the resulting model can be used to predict the probability that a new sample is a member of the training set.

We propose two slight alterations to this method, to better address real data. First, given that many data sets contain different types of predictors, we recommend randomly permuting predictors rather than sampling from a uniform distribution across the range of predictors. By doing this, we achieve a random distribution across the entire space, while keeping within the permissible values of each predictor. Therefore categorical predictors will only receive appropriate categorical values. Second, given that data are large both in terms of predictors and dimensions, we recommend building the categorical model on a subset of the original predictors. Specifically, we suggest selecting the top 20 (or some reasonable fraction based on the context of the problem and model) important predictors from the original model of the training data. This will greatly reduce model building time, while still generating a model that can assist in assessing if the model is producing an extrapolated prediction. The steps of this process are listed in Algorithm 20.1.

To illustrate this method, we return to the two-dimensional example originally displayed in Fig. 4.1. Of course, here we omit variable selection and proceed to step 2. We augmented the original data with randomly permuted values of the original predictors (Fig. 20.8) and built a bagged classification tree. We then generated 50 random samples and moved them further away from the original data in sequential steps and used the bagged classification tree to predict the probability that the samples were from the training data.

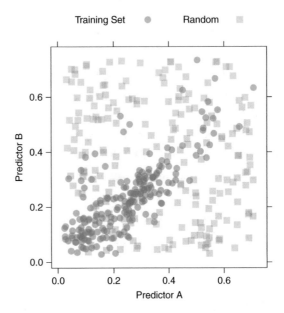

Fig. 20.8: Random uniform data have been added to the example data originally displayed in Fig. 4.1 in order to cover the range of space of the two predictors

The placement of the new samples as well as the probability of the samples being members of the training set are illustrated in Fig. 20.9. Clearly, as samples move farther from the original training data, the likelihood of training set membership decreases.

20.6 The Impact of a Large Sample

Our focus on performance thus far has been through the lens of the predictors and the response. Now we turn to the impact of the number of samples on model performance. An underlying presumption is that the more samples we have, the better model we can produce. This presumption is certainly fueled by our ability to now easily attain as many samples as we desire. As an example of the ease at which data can be obtained, consider Ayres (2007), who described the process he followed for naming his book *Super Crunchers*. To understand the reader population's opinion on his choices of titles, he used several variations of targeted Google Ads, each with a different candidate name for the book. After a short period of time, he collected a quarter of a million samples related to which ad was clicked on most. Since the ads were

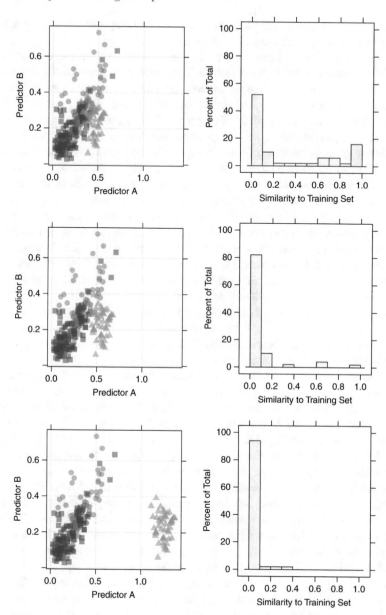

Fig. 20.9: An illustration for detecting model extrapolation. The *left column* of figures depicts three test set scenarios with the proximity ranging from near the training data (*top*) to far from the training data (*bottom*). The *right column* of figures present the probability that the test set samples are members of the original training data

served at random, this large-scale test provided strong evidence of which book name the reader population liked best.

This straightforward and clever approach to understanding a population provides a positive example of how a large number of samples can be beneficially used. But as we have seen from previous sections, noise in the predictors or the response can minimize any advantages that may be brought by an increase in the number of samples. Furthermore, an increase in the number of samples can have less positive consequences. First, many of the predictive models have significant computational burdens as the number of samples (and predictors) grows. For example, a single classification tree does many exhaustive searches across the samples and predictors to find optimal splits of the data. As the dimensions of the data increase, computation time likewise increases. Moreover the computational burden for ensembles of trees is even greater, often requiring more expensive hardware and/or special implementations of models that make the computations feasible. Second, there are diminishing returns on adding more *of the same data* from the same population. Since models stabilize with a sufficiently large number of samples, garnering more samples is less likely to change the model fit.

For example, web search technology initially used the content of a web site to rank search results. If one searched on a term such as "`predictive modeling`", the search algorithm would focus on terms in the collection of web sites in their collection and use these to predict which web pages were relevant. For this particular search term, web sites related to "`machine learning`", "`pattern recognition`", "`data mining`", and others may also be relevant and the algorithm would need to understand. For these algorithms, adding more web sites to their collection is unlikely to substantially improve the search results, but adding different data may. A web search portal like Google can also track user interaction. This leverages more direct, and higher quality, information for each search. For example, if a large proportion of users who searched for "`predictive modeling`" clicked on web site A, this should raise the likelihood that it is relevant. In this example, adding *different* data is more effective than adding more realizations of the same data attributes. In short, "Big P" usually helps more than "Big n". There are cases where adding more samples may materially improve the quality of predictions, but one should remember that *big data* may not mean *better data*.

In summary, a large number of samples can be beneficial, especially if the samples contain information throughout the predictor space, the noise in the predictors and the response can be minimized, or new content is being added. At the same time, the cost of these samples increases computational burden.

20.7 Computing

Computing details for training models discussed in this chapter can be found in the earlier sections of the book. One new computing thread presented here addresses the implementation of Algorithm 20.1. To illustrate this method, the R caret package will be referenced.

To illustrate the implementation of the similarity algorithm, first load the solubility data and define the control structure for training. Here we will use the training structure used throughout the text for these data.

```
> library(AppliedPredictiveModeling)
> data(solubility)
> set.seed(100)
> indx <- createFolds(solTrainY, returnTrain = TRUE)
> ctrl <- trainControl(method = "cv", index = indx)
```

Next, tune the desired model and compute variable importance, since the similarity algorithm can be made more efficient by working with the most important predictors. Here we tune a random forests model and create a subset of the training and test data using the top 20 predictors (step 1) for inclusion in the similarity algorithm:

```
> set.seed(100)
> mtryVals <- floor(seq(10, ncol(solTrainXtrans), length = 10))
> mtryGrid <- data.frame(.mtry = mtryVals)
> rfTune <- train(x = solTrainXtrans, y = solTrainY,
+                  method = "rf",
+                  tuneGrid = mtryGrid,
+                  ntree = 1000,
+                  importance = TRUE,
+                  trControl = ctrl)
> ImportanceOrder <- order(rfTune$finalModel$importance[,1],
+                           decreasing = TRUE)
> top20 <- rownames(rfTune$finalModel$importance[ImportanceOrder,])[1:20]
> solTrainXimp <- subset(solTrainX, select = top20)
> solTestXimp <- subset(solTestX, select = top20)
```

The subset of predictors are then permuted to create the random set. There are many ways to permute data in R; a simple and direct way is by using the apply and sample functions together. The original subset of data and permuted set are then combined and a new classification variable is created to identify each row's membership. This defines steps 2–4 of the algorithm which can be implemented as follows:

```
> permutesolTrainXimp <- apply(solTrainXimp, 2, function(x) sample(x))
> solSimX <- rbind(solTrainXimp, permutesolTrainXimp)
> groupVals <- c("Training", "Random")
> groupY <- factor(rep(groupVals, each = nrow(solTrainX)))
```

Finally, we tune a model on the newly created classification data and use the model to predict the training set membership probability.

```
> rfSolClass <- train(x = solSimX, y = groupY,
+                     method = "rf",
+                     tuneLength = 5,
+                     ntree = 1000,
+                     control = trainControl(method = "LGOCV"))
> solTestGroupProbs <- predict(rfSolClass, solTestXimp, type = "prob")
```

Exercises

20.1. Figure 20.10 provides a comparison across several models when the response is modeled as both a continuous and categorical value. The x-axis represents the observed test set solubility value, and the y-axis represents the predicted solubility value or predicted solubility probability.

(a) Based on the figure, which continuous model performs best (and worst) on the test set? Which categorical model performs best (and worst)?

(b) Examine the results from the neural net models. If the predicted probability for a compound is close to zero, what is the range of actual solubility values for the test set? If the predicted solubility value (from the continuous model) is close to -10, what is the range of actual solubility values? Which model (categorical or continuous) gives more precise results at this extreme?

(c) Are any of the categorical models better than the corresponding regression models? If yes, then explain.

20.2. As discussed in Sect. 20.4, categorizing a continuous outcome can have detrimental impacts on model performance especially when the distribution does not have distinct groupings. Sometimes, however, there may be a plausible rationale for binning continuous data. If this is the case, but the data have a distribution like the solubility data (Fig. 20.5), then a possible option for the modeler is to construct a response that partitions data into three groups for which there is higher confidence in the data at the extremes. For example, the solubility data could be partitioned into groups such as "Insoluble," "Soluble," and "Indeterminate," where the indeterminate group is the data centered around the mean of the response.

Load the solubility data and create two training sets. For the first set, split the data at the mean of the response. For the second set, define compounds to be indeterminate if they are within one standard deviation of the mean of the response. This can be done with the following code:

```
> library(AppliedPredictiveModeling)
> data(solubility)
```

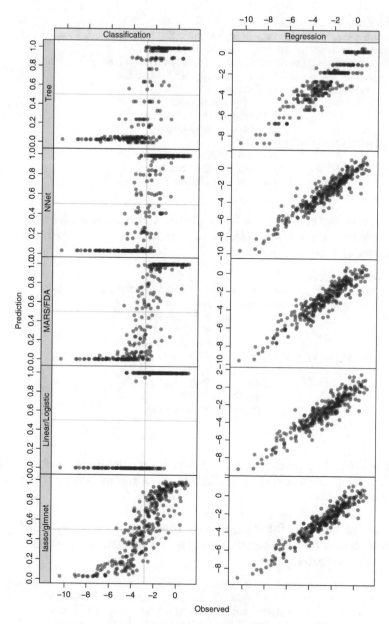

Fig. 20.10: Test set performance comparison of solubility models when the response is modeled as a continuous and categorical value

```
> trainData <- solTrainXtrans
> lowcut <- mean(solTrainY) - sd(solTrainY)
> highcut <- mean(solTrainY) + sd(solTrainY)
> breakpoints <- c(min(solTrainY), lowcut, highcut, max(solTrainY))
> groupNames <- c("Insoluble", "MidRange", "Soluble")
> solTrainY3bin <- cut(solTrainY,
+                            breaks = breakpoints,
+                            include.lowest = TRUE,
+                            labels = groupNames)
> solTestY3bin <- cut(solTestY,
+                            breaks = breakpoints,
+                            include.lowest = TRUE,
+                            labels = groupNames)
```

(a) Fit a linear model, a nonlinear model, and a tree-based model to the three-bin data. For example, the following code could be used to generate a recursive partitioning model:

```
> set.seed(100)
> indx3bin <- createFolds(solTrainY3bin, returnTrain = TRUE)
> ctrl3bin <- trainControl(method = "cv",
+                               index = indx3bin,
+                               classProbs = TRUE,
+                               savePredictions = TRUE)
> Rpart3bin <- train(x = trainXfiltered, y = solTrainY3bin,
+                          method = "rpart",
+                          metric = "Kappa",
+                          tuneLength = 30,
+                          trControl = ctrl3bin)
>
```

(b) Predict test set performance using the performance measure of your choice for each of the models in (a). Which model performs best for the three-bin data?

(c) Now exclude the "MidRange" data from the training set, rebuild each model, and predict the test set. This can be done with recursive partitioning as follows:

```
> trainXfiltered2bin <- trainXfiltered[solTrainY3bin != "MidRange",]
> solTrainY2bin <- solTrainY3bin[solTrainY3bin != "MidRange"]
> testXfiltered2bin <- testXfiltered[solTestY3bin != "MidRange",]
> solTestY2bin <- solTestY3bin[solTestY3bin != "MidRange"]
> set.seed(100)
> indx2bin <- createFolds(solTrainY2bin, returnTrain = TRUE)
> ctrl2bin <- trainControl(method = "cv",
+                               index = indx2bin,
+                               classProbs = TRUE,
+                               savePredictions = TRUE)
> Rpart2bin <- train(x = trainXfiltered2bin, y = solTrainY2bin,
+                          method = "rpart",
```

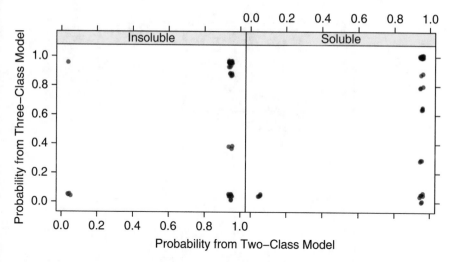

Fig. 20.11: Predicted probabilities from the two- and three-class models for the test set from the recursive partitioning model. Probabilities have been slightly jittered in order to see relative numbers of samples

```
+                           metric = "Kappa",
+                           tuneLength = 30,
+                           trControl = ctrl2bin)
> Rpart2binPred <- predict(Rpart2bin, newdata = testXfiltered)
> Rpart2binCM <- confusionMatrix(Rpart2binPred, solTestY3bin)
```

(d) How do sensitivity and specificity compare for the insoluble and soluble classes for the binning approaches in (b) and (c) within each model and between models?

(e) Figure 20.11 compares the predicted class probabilities from the two-bin and three-bin models for both the insoluble and soluble test set compounds. Based on class probabilities, does the two- or three-class model provide any distinct prediction advantages for the insoluble and/or soluble compounds? How do the predicted class probabilities within the insoluble and soluble groups compare for the other models you have developed?

20.3. Computing details for Algorithm 20.1 applied to the solubility data are presented in Sect. 20.7. Run this code and plot the distribution of the test set samples' probability of training set membership. How many test set samples are unlikely to have been part of the training set distribution?

20.4. Exercise 4.4 describes a data set in which food oils were analyzed for the content of seven types of fatty acids. Load the data and create a training and testing set as follows:

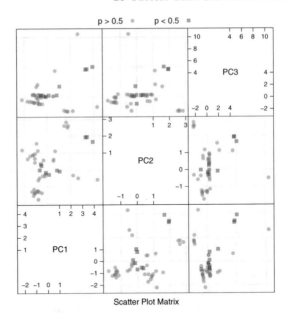

Fig. 20.12: The projection of the oil test set onto the first three principal components. Samples are colored and shaped by their probability of membership in the training set

```
> data(oil)
> set.seed(314)
> sampleRows <- sample.int(nrow(fattyAcids), size = 0.5*nrow(fattyAcids))
> fattyAcidsTrain <- fattyAcids[sampleRows,]
> fattyAcidsTest <- fattyAcids[-sampleRows,]
```

(a) Run Algorithm 20.1 using the training set. Which test set samples are not likely to be members of the training set? Why are these samples not likely to be members of the training set?

(b) Figure 20.12 presents the projections of the test set data onto the first three PCA components as determined by the training set. Samples are colored and shaped by their probability of membership in the training set. What does this plot reveal about the location of the samples that are not likely to be members of the training set?

(c) What steps could be taken to better ensure that the training and test sets cover the same region of predictor space?

Appendix

Appendix A
A Summary of Various Models

Table A.1 shows a short summary of several characteristics of the models discussed here. These properties generally hold, but are not always true for every problem. For example, linear discriminant analysis models do not perform feature selection, but there are specialized versions of the model that use regularization to eliminate predictors. Also, the interpretability of a model is subjective. A single tree might be understandable if it is not excessively large and the splits do not involve a large number of categories.

As stated in Chap. 2, no one model is uniformly better than the others. The applicability of a technique is dependent on the type of data being analyzed, the needs of the modeler, and the context of how the model will be used.

M. Kuhn and K. Johnson, *Applied Predictive Modeling*,
DOI 10.1007/978-1-4614-6849-3,
© Springer Science+Business Media New York 2013

Table A.1: A summary of models and some of their characteristics

Model	Allows $n < p$	Pre-processing	Interpretable	Automatic feature selection	# Tuning parameters	Robust to predictor noise	Computation time
Linear regression†	×	CS, NZV, Corr	✓	×	0	×	✓
Partial least squares	✓	CS	✓	○	1	×	✓
Ridge regression	×	CS, NZV	✓	×	1	×	✓
Elastic net/lasso	✓	CS, NZV	✓	✓	1–2	×	✓
Neural networks	✓	CS, NZV, Corr	×	×	2	×	×
Support vector machines	✓	CS	×	×	1–3	×	×
MARS/FDA	✓		○	✓	1–2	○	○
K-nearest neighbors	✓	CS, NZV	×	×	1	○	✓
Single trees	✓		○	✓	1	✓	✓
Model trees/rules†	✓		○	✓	1–2	✓	✓
Bagged trees	✓		×	✓	0	✓	○
Random forest	✓		×	○	0–1	✓	×
Boosted trees	✓		×	✓	3	✓	×
Cubist†	✓		×	○	2	✓	×
Logistic regression*	×	CS, NZV, Corr	✓	×	0	×	✓
{LQRM}DA*	×	NZV	○	×	0–2	×	✓
Nearest shrunken centroids*	✓	NZV	○	✓	1	×	✓
Naïve Bayes*	✓	NZV	×	×	0–1	○	○
C5.0*	✓		○	✓	0–3	✓	×

Symbols represent affirmative (✓), negative (×), and somewhere in between (○)

†regression only *classification only

- CS = centering and scaling
- NZV = remove near-zero predictors
- Corr = remove highly correlated predictors

Appendix B
An Introduction to R

The R language (Ihaka and Gentleman 1996; R Development Core Team 2010) is a platform for mathematical and statistical computations. It is free in two senses. First, R can be obtained free of charge (although commercial versions exist). Second, anyone can examine or modify the source code. R is released under the *General Public License* (Free Software Foundation June 2007), which outlines how the program can be redistributed.

R is used extensively in this book for several reasons. As just mentioned, anyone can download and use the program. Second, R is an extremely powerful and flexible tool for data analysis, and it contains extensive capabilities for predictive modeling.

The Comprehensive R Archive Network (CRAN) web site contains the source code for the program, as well as compiled versions that are ready to use:

http://cran.r-project.org/

This appendix is intended to be a crash course in basic concepts and syntax for R. More in-depth guides to the language basics are Spector (2008) and Gentleman (2008). The software development life cycle is detailed in R Development Core Team (2008).

B.1 Start-Up and Getting Help

CRAN contains pre-compiled versions of R for Microsoft Windows, Apple OS X, and several versions of Linux. For Windows and OS X, the program comes with a graphical user interface (GUI). When installing complied versions of R for these two operating systems, an icon for R is installed on the computer. To start an interactive session, launch the program using the icon. Alternatively, R can be started at the command line by typing R.

Once the program is started, the q function (for quit) ends the session.

M. Kuhn and K. Johnson, *Applied Predictive Modeling*,
DOI 10.1007/978-1-4614-6849-3,
© Springer Science+Business Media New York 2013

```
> # Comments occur after '#' symbols and are not executed
> # Use this command to quit
> q()
```

When quitting, the user will be prompted for options for saving their current work. Note the language is case-sensitive: `Q` could not be used to quit the session.

To get help on a specific topic, such as a function, put a question mark before the function and press enter:

```
> # Get help on the Sweave function
> ?Sweave
```

This opens the `Sweave` help page. One common challenge with R is finding an appropriate function. To search within all the local R functions on your computer, `apropos` will match a keyword against the available functions:

```
> apropos("prop")
   [1] "apropos"                "getProperties"
   [3] "pairwise.prop.test"     "power.prop.test"
   [5] "prop.table"             "prop.test"
   [7] "prop.trend.test"        "reconcilePropertiesAndPrototype"
```

Alternatively, the `RSiteSearch` function conducts an online search of all functions, manuals, contributed documentation, the R-Help newsgroup, and other sources for a keyword. For example, to search for different methods to produce ROC curves,

```
> RSiteSearch("roc")
```

will open a web browser and show the matches. The `restrict` argument of this function widens the search (see `?RSiteSearch` for more details).

B.2 Packages

Base R is the nominal system that encompasses the core language features (e.g., the executable program, the fundamental programming framework). Most of the actual R code is contained in distinct modules called *packages*. When R is installed, a small set of core packages is also installed (see R Development Core Team (2008) for the definitive list). However, a large number of packages exist outside of this set. The CRAN web site contains over 4,150 packages for download while the Bioconductor project (Gentleman et al. 2004), an R-based system for computational biology, includes over 600 R packages.

To load a package, the `library` function is used:

```
> # Load the random forests package
> library(randomForest)
> # Show the list of currently loaded packages and other information
> sessionInfo()
```

```
R version 2.15.2 (2012-10-26)
Platform: x86_64-apple-darwin9.8.0/x86_64 (64-bit)

locale:
[1] C

attached base packages:
[1] splines    tools      stats    graphics  grDevices utils    datasets
[8] methods    base

other attached packages:
 [1] randomForest_4.6-7  BiocInstaller_1.8.3  caret_5.15-045
 [4] foreach_1.4.0       cluster_1.14.3       reshape_0.8.4
 [7] plyr_1.7.1          lattice_0.20-10      Hmisc_3.10-1
[10] survival_2.36-14    weaver_1.24.0        codetools_0.2-8
[13] digest_0.6.0

loaded via a namespace (and not attached):
[1] grid_2.15.2     iterators_1.0.6
```

The function install.packages can be used to install additional modules. For example, to install the rpart package for classification and regression trees discussed in Sects. 8.1 and 14.1, the code

```
> install.packages("rpart")
```

can be used. Alternatively, the CRAN web site includes "task views" which group similar packages together. For example, the task view for "Machine Learning" would install a set of predictive modeling packages:

```
> # First install the task view package
> install.packages("ctv")
> # Load the library prior to first use
> library(ctv)
> install.views("MachineLearning")
```

Some packages depend on other packages (or specific versions). The functions install.packages and install.views will determine additional package requirements and install the necessary dependencies.

B.3 Creating Objects

Anything created in R is an *object*. Objects can be assigned values using "<-". For example:

```
> pages <- 97
> town <- "Richmond"
> ## Equals also works, but see Section B.9 below
```

To see the value of an object, simply type it and hit enter. Also, you can explicitly tell R to print the value of the object

```
> pages
  [1] 97
> print(town)
  [1] "Richmond"
```

Another helpful function for understanding the contents of an object is `str` (for structure). As an example, R automatically comes with an object that contains the abbreviated month names.

```
> month.abb
  [1] "Jan" "Feb" "Mar" "Apr" "May" "Jun" "Jul" "Aug" "Sep" "Oct" "Nov"
  [12] "Dec"
> str(month.abb)
  chr [1:12] "Jan" "Feb" "Mar" "Apr" "May" "Jun" "Jul" ...
```

This shows that `month.abb` is a character object with twelve elements. We can also determine the structure of objects that do not contain data, such as the `print` function discussed earlier:

```
> str(print)
  function (x, ...)
> str(sessionInfo)
  function (package = NULL)
```

This is handy for looking up the names of the function arguments. Functions will be discussed in more detail below.

B.4 Data Types and Basic Structures

There are many different core data types in R. The relevant types are numeric, character, factor, and logical types. Logical data can take on value of TRUE or FALSE. For example, these values can be used to make comparisons or can be assigned to an object:

```
> if(3 > 2) print("greater") else print("less")
  [1] "greater"
> isGreater <- 3 > 2
> isGreater
  [1] TRUE
> is.logical(isGreater)
  [1] TRUE
```

Numeric data encompass integers and double precision (i.e., decimal valued) numbers. To assign a single numeric value to an R object:

```
> x <- 3.6
> is.numeric(x)
```

```
    [1] TRUE
> is.integer(x)
    [1] FALSE
> is.double(x)
    [1] TRUE
> typeof(x)
    [1] "double"
```

Character strings can be created by putting text inside of quotes:

```
> y <- "your ad here"
> typeof(y)
    [1] "character"
> z <- "you can also 'quote' text too"
> z
    [1] "you can also 'quote' text too"
```

Note that R does not restrict the length of character strings.

There are several helpful functions that work on strings. First, char counts the number of characters:

```
> nchar(y)
    [1] 12
> nchar(z)
    [1] 29
```

The grep function can be used to determine if a substring exists in the character string

```
> grep("ad", y)
    [1] 1
> grep("my", y)
    integer(0)
> # If the string is present, return the whole value
> grep("too", z, value = TRUE)
    [1] "you can also 'quote' text too"
```

So far, the R objects shown have a single value or element. The most basic data structure for holding multiple values of the same type of data is a vector. The most basic method of creating a vector is to use the c function (for *combine*). To create a vector of numeric data:

```
> weights <- c(90, 150, 111, 123)
> is.vector(weights)
    [1] TRUE
> typeof(weights)
    [1] "double"
> length(weights)
    [1] 4
```

```
> weights + .25
   [1]   90.25 150.25 111.25 123.25
```

Note that the last command is an example of *vector operations*. Instead of looping over the elements of the vector, vector operations are more concise and efficient operations.

Many functions work on vectors:

```
> mean(weights)
   [1] 118.5
> colors <- c("green", "red", "blue", "red", "white")
> grep("red", colors)
   [1] 2 4
> nchar(colors)
   [1] 5 3 4 3 5
```

An alternate method for storing character data in a vector is to use *factors*. Factors store character data by first determining all unique values in the data, called the factor levels. The character data is then stored as integers that correspond to the factor levels:

```
> colors2 <- as.factor(colors)
> colors2
   [1] green red   blue  red   white
   Levels: blue green red white
> levels(colors2)
   [1] "blue"  "green" "red"   "white"
> as.numeric(colors2)
   [1] 2 3 1 3 4
```

There are a few advantages to storing data in factors. First, less memory is required to store the values since potentially long character strings are saved only once (in the levels) and their occurrences are saved as vectors. Second, the factor vector "remembers" all of the possible values. Suppose we subset the factor vector by removing the first value using a negative integer value:

```
> colors2[-1]
   [1] red   blue  red   white
   Levels: blue green red white
```

Even though the element with a value of "green" was removed, the factor still keeps the same levels. Factors are the primary means of storing discrete variables in R and many classification models use them to specify the outcome data.

To work with a subset of a vector, single brackets can be used in different ways:

```
> weights
   [1]   90 150 111 123
```

```
> # positive integers indicate which elements to keep
> weights[c(1, 4)]
   [1]  90 123
> # negative integers correspond to elements to exclude
> weights[-c(1, 4)]
   [1] 150 111
> # A vector of logical values can be used also but there should
> # be as many logical values as elements
> weights[c(TRUE, TRUE, FALSE, TRUE)]
   [1]  90 150 123
```

Vectors must store the same type of data. An alternative is a list; this is a type of vector that can store objects of any type as elements:

```
> both <- list(colors = colors2, weight = weights)
> is.vector(both)
   [1] TRUE
> is.list(both)
   [1] TRUE
> length(both)
   [1] 2
> names(both)
   [1] "colors" "weight"
```

Lists can be filtered in a similar manner as vectors. However, double brackets return only the element, while single brackets return another list:

```
> both[[1]]
   [1] green red    blue   red    white
   Levels: blue green red white
> is.list(both[[1]])
   [1] FALSE
> both[1]
   $colors
   [1] green red    blue   red    white
   Levels: blue green red white
> is.list(both[1])
   [1] TRUE
> # We can also subset using the name of the list
> both[["colors"]]
   [1] green red    blue   red    white
   Levels: blue green red white
```

Missing values in R are encoded as NA values:

```
> probabilities <- c(.05, .67, NA, .32, .90)
> is.na(probabilities)
   [1] FALSE FALSE  TRUE FALSE FALSE
```

```
> # NA is not treated as a character string
> probabilities == "NA"
  [1] FALSE FALSE    NA FALSE FALSE
> # Most functions propagate missing values...
> mean(probabilities)
  [1] NA
> # ... unless told otherwise
> mean(probabilities, na.rm = TRUE)
  [1] 0.485
```

B.5 Working with Rectangular Data Sets

Rectangular data sets usually refer to situations where samples are in rows of a data set while columns correspond to variables (in some domains, this convention is reversed). There are two main structures for rectangular data: matrices and data frames. The main difference between these two types of objects is the type of data that can be stored within them. A matrix can only contain data of the same type (e.g., character or numeric) while data frames must contain columns of the same data type. Matrices are more computationally efficient but are obviously limited.

We can create a matrix using the matrix function. Here, we create a numeric vector of integers from one to twelve and use three rows and four columns:

```
> mat <- matrix(1:12, nrow = 3)
> mat
     [,1] [,2] [,3] [,4]
[1,]    1    4    7   10
[2,]    2    5    8   11
[3,]    3    6    9   12
```

The rows and columns can be given names:

```
> rownames(mat) <- c("row 1", "row 2", "row 3")
> colnames(mat) <- c("col1", "col2", "col3", "col4")
> mat
      col1 col2 col3 col4
row 1    1    4    7   10
row 2    2    5    8   11
row 3    3    6    9   12
> rownames(mat)
  [1] "row 1" "row 2" "row 3"
```

Matrices can be subset using method similar to vectors, but rows and columns can be subset separately:

```
> mat[1, 2:3]
```

```
col2 col3
   4    7
> mat["row 1", "col3"]
  [1] 7
> mat[1,]
  col1 col2 col3 col4
     1    4    7   10
```

One difficulty with subsetting matrices is that dimensions can be *dropped*; if either a single row or column is produced by subsetting a matrix, then a vector is the result:

```
> is.matrix(mat[1,])
  [1] FALSE
> is.vector(mat[1,])
  [1] TRUE
```

One method for avoiding this is to pass the `drop` option to the matrix when subsetting:

```
> mat[1,]
  col1 col2 col3 col4
     1    4    7   10
> mat[1,,drop = FALSE]
        col1 col2 col3 col4
  row 1    1    4    7   10
> is.matrix(mat[1,,drop = FALSE])
  [1] TRUE
> is.vector(mat[1,,drop = FALSE])
  [1] FALSE
```

Data frames can be created using the `data.frame` function:

```
> df <- data.frame(colors = colors2,
+                  time = 1:5)
> df
    colors time
  1  green    1
  2    red    2
  3   blue    3
  4    red    4
  5  white    5
> dim(df)
  [1] 5 2
> colnames(df)
  [1] "colors" "time"
> rownames(df)
  [1] "1" "2" "3" "4" "5"
```

In addition to the subsetting techniques previously shown for matrices, the $ operator can be used to return single columns while the subset function can be used to return more complicated subsets of rows:

```
> df$colors
  [1] green red    blue   red    white
  Levels: blue green red white
> subset(df, colors %in% c("red", "green") & time <= 2)
    colors time
  1  green    1
  2    red    2
```

A helpful function for determining if there are any missing values in a row of a matrix or data frame is the complete.cases function, which returns TRUE if there are no missing values:

```
> df2 <- df
> # Add missing values to the data frame
> df2[1, 1] <- NA
> df2[5, 2] <- NA
> df2
    colors time
  1   <NA>    1
  2    red    2
  3   blue    3
  4    red    4
  5  white   NA
> complete.cases(df2)
  [1] FALSE  TRUE  TRUE  TRUE FALSE
```

B.6 Objects and Classes

Each object has at least one type or *class* associated with it. The class of an object declares what it is (e.g., a character string, linear model, web site URL). The class defines the structure of an object (i.e., how it is stored) and the possible operations associated with this type of object (called *methods* for the class). For example, if some sort of model object is created, it may be of interest to:

- *Print* the model details for understanding
- *Plot* the model for visualization, or
- *Predict* new samples

In this case, print, plot, and predict are some of the possible methods for that particular type of model (as determined by its class). This paradigm is called object-oriented programming.

We can quickly determine the class of the previous objects:

```
> pages
 [1] 97
> class(pages)
 [1] "numeric"
> town
 [1] "Richmond"
> class(town)
 [1] "character"
```

When the user directs R to perform some operation, such as creating predictions from a model object, the class determines the specific code for the prediction equation. This is called *method dispatch*. There are two main techniques for object-oriented programming in R: S3 classes and S4 classes. The S3 approach is more simplistic than S4 and is used by many packages. S4 methods are more powerful than S3 methods but are too complex to adequately describe in this overview. Chambers (2008) describes these techniques in greater detail.

With S3 methods, the naming convention is to use dots to separate classes and methods. For example, summary.lm is the function that is used to compute summary values for an object that has the lm class (this class is to fit linear models, such as linear regression analysis). Suppose a user created an object called myModel using the lm function. The command

```
modelSummary <- summary(myModel)
```

calculates the common descriptive statistics for the model. R sees that myModel has class lm, so it executes the code in the function summary.lm.

For this text, it is important to understand the concept of objects, classes, and methods. However, these concepts will be used at a high level; the code contained in the book rarely delves into the technical minutia "under the hood." For example, the predict function will be used extensively, but the use will not be required to know which specific method is executed.

B.7 R Functions

In R, modular pieces of code can be collected in functions. Many functions have already been used in this section, such as the library function that loads packages. Functions have *arguments*: specific slots that are used to pass objects into the function. In R, arguments are named (unlike other languages, such as matlab). For example, the function for reading data stored in comma delimited format (CSV) into an R object has these arguments:

```
> str(read.csv)
function (file, header = TRUE, sep = ",", quote = "\"", dec = ".",
    fill = TRUE, comment.char = "", ...)
```

where `file` is a character string that points to the CSV file and `header` indicates whether the initial row corresponds to variable names. The `file` argument has no default value and the function will result in an error if no file name is specified. Since these functions are named, they can be called in several different ways:

```
> read.csv("data.csv")
> read.csv(header = FALSE, file = "data.csv")
```

Notice that the `read.csv` function has an argument at the end with three dots. This means that other arguments can be added to the `read.csv` function call that are passed to a specific function within the code for `read.csv`. In this case, the code uses another function called `read.table` that is more general. The `read.table` contains an argument called `na.strings` that is absent from `read.csv`. This argument tells R which character values indicate a missing value in the file. Using

```
> read.csv("data.csv", na.strings = "?")
```

has the effect of passing the argument `na.strings = "?"` from the `read.csv` function to the `read.table` function. Note that this argument must be named if it is to be passed through. The three dots are used extensively in the computing sections of each chapter.

B.8 The Three Faces of =

So far, the = symbol has been used in several different contexts:

1. Creating objects, such as `x = 3`
2. Testing for equivalence: `x == 4`
3. Specifying values to function arguments: `read.csv(header = FALSE)`

This can be confusing for newcomers. For example:

```
> new = subset(old, subset = value == "blue", drop = FALSE)
```

uses the symbol four times across all three cases. One method for avoiding confusion is to use `<-` as the assignment operator.

B.9 The **AppliedPredictiveModeling** Package

This package serves as a companion to the book and includes many of the data sets used here that are not already available in other R packages. It also includes the R code used throughout the chapters and R functions. The package is available on CRAN.

Table B.1: A survey of commands to produce class probabilities across different packages

Object class	Package	predict Function syntax
lda	MASS	predict(object) (no options needed)
glm	stats	predict(object, type = "response")
gbm	gbm	predict(object, type = "response", n.trees)
mda	mda	predict(object, type = "posterior")
rpart	rpart	predict(object, type = "prob")
Weka_classifier	RWeka	predict(object, type = "probability")
LogitBoost	caTools	predict(object, type = "raw", nIter)

The train function in the caret package uses a common syntax of `predict(object, type = "prob")`

B.10 The caret Package

The caret package (short for **C**lassification **A**nd **RE**gression **T**raining) was created to streamline the process for building and evaluating predictive models. Using the package, a practitioner can quickly evaluate many different types of models to find the more appropriate tool for their data.

The beauty of R is that it provides a large and diverse set of modeling packages. However, since these packages are created by many different people over time, there are a minimal set of conventions that are common to each model. For example, Table B.1 shows the syntax for calculating class probabilities for several different types of classification models. Remembering the syntactical variations can be difficult and this discourages users from evaluating a variety of models. One method to reduce this complexity is to provide a unified interface to functions for model building and prediction. caret provides such an interface for across a wide vary of models (over 140). The package also provides many options for data pre-processing and resampling-based parameter tuning techniques (Chaps. 3 and 4).

In this text, resampling is the primary approach for optimizing predictive models with tuning parameters. To do this, many alternate versions of the training set are used to train the model and predict a holdout set. This process is repeated many times to get performance estimates that generalize to new data sets. Each of the resampled data sets is independent of the others, so there is no formal requirement that the models must be run sequentially. If a computer with multiple processors or cores is available, the computations could be spread across these "workers" to increase the computational efficiency. caret leverages one of the parallel processing frameworks in R to do just this. The foreach package allows R code to be run either sequentially or in parallel using several different technologies, such as the multicore or Rmpi packages (see Schmidberger et al. (2009) for summaries and descriptions of the available options). There are several R packages that work with foreach to implement these techniques, such as doMC (for multicore) or doMPI (for Rmpi).

To tune a predictive model using multiple workers, the syntax in the caret package functions (e.g., train, rfe or sbf) does not change. A separate function is used to "register" the parallel processing technique and specify the number of workers to use. For example, to use the multicore package (not available on Windows) with five cores on the same machine, the package is loaded and then registered:

```
> library(doMC)
> registerDoMC(cores = 5)
> ## All subsequent models are then run in parallel
> model <- train(y ~ ., data = training, method = "rf")
```

The syntax for other packages associated with foreach is very similar. Note that as the number of workers increases, the memory required also increases. For example, using five workers would keep a total of six versions of the data in memory. If the data are large or the computational model is demanding, performance can be affected if the amount of required memory exceeds the physical amount available.

Does this help reduce the time to fit models? The job scheduling data (Chap. 17) was modeled multiple times with different number of workers for several models. Random forest was used with 2,000 trees and tuned over 10 values of m_{try}. Variable importance calculations were also conducted during each model fit. Linear discriminant analysis was also run, as was a cost-sensitive radial basis function support vector machine (tuned over 15 cost values). All models were tuned using five repeats of 10-fold cross-validation. The results are shown in Fig. B.1. The y-axis corresponds to the total execution time (encompassing model tuning and the final model fit) versus the number of workers. Random forest clearly took the longest to train and the LDA models were very computationally efficient. The total time (in minutes) decreased as the number of workers increase but stabilized around seven workers. The data for this plot were generated in a randomized fashion so that there should be no bias in the run order. The bottom right panel shows the *speedup* which is the sequential time divided by the parallel time. For example, a speedup of three indicates that the parallel version was three times faster than the sequential version. At best, parallelization can achieve linear speedups; that is, for M workers, the parallel time is $1/M$. For these models, the speedup is close to linear until four or five workers are used. After this, there is a small improvement in performance. Since LDA is already computationally efficient, the speed-up levels off more rapidly than the other models. While not linear, the decrease in execution time is helpful—a nearly 10 h model fit was decreased to about 90 min.

Note that some models, especially those using the RWeka package, may not be able to be run in parallel due to the underlying code structure.

One additional "trick" that train exploits to increase computational efficiency is to use sub-models; a single model fit can produce predictions for

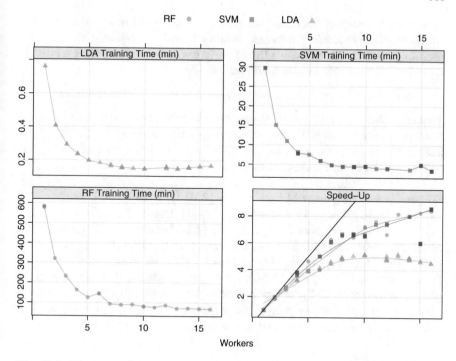

Fig. B.1: Three models run using different numbers of workers. The y-axis is either the execution time in minutes or the speed-up (in the *bottom right panel*)

multiple tuning parameters. For example, in most implementations of boosted models, a model trained on B boosting iterations can produce predictions for models for iterations less than B. For the grant data, a gbm model was fit that evaluated 200 distinct combinations of the three tuning parameters (see Fig. 14.10). In reality, train only created objects for 40 models and derived the other predictions from these objects.

More detail on the caret package can be found in Kuhn (2008) or the four extended manuals (called "vignettes") on the package web site (Kuhn 2010).

B.11 Software Used in this Text

The excellent Sweave function (Leisch 2002a,b) in R enabled data analysis code to be integrated within the content of this text. The function executed the R code and replaced the code with the items produced by the code, such as text, figures, and tables. All the software and data used here are publicly available at the time of this writing. The R packages AppliedPredictiveModeling and caret include many of the data sets. For data that could not be included, the AppliedPredictiveModeling package includes R code to recreate the data set used in this text. An extensive list of packages and functions in R related to reproducible research can be found on CRAN:

http://cran.r-project.org/web/views/ReproducibleResearch.html

Version 2.15.2 (2012-10-26) of R was used in conjunction with the following package versions: AppliedPredictiveModeling (1.01), arules (1.0-12), C50 (0.1.0-013), caret (5.15-045), coin (1.0-21), CORElearn (0.9.40), corrplot (0.70), ctv (0.7-4), Cubist (0.0.12), desirability (1.05), DMwR (0.2.3), doBy (4.5-5), doMC (1.2.5), DWD (0.10), e1071 (1.6-1), earth (3.2-3), elasticnet (1.1), ellipse (0.3-7), gbm (1.6-3.2), glmnet (1.8-2), Hmisc (3.10-1), ipred (0.9-1), kernlab (0.9-15), klaR (0.6-7), lars (1.1), latticeExtra (0.6-24), lattice (0.20-10), MASS (7.3-22), mda (0.4-2), minerva (1.2), mlbench (2.1-1), nnet (7.3-5), pamr (1.54), partykit (0.1-4), party (1.0-3), pls (2.3-0), plyr (1.7.1), pROC (1.5.4), proxy (0.4-9), QSARdata (1.02), randomForest (4.6-7), RColorBrewer (1.0-5), reshape2 (1.2.1), reshape (0.8.4), rms (3.6-0), rpart (4.0-3), RWeka (0.4-12), sparseLDA (0.1-6), subselect (0.12-2), svmpath (0.952), and tabplot (0.12). Some of these packages are not directly related to predictive modeling but were used to compile or format the content or for visualization.

Appendix C
Interesting Web Sites

Software

http://www.r-project.org
This is the main R web site with links to announcements, manuals, books, conference, and other information.

http://cran.r-project.org
CRAN, or the Comprehensive R Archive Network, is the primary repository for R and numerous add-on packages.

http://cran.r-project.org/web/views/MachineLearning.html
The machine learning Task View is a list of many predictive modeling packages in R.

http://caret.r-forge.r-project.org
The caret package is hosted here.

http://www.rulequest.com
RuleQuest releases commercial and open-source versions of Cubist and C5.0.

http://rattle.togaware.com
Rattle (Williams 2011) is a graphical user interface for R predictive models.

http://www.cs.waikato.ac.nz/ml/weka/
Weka is collection of Java programs for data mining.

http://orange.biolab.si
Orange is an open-source, cross-platform graphical user interface to many machine learning tools. The interface is a "pipeline" where users piece together components to create a workflow.

http://www.knime.org
"KNIME (Konstanz Information Miner) is a user-friendly and comprehensive open-source data integration, processing, analysis, and exploration platform."

M. Kuhn and K. Johnson, *Applied Predictive Modeling*,
DOI 10.1007/978-1-4614-6849-3,
© Springer Science+Business Media New York 2013

http://www.spss.com/software/modeler
The IBM SPSS Modeler, formerly called Clemintine, is a visual platform for model building.

http://www.sas.com/technologies/analytics/datamining/miner
A SAS product for data mining.

Other programs are listed at http://www.kdnuggets.com/software/suites. html.

Competitions

http://www.kaggle.com

http://tunedit.org

Data Sets

http://archive.ics.uci.edu/ml
The University of California (Irvine) is a well-known location for classification and regression data sets.

http://www.kdnuggets.com/datasets
The Association For Computing Machinery (ACM) has a special interest group on Knowledge Discovery in Data (KDD). The KDD group organizes annual machine learning competitions.

http://fueleconomy.gov
A web site run by the U.S. Department of Energy's Office of Energy Efficiency and Renewable Energy and the U.S. Environmental Protection Agency that lists different estimates of fuel economy for passenger cars and trucks.

http://www.cheminformatics.org
This web site contains many examples of computational chemistry data sets.

http://www.ncbi.nlm.nih.gov/geo
The NCBI GEO web site is "a public repository that archives and freely distributes microarray, next-generation sequencing, and other forms of high-throughput functional genomic data submitted by the scientific community."

References

Abdi H, Williams L (2010). "Principal Component Analysis." *Wiley Interdisciplinary Reviews: Computational Statistics*, **2**(4), 433–459.

Agresti A (2002). *Categorical Data Analysis*. Wiley–Interscience.

Ahdesmaki M, Strimmer K (2010). "Feature Selection in Omics Prediction Problems Using CAT Scores and False Nondiscovery Rate Control." *The Annals of Applied Statistics*, **4**(1), 503–519.

Alin A (2009). "Comparison of PLS Algorithms when Number of Objects is Much Larger than Number of Variables." *Statistical Papers*, **50**, 711–720.

Altman D, Bland J (1994). "Diagnostic Tests 3: Receiver Operating Characteristic Plots." *British Medical Journal*, **309**(6948), 188.

Ambroise C, McLachlan G (2002). "Selection Bias in Gene Extraction on the Basis of Microarray Gene–Expression Data." *Proceedings of the National Academy of Sciences*, **99**(10), 6562–6566.

Amit Y, Geman D (1997). "Shape Quantization and Recognition with Randomized Trees." *Neural Computation*, **9**, 1545–1588.

Armitage P, Berry G (1994). *Statistical Methods in Medical Research*. Blackwell Scientific Publications, Oxford, 3rd edition.

Artis M, Ayuso M, Guillen M (2002). "Detection of Automobile Insurance Fraud with Discrete Choice Models and Misclassified Claims." *The Journal of Risk and Insurance*, **69**(3), 325–340.

Austin P, Brunner L (2004). "Inflation of the Type I Error Rate When a Continuous Confounding Variable Is Categorized in Logistic Regression Analyses." *Statistics in Medicine*, **23**(7), 1159–1178.

Ayres I (2007). *Super Crunchers: Why Thinking–By–Numbers Is The New Way To Be Smart*. Bantam.

Barker M, Rayens W (2003). "Partial Least Squares for Discrimination." *Journal of Chemometrics*, **17**(3), 166–173.

Batista G, Prati R, Monard M (2004). "A Study of the Behavior of Several Methods for Balancing Machine Learning Training Data." *ACM SIGKDD Explorations Newsletter*, **6**(1), 20–29.

Bauer E, Kohavi R (1999). "An Empirical Comparison of Voting Classification Algorithms: Bagging, Boosting, and Variants." *Machine Learning*, **36**, 105–142.

Becton Dickinson and Company (1991). *ProbeTec ET Chlamydia trachomatis and Neisseria gonorrhoeae Amplified DNA Assays (Package Insert)*.

Ben-Dor A, Bruhn L, Friedman N, Nachman I, Schummer M, Yakhini Z (2000). "Tissue Classification with Gene Expression Profiles." *Journal of Computational Biology*, **7**(3), 559–583.

Bentley J (1975). "Multidimensional Binary Search Trees Used for Associative Searching." *Communications of the ACM*, **18**(9), 509–517.

Berglund A, Kettaneh N, Uppgård L, Wold S, DR NB, Cameron (2001). "The GIFI Approach to Non–Linear PLS Modeling." *Journal of Chemometrics*, **15**, 321–336.

Berglund A, Wold S (1997). "INLR, Implicit Non–Linear Latent Variable Regression." *Journal of Chemometrics*, **11**, 141–156.

Bergmeir C, Benitez JM (2012). "Neural Networks in R Using the Stuttgart Neural Network Simulator: RSNNS." *Journal of Statistical Software*, **46**(7), 1–26.

Bergstra J, Casagrande N, Erhan D, Eck D, Kégl B (2006). "Aggregate Features and AdaBoost for Music Classification." *Machine Learning*, **65**, 473–484.

Berntsson P, Wold S (1986). "Comparison Between X-ray Crystallographic Data and Physiochemical Parameters with Respect to Their Information About the Calcium Channel Antagonist Activity of 4-Phenyl-1,4-Dihydropyridines." *Quantitative Structure-Activity Relationships*, **5**, 45–50.

Bhanu B, Lin Y (2003). "Genetic Algorithm Based Feature Selection for Target Detection in SAR Images." *Image and Vision Computing*, **21**, 591–608.

Bishop C (1995). *Neural Networks for Pattern Recognition*. Oxford University Press, Oxford.

Bishop C (2006). *Pattern Recognition and Machine Learning*. Springer.

Bland J, Altman D (1995). "Statistics Notes: Multiple Significance Tests: The Bonferroni Method." *British Medical Journal*, **310**(6973), 170–170.

Bland J, Altman D (2000). "The Odds Ratio." *British Medical Journal*, **320**(7247), 1468.

Bohachevsky I, Johnson M, Stein M (1986). "Generalized Simulated Annealing for Function Optimization." *Technometrics*, **28**(3), 209–217.

Bone R, Balk R, Cerra F, Dellinger R, Fein A, Knaus W, Schein R, Sibbald W (1992). "Definitions for Sepsis and Organ Failure and Guidelines for the Use of Innovative Therapies in Sepsis." *Chest*, **101**(6), 1644–1655.

Boser B, Guyon I, Vapnik V (1992). "A Training Algorithm for Optimal Margin Classifiers." In "Proceedings of the Fifth Annual Workshop on Computational Learning Theory," pp. 144–152.

Boulesteix A, Strobl C (2009). "Optimal Classifier Selection and Negative Bias in Error Rate Estimation: An Empirical Study on High–Dimensional Prediction." *BMC Medical Research Methodology*, **9**(1), 85.

Box G, Cox D (1964). "An Analysis of Transformations." *Journal of the Royal Statistical Society. Series B (Methodological)*, pp. 211–252.

Box G, Hunter W, Hunter J (1978). *Statistics for Experimenters*. Wiley, New York.

Box G, Tidwell P (1962). "Transformation of the Independent Variables." *Technometrics*, **4**(4), 531–550.

Breiman L (1996a). "Bagging Predictors." *Machine Learning*, **24**(2), 123–140.

Breiman L (1996b). "Heuristics of Instability and Stabilization in Model Selection." *The Annals of Statistics*, **24**(6), 2350–2383.

Breiman L (1996c). "Technical Note: Some Properties of Splitting Criteria." *Machine Learning*, **24**(1), 41–47.

Breiman L (1998). "Arcing Classifiers." *The Annals of Statistics*, **26**, 123–140.

Breiman L (2000). "Randomizing Outputs to Increase Prediction Accuracy." *Mach. Learn.*, **40**, 229–242. ISSN 0885-6125.

Breiman L (2001). "Random Forests." *Machine Learning*, **45**, 5–32.

Breiman L, Friedman J, Olshen R, Stone C (1984). *Classification and Regression Trees*. Chapman and Hall, New York.

Bridle J (1990). "Probabilistic Interpretation of Feedforward Classification Network Outputs, with Relationships to Statistical Pattern Recognition." In "Neurocomputing: Algorithms, Architectures and Applications," pp. 227–236. Springer–Verlag.

Brillinger D (2004). "Some Data Analyses Using Mutual Information." *Brazilian Journal of Probability and Statistics*, **18**(6), 163–183.

Brodnjak-Vonina D, Kodba Z, Novi M (2005). "Multivariate Data Analysis in Classification of Vegetable Oils Characterized by the Content of Fatty Acids." *Chemometrics and Intelligent Laboratory Systems*, **75**(1), 31–43.

Brown C, Davis H (2006). "Receiver Operating Characteristics Curves and Related Decision Measures: A Tutorial." *Chemometrics and Intelligent Laboratory Systems*, **80**(1), 24–38.

Bu G (2009). "Apolipoprotein E and Its Receptors in Alzheimer's Disease: Pathways, Pathogenesis and Therapy." *Nature Reviews Neuroscience*, **10**(5), 333–344.

Buckheit J, Donoho DL (1995). "WaveLab and Reproducible Research." In A Antoniadis, G Oppenheim (eds.), "Wavelets in Statistics," pp. 55–82. Springer-Verlag, New York.

Burez J, Van den Poel D (2009). "Handling Class Imbalance In Customer Churn Prediction." *Expert Systems with Applications*, **36**(3), 4626–4636.

Cancedda N, Gaussier E, Goutte C, Renders J (2003). "Word–Sequence Kernels." *The Journal of Machine Learning Research*, **3**, 1059–1082.

Caputo B, Sim K, Furesjo F, Smola A (2002). "Appearance–Based Object Recognition Using SVMs: Which Kernel Should I Use?" In "Proceedings of NIPS Workshop on Statistical Methods for Computational Experiments in Visual Processing and Computer Vision," .

Strobl C, Carolin C, Boulesteix A-L, Augustin T (2007). "Unbiased Split Selection for Classification Trees Based on the Gini Index." *Computational Statistics & Data Analysis*, **52**(1), 483–501.

Castaldi P, Dahabreh I, Ioannidis J (2011). "An Empirical Assessment of Validation Practices for Molecular Classifiers." *Briefings in Bioinformatics*, **12**(3), 189–202.

Chambers J (2008). *Software for Data Analysis: Programming with R.* Springer.

Chan K, Loh W (2004). "LOTUS: An Algorithm for Building Accurate and Comprehensible Logistic Regression Trees." *Journal of Computational and Graphical Statistics*, **13**(4), 826–852.

Chang CC, Lin CJ (2011). "LIBSVM: A Library for Support Vector Machines." *ACM Transactions on Intelligent Systems and Technology*, **2**, 27: 1–27:27.

Chawla N, Bowyer K, Hall L, Kegelmeyer W (2002). "SMOTE: Synthetic Minority Over–Sampling Technique." *Journal of Artificial Intelligence Research*, **16**(1), 321–357.

Chun H, Keleş S (2010). "Sparse Partial Least Squares Regression for Simultaneous Dimension Reduction and Variable Selection." *Journal of the Royal Statistical Society: Series B (Statistical Methodology)*, **72**(1), 3–25.

Chung D, Keles S (2010). "Sparse Partial Least Squares Classification for High Dimensional Data." *Statistical Applications in Genetics and Molecular Biology*, **9**(1), 17.

Clark R (1997). "OptiSim: An Extended Dissimilarity Selection Method for Finding Diverse Representative Subsets." *Journal of Chemical Information and Computer Sciences*, **37**(6), 1181–1188.

Clark T (2004). "Can Out–of–Sample Forecast Comparisons Help Prevent Overfitting?" *Journal of Forecasting*, **23**(2), 115–139.

Clemmensen L, Hastie T, Witten D, Ersboll B (2011). "Sparse Discriminant Analysis." *Technometrics*, **53**(4), 406–413.

Cleveland W (1979). "Robust Locally Weighted Regression and Smoothing Scatterplots." *Journal of the American Statistical Association*, **74**(368), 829–836.

Cleveland W, Devlin S (1988). "Locally Weighted Regression: An Approach to Regression Analysis by Local Fitting." *Journal of the American Statistical Association*, pp. 596–610.

Cohen G, Hilario M, Pellegrini C, Geissbuhler A (2005). "SVM Modeling via a Hybrid Genetic Strategy. A Health Care Application." In R Engelbrecht, AGC Lovis (eds.), "Connecting Medical Informatics and Bio–Informatics," pp. 193–198. IOS Press.

Cohen J (1960). "A Coefficient of Agreement for Nominal Data." *Educational and Psychological Measurement*, **20**, 37–46.

Cohn D, Atlas L, Ladner R (1994). "Improving Generalization with Active Learning." *Machine Learning*, **15**(2), 201–221.

Cornell J (2002). *Experiments with Mixtures: Designs, Models, and the Analysis of Mixture Data.* Wiley, New York, NY.

Cortes C, Vapnik V (1995). "Support–Vector Networks." *Machine Learning*, **20**(3), 273–297.

Costa N, Lourenco J, Pereira Z (2011). "Desirability Function Approach: A Review and Performance Evaluation in Adverse Conditions." *Chemometrics and Intelligent Lab Systems*, **107**(2), 234–244.

Cover TM, Thomas JA (2006). *Elements of Information Theory.* Wiley–Interscience.

Craig-Schapiro R, Kuhn M, Xiong C, Pickering E, Liu J, Misko TP, Perrin R, Bales K, Soares H, Fagan A, Holtzman D (2011). "Multiplexed Immunoassay Panel Identifies Novel CSF Biomarkers for Alzheimer's Disease Diagnosis and Prognosis." *PLoS ONE*, **6**(4), e18850.

Cruz-Monteagudo M, Borges F, Cordeiro MND (2011). "Jointly Handling Potency and Toxicity of Antimicrobial Peptidomimetics by Simple Rules from Desirability Theory and Chemoinformatics." *Journal of Chemical Information and Modeling*, **51**(12), 3060–3077.

Davison M (1983). *Multidimensional Scaling.* John Wiley and Sons, Inc.

Dayal B, MacGregor J (1997). "Improved PLS Algorithms." *Journal of Chemometrics*, **11**, 73–85.

de Jong S (1993). "SIMPLS: An Alternative Approach to Partial Least Squares Regression." *Chemometrics and Intelligent Laboratory Systems*, **18**, 251–263.

de Jong S, Ter Braak C (1994). "Short Communication: Comments on the PLS Kernel Algorithm." *Journal of Chemometrics*, **8**, 169–174.

de Leon M, Klunk W (2006). "Biomarkers for the Early Diagnosis of Alzheimer's Disease." *The Lancet Neurology*, **5**(3), 198–199.

Defernez M, Kemsley E (1997). "The Use and Misuse of Chemometrics for Treating Classification Problems." *TrAC Trends in Analytical Chemistry*, **16**(4), 216–221.

DeLong E, DeLong D, Clarke-Pearson D (1988). "Comparing the Areas Under Two Or More Correlated Receiver Operating Characteristic Curves: A Nonparametric Approach." *Biometrics*, **44**(3), 837–45.

Derksen S, Keselman H (1992). "Backward, Forward and Stepwise Automated Subset Selection Algorithms: Frequency of Obtaining Authentic and Noise Variables." *British Journal of Mathematical and Statistical Psychology*, **45**(2), 265–282.

Derringer G, Suich R (1980). "Simultaneous Optimization of Several Response Variables." *Journal of Quality Technology*, **12**(4), 214–219.

Dietterich T (2000). "An Experimental Comparison of Three Methods for Constructing Ensembles of Decision Trees: Bagging, Boosting, and Randomization." *Machine Learning*, **40**, 139–158.

Dillon W, Goldstein M (1984). *Multivariate Analysis: Methods and Applications.* Wiley, New York.

Dobson A (2002). *An Introduction to Generalized Linear Models*. Chapman & Hall/CRC.

Drucker H, Burges C, Kaufman L, Smola A, Vapnik V (1997). "Support Vector Regression Machines." *Advances in Neural Information Processing Systems*, pp. 155–161.

Drummond C, Holte R (2000). "Explicitly Representing Expected Cost: An Alternative to ROC Representation." In "Proceedings of the Sixth ACM SIGKDD International Conference on Knowledge Discovery and Data Mining," pp. 198–207.

Duan K, Keerthi S (2005). "Which is the Best Multiclass SVM Method? An Empirical Study." *Multiple Classifier Systems*, pp. 278–285.

Dudoit S, Fridlyand J, Speed T (2002). "Comparison of Discrimination Methods for the Classification of Tumors Using Gene Expression Data." *Journal of the American Statistical Association*, **97**(457), 77–87.

Duhigg C (2012). "How Companies Learn Your Secrets." *The New York Times*. URL http://www.nytimes.com/2012/02/19/magazine/shopping-habits.html.

Dunn W, Wold S (1990). "Pattern Recognition Techniques in Drug Design." In C Hansch, P Sammes, J Taylor (eds.), "Comprehensive Medicinal Chemistry," pp. 691–714. Pergamon Press, Oxford.

Dwyer D (2005). "Examples of Overfitting Encountered When Building Private Firm Default Prediction Models." *Technical report*, Moody's KMV.

Efron B (1983). "Estimating the Error Rate of a Prediction Rule: Improvement on Cross–Validation." *Journal of the American Statistical Association*, pp. 316–331.

Efron B, Hastie T, Johnstone I, Tibshirani R (2004). "Least Angle Regression." *The Annals of Statistics*, **32**(2), 407–499.

Efron B, Tibshirani R (1986). "Bootstrap Methods for Standard Errors, Confidence Intervals, and Other Measures of Statistical Accuracy." *Statistical Science*, pp. 54–75.

Efron B, Tibshirani R (1997). "Improvements on Cross–Validation: The 632+ Bootstrap Method." *Journal of the American Statistical Association*, **92**(438), 548–560.

Eilers P, Boer J, van Ommen G, van Houwelingen H (2001). "Classification of Microarray Data with Penalized Logistic Regression." In "Proceedings of SPIE," volume 4266, p. 187.

Eugster M, Hothorn T, Leisch F (2008). "Exploratory and Inferential Analysis of Benchmark Experiments." *Ludwigs-Maximilians-Universität München, Department of Statistics, Tech. Rep*, **30**.

Everitt B, Landau S, Leese M, Stahl D (2011). *Cluster Analysis*. Wiley.

Ewald B (2006). "Post Hoc Choice of Cut Points Introduced Bias to Diagnostic Research." *Journal of clinical epidemiology*, **59**(8), 798–801.

Fanning K, Cogger K (1998). "Neural Network Detection of Management Fraud Using Published Financial Data." *International Journal of Intelligent Systems in Accounting, Finance & Management*, **7**(1), 21–41.

Faraway J (2005). *Linear Models with R*. Chapman & Hall/CRC, Boca Raton.

Fawcett T (2006). "An Introduction to ROC Analysis." *Pattern Recognition Letters*, **27**(8), 861–874.

Fisher R (1936). "The Use of Multiple Measurements in Taxonomic Problems." *Annals of Eugenics*, **7**(2), 179–188.

Forina M, Casale M, Oliveri P, Lanteri S (2009). "CAIMAN brothers: A Family of Powerful Classification and Class Modeling Techniques." *Chemometrics and Intelligent Laboratory Systems*, **96**(2), 239–245.

Frank E, Wang Y, Inglis S, Holmes G (1998). "Using Model Trees for Classification." *Machine Learning*.

Frank E, Witten I (1998). "Generating Accurate Rule Sets Without Global Optimization." *Proceedings of the Fifteenth International Conference on Machine Learning*, pp. 144–151.

Free Software Foundation (June 2007). *GNU General Public License*.

Freund Y (1995). "Boosting a Weak Learning Algorithm by Majority." *Information and Computation*, **121**, 256–285.

Freund Y, Schapire R (1996). "Experiments with a New Boosting Algorithm." *Machine Learning: Proceedings of the Thirteenth International Conference*, pp. 148–156.

Friedman J (1989). "Regularized Discriminant Analysis." *Journal of the American Statistical Association*, **84**(405), 165–175.

Friedman J (1991). "Multivariate Adaptive Regression Splines." *The Annals of Statistics*, **19**(1), 1–141.

Friedman J (2001). "Greedy Function Approximation: A Gradient Boosting Machine." *Annals of Statistics*, **29**(5), 1189–1232.

Friedman J (2002). "Stochastic Gradient Boosting." *Computational Statistics and Data Analysis*, **38**(4), 367–378.

Friedman J, Hastie T, Tibshirani R (2000). "Additive Logistic Regression: A Statistical View of Boosting." *Annals of Statistics*, **38**, 337–374.

Friedman J, Hastie T, Tibshirani R (2010). "Regularization Paths for Generalized Linear Models via Coordinate Descent." *Journal of Statistical Software*, **33**(1), 1–22.

Geisser S (1993). *Predictive Inference: An Introduction*. Chapman and Hall.

Geladi P, Kowalski B (1986). "Partial Least-Squares Regression: A Tutorial." *Analytica Chimica Acta*, **185**, 1–17.

Geladi P, Manley M, Lestander T (2003). "Scatter Plotting in Multivariate Data Analysis." *Journal of Chemometrics*, **17**(8–9), 503–511.

Gentleman R (2008). *R Programming for Bioinformatics*. CRC Press.

Gentleman R, Carey V, Bates D, Bolstad B, Dettling M, Dudoit S, Ellis B, Gautier L, Ge Y, Gentry J, Hornik K, Hothorn T, Huber M, Iacus S, Irizarry R, Leisch F, Li C, Mächler M, Rossini A, Sawitzki G, Smith C, Smyth G, Tierney L, Yang JY, Zhang J (2004). "Bioconductor: Open Software Development for Computational Biology and Bioinformatics." *Genome Biology*, **5**(10), R80.

Giuliano K, DeBiasio R, Dunlay R, Gough A, Volosky J, Zock J, Pavlakis G, Taylor D (1997). "High–Content Screening: A New Approach to Easing Key Bottlenecks in the Drug Discovery Process." *Journal of Biomolecular Screening*, **2**(4), 249–259.

Goldberg D (1989). *Genetic Algorithms in Search, Optimization, and Machine Learning*. Addison–Wesley, Boston.

Golub G, Heath M, Wahba G (1979). "Generalized Cross–Validation as a Method for Choosing a Good Ridge Parameter." *Technometrics*, **21**(2), 215–223.

Good P (2000). *Permutation Tests: A Practical Guide to Resampling Methods for Testing Hypotheses*. Springer.

Gowen A, Downey G, Esquerre C, O'Donnell C (2010). "Preventing Over–Fitting in PLS Calibration Models of Near-Infrared (NIR) Spectroscopy Data Using Regression Coefficients." *Journal of Chemometrics*, **25**, 375–381.

Graybill F (1976). *Theory and Application of the Linear Model*. Wadsworth & Brooks, Pacific Grove, CA.

Guo Y, Hastie T, Tibshirani R (2007). "Regularized Linear Discriminant Analysis and its Application in Microarrays." *Biostatistics*, **8**(1), 86–100.

Gupta S, Hanssens D, Hardie B, Kahn W, Kumar V, Lin N, Ravishanker N, Sriram S (2006). "Modeling Customer Lifetime Value." *Journal of Service Research*, **9**(2), 139–155.

Guyon I, Elisseeff A (2003). "An Introduction to Variable and Feature Selection." *The Journal of Machine Learning Research*, **3**, 1157–1182.

Guyon I, Weston J, Barnhill S, Vapnik V (2002). "Gene Selection for Cancer Classification Using Support Vector Machines." *Machine Learning*, **46**(1), 389–422.

Hall M, Smith L (1997). "Feature Subset Selection: A Correlation Based Filter Approach." *International Conference on Neural Information Processing and Intelligent Information Systems*, pp. 855–858.

Hall P, Hyndman R, Fan Y (2004). "Nonparametric Confidence Intervals for Receiver Operating Characteristic Curves." *Biometrika*, **91**, 743–750.

Hampel H, Frank R, Broich K, Teipel S, Katz R, Hardy J, Herholz K, Bokde A, Jessen F, Hoessler Y (2010). "Biomarkers for Alzheimer's Disease: Academic, Industry and Regulatory Perspectives." *Nature Reviews Drug Discovery*, **9**(7), 560–574.

Hand D, Till R (2001). "A Simple Generalisation of the Area Under the ROC Curve for Multiple Class Classification Problems." *Machine Learning*, **45**(2), 171–186.

Hanley J, McNeil B (1982). "The Meaning and Use of the Area under a Receiver Operating (ROC) Curvel Characteristic." *Radiology*, **143**(1), 29–36.

Hardle W, Werwatz A, Müller M, Sperlich S, Hardle W, Werwatz A, Müller M, Sperlich S (2004). "Nonparametric Density Estimation." In "Nonparametric and Semiparametric Models," pp. 39–83. Springer Berlin Heidelberg.

Harrell F (2001). *Regression Modeling Strategies: With Applications to Linear Models, Logistic Regression, and Survival Analysis.* Springer, New York.

Hastie T, Pregibon D (1990). "Shrinking Trees." *Technical report*, AT&T Bell Laboratories Technical Report.

Hastie T, Tibshirani R (1990). *Generalized Additive Models.* Chapman & Hall/CRC.

Hastie T, Tibshirani R (1996). "Discriminant Analysis by Gaussian Mixtures." *Journal of the Royal Statistical Society. Series B*, pp. 155–176.

Hastie T, Tibshirani R, Buja A (1994). "Flexible Discriminant Analysis by Optimal Scoring." *Journal of the American Statistical Association*, **89**(428), 1255–1270.

Hastie T, Tibshirani R, Friedman J (2008). *The Elements of Statistical Learning: Data Mining, Inference and Prediction.* Springer, 2 edition.

Hawkins D (2004). "The Problem of Overfitting." *Journal of Chemical Information and Computer Sciences*, **44**(1), 1–12.

Hawkins D, Basak S, Mills D (2003). "Assessing Model Fit by Cross–Validation." *Journal of Chemical Information and Computer Sciences*, **43**(2), 579–586.

Henderson H, Velleman P (1981). "Building Multiple Regression Models Interactively." *Biometrics*, pp. 391–411.

Hesterberg T, Choi N, Meier L, Fraley C (2008). "Least Angle and L_1 Penalized Regression: A Review." *Statistics Surveys*, **2**, 61–93.

Heyman R, Slep A (2001). "The Hazards of Predicting Divorce Without Cross-validation." *Journal of Marriage and the Family*, **63**(2), 473.

Hill A, LaPan P, Li Y, Haney S (2007). "Impact of Image Segmentation on High–Content Screening Data Quality for SK–BR-3 Cells." *BMC Bioinformatics*, **8**(1), 340.

Ho T (1998). "The Random Subspace Method for Constructing Decision Forests." *IEEE Transactions on Pattern Analysis and Machine Intelligence*, **13**, 340–354.

Hoerl A (1970). "Ridge Regression: Biased Estimation for Nonorthogonal Problems." *Technometrics*, **12**(1), 55–67.

Holland J (1975). *Adaptation in Natural and Artificial Systems.* University of Michigan Press, Ann Arbor, MI.

Holland J (1992). *Adaptation in Natural and Artificial Systems.* MIT Press, Cambridge, MA.

Holmes G, Hall M, Frank E (1993). "Generating Rule Sets from Model Trees." In "Australian Joint Conference on Artificial Intelligence," .

Hothorn T, Hornik K, Zeileis A (2006). "Unbiased Recursive Partitioning: A Conditional Inference Framework." *Journal of Computational and Graphical Statistics*, **15**(3), 651–674.

Hothorn T, Leisch F, Zeileis A, Hornik K (2005). "The Design and Analysis of Benchmark Experiments." *Journal of Computational and Graphical Statistics*, **14**(3), 675–699.

Hsieh W, Tang B (1998). "Applying Neural Network Models to Prediction and Data Analysis in Meteorology and Oceanography." *Bulletin of the American Meteorological Society*, **79**(9), 1855–1870.

Hsu C, Lin C (2002). "A Comparison of Methods for Multiclass Support Vector Machines." *IEEE Transactions on Neural Networks*, **13**(2), 415–425.

Huang C, Chang B, Cheng D, Chang C (2012). "Feature Selection and Parameter Optimization of a Fuzzy-Based Stock Selection Model Using Genetic Algorithms." *International Journal of Fuzzy Systems*, **14**(1), 65–75.

Huuskonen J (2000). "Estimation of Aqueous Solubility for a Diverse Set of Organic Compounds Based on Molecular Topology." *Journal of Chemical Information and Computer Sciences*, **40**(3), 773–777.

Ihaka R, Gentleman R (1996). "R: A Language for Data Analysis and Graphics." *Journal of Computational and Graphical Statistics*, **5**(3), 299–314.

Jeatrakul P, Wong K, Fung C (2010). "Classification of Imbalanced Data By Combining the Complementary Neural Network and SMOTE Algorithm." *Neural Information Processing. Models and Applications*, pp. 152–159.

Jerez J, Molina I, Garcia-Laencina P, Alba R, Ribelles N, Martin M, Franco L (2010). "Missing Data Imputation Using Statistical and Machine Learning Methods in a Real Breast Cancer Problem." *Artificial Intelligence in Medicine*, **50**, 105–115.

John G, Kohavi R, Pfleger K (1994). "Irrelevant Features and the Subset Selection Problem." *Proceedings of the Eleventh International Conference on Machine Learning*, **129**, 121–129.

Johnson K, Rayens W (2007). "Modern Classification Methods for Drug Discovery." In A Dmitrienko, C Chuang-Stein, R D'Agostino (eds.), "Pharmaceutical Statistics Using SAS: A Practical Guide," pp. 7–43. Cary, NC: SAS Institute Inc.

Johnson R, Wichern D (2001). *Applied Multivariate Statistical Analysis*. Prentice Hall.

Jolliffe I, Trendafilov N, Uddin M (2003). "A Modified Principal Component Technique Based on the lasso." *Journal of Computational and Graphical Statistics*, **12**(3), 531–547.

Kansy M, Senner F, Gubernator K (1998). "Physiochemical High Throughput Screening: Parallel Artificial Membrane Permeation Assay in the Description of Passive Absorption Processes." *Journal of Medicinal Chemistry*, **41**, 1007–1010.

Karatzoglou A, Smola A, Hornik K, Zeileis A (2004). "kernlab - An S4 Package for Kernel Methods in R." *Journal of Statistical Software*, **11**(9), 1–20.

Kearns M, Valiant L (1989). "Cryptographic Limitations on Learning Boolean Formulae and Finite Automata." In "Proceedings of the Twenty-First Annual ACM Symposium on Theory of Computing," .

Kim J, Basak J, Holtzman D (2009). "The Role of Apolipoprotein E in Alzheimer's Disease." *Neuron*, **63**(3), 287–303.

Kim JH (2009). "Estimating Classification Error Rate: Repeated Cross–Validation, Repeated Hold–Out and Bootstrap." *Computational Statistics & Data Analysis*, **53**(11), 3735–3745.

Kimball A (1957). "Errors of the Third Kind in Statistical Consulting." *Journal of the American Statistical Association*, **52**, 133–142.

Kira K, Rendell L (1992). "The Feature Selection Problem: Traditional Methods and a New Algorithm." *Proceedings of the National Conference on Artificial Intelligence*, pp. 129–129.

Kline DM, Berardi VL (2005). "Revisiting Squared–Error and Cross–Entropy Functions for Training Neural Network Classifiers." *Neural Computing and Applications*, **14**(4), 310–318.

Kohavi R (1995). "A Study of Cross–Validation and Bootstrap for Accuracy Estimation and Model Selection." *International Joint Conference on Artificial Intelligence*, **14**, 1137–1145.

Kohavi R (1996). "Scaling Up the Accuracy of Naive–Bayes Classifiers: A Decision–Tree Hybrid." In "Proceedings of the second international conference on knowledge discovery and data mining," volume 7.

Kohonen T (1995). *Self–Organizing Maps*. Springer.

Kononenko I (1994). "Estimating Attributes: Analysis and Extensions of Relief." In F Bergadano, L De Raedt (eds.), "Machine Learning: ECML–94," volume 784, pp. 171–182. Springer Berlin / Heidelberg.

Kuhn M (2008). "Building Predictive Models in R Using the caret Package." *Journal of Statistical Software*, **28**(5).

Kuhn M (2010). "The caret Package Homepage." URL http://caret.r-forge.r-project.org/.

Kuiper S (2008). "Introduction to Multiple Regression: How Much Is Your Car Worth?" *Journal of Statistics Education*, **16**(3).

Kvålseth T (1985). "Cautionary Note About R^2." *American Statistician*, **39**(4), 279–285.

Lachiche N, Flach P (2003). "Improving Accuracy and Cost of Two–Class and Multi–Class Probabilistic Classifiers using ROC Curves." In "Proceedings of the Twentieth International Conference on Machine Learning," volume 20, pp. 416–424.

Larose D (2006). *Data Mining Methods and Models*. Wiley.

Lavine B, Davidson C, Moores A (2002). "Innovative Genetic Algorithms for Chemoinformatics." *Chemometrics and Intelligent Laboratory Systems*, **60**(1), 161–171.

Leach A, Gillet V (2003). *An Introduction to Chemoinformatics*. Springer.

Leisch F (2002a). "Sweave: Dynamic Generation of Statistical Reports Using Literate Data Analysis." In W Härdle, B Rönz (eds.), "Compstat 2002 — Proceedings in Computational Statistics," pp. 575–580. Physica Verlag, Heidelberg.

Leisch F (2002b). "Sweave, Part I: Mixing R and LATEX." *R News*, **2**(3), 28–31.

Levy S (2010). "The AI Revolution is On." *Wired*.

Li J, Fine JP (2008). "ROC Analysis with Multiple Classes and Multiple Tests: Methodology and Its Application in Microarray Studies." *Biostatistics*, **9**(3), 566–576.

Lindgren F, Geladi P, Wold S (1993). "The Kernel Algorithm for PLS." *Journal of Chemometrics*, **7**, 45–59.

Ling C, Li C (1998). "Data Mining for Direct Marketing: Problems and solutions." In "Proceedings of the Fourth International Conference on Knowledge Discovery and Data Mining," pp. 73–79.

Lipinski C, Lombardo F, Dominy B, Feeney P (1997). "Experimental and Computational Approaches To Estimate Solubility and Permeability In Drug Discovery and Development Settings." *Advanced Drug Delivery Reviews*, **23**, 3–25.

Liu B (2007). *Web Data Mining*. Springer Berlin / Heidelberg.

Liu Y, Rayens W (2007). "PLS and Dimension Reduction for Classification." *Computational Statistics*, pp. 189–208.

Lo V (2002). "The True Lift Model: A Novel Data Mining Approach To Response Modeling in Database Marketing." *ACM SIGKDD Explorations Newsletter*, **4**(2), 78–86.

Lodhi H, Saunders C, Shawe-Taylor J, Cristianini N, Watkins C (2002). "Text Classification Using String Kernels." *The Journal of Machine Learning Research*, **2**, 419–444.

Loh WY (2002). "Regression Trees With Unbiased Variable Selection and Interaction Detection." *Statistica Sinica*, **12**, 361–386.

Loh WY (2010). "Tree–Structured Classifiers." *Wiley Interdisciplinary Reviews: Computational Statistics*, **2**, 364–369.

Loh WY, Shih YS (1997). "Split Selection Methods for Classification Trees." *Statistica Sinica*, **7**, 815–840.

Mahé P, Ueda N, Akutsu T, Perret J, Vert J (2005). "Graph Kernels for Molecular Structure–Activity Relationship Analysis with Support Vector Machines." *Journal of Chemical Information and Modeling*, **45**(4), 939–951.

Mahé P, Vert J (2009). "Graph Kernels Based on Tree Patterns for Molecules." *Machine Learning*, **75**(1), 3–35.

Maindonald J, Braun J (2007). *Data Analysis and Graphics Using R*. Cambridge University Press, 2nd edition.

Mandal A, Johnson K, Wu C, Bornemeier D (2007). "Identifying Promising Compounds in Drug Discovery: Genetic Algorithms and Some New Statistical Techniques." *Journal of Chemical Information and Modeling*, **47**(3), 981–988.

Mandal A, Wu C, Johnson K (2006). "SELC: Sequential Elimination of Level Combinations by Means of Modified Genetic Algorithms." *Technometrics*, **48**(2), 273–283.

Martin J, Hirschberg D (1996). "Small Sample Statistics for Classification Error Rates I: Error Rate Measurements." *Department of Informatics and Computer Science Technical Report*.

Martin T, Harten P, Young D, Muratov E, Golbraikh A, Zhu H, Tropsha A (2012). "Does Rational Selection of Training and Test Sets Improve the Outcome of QSAR Modeling?" *Journal of Chemical Information and Modeling*, **52**(10), 2570–2578.

Massy W (1965). "Principal Components Regression in Exploratory Statistical Research." *Journal of the American Statistical Association*, **60**, 234–246.

McCarren P, Springer C, Whitehead L (2011). "An Investigation into Pharmaceutically Relevant Mutagenicity Data and the Influence on Ames Predictive Potential." *Journal of Cheminformatics*, **3**(51).

McClish D (1989). "Analyzing a Portion of the ROC Curve." *Medical Decision Making*, **9**, 190–195.

Melssen W, Wehrens R, Buydens L (2006). "Supervised Kohonen Networks for Classification Problems." *Chemometrics and Intelligent Laboratory Systems*, **83**(2), 99–113.

Mente S, Lombardo F (2005). "A Recursive–Partitioning Model for Blood–Brain Barrier Permeation." *Journal of Computer–Aided Molecular Design*, **19**(7), 465–481.

Menze B, Kelm B, Splitthoff D, Koethe U, Hamprecht F (2011). "On Oblique Random Forests." *Machine Learning and Knowledge Discovery in Databases*, pp. 453–469.

Mevik B, Wehrens R (2007). "The pls Package: Principal Component and Partial Least Squares Regression in R." *Journal of Statistical Software*, **18**(2), 1–24.

Michailidis G, de Leeuw J (1998). "The Gifi System Of Descriptive Multivariate Analysis." *Statistical Science*, **13**, 307–336.

Milborrow S (2012). *Notes On the earth Package*. URL http://cran.r-project.org/package=earth.

Min S, Lee J, Han I (2006). "Hybrid Genetic Algorithms and Support Vector Machines for Bankruptcy Prediction." *Expert Systems with Applications*, **31**(3), 652–660.

Mitchell M (1998). *An Introduction to Genetic Algorithms*. MIT Press.

Molinaro A (2005). "Prediction Error Estimation: A Comparison of Resampling Methods." *Bioinformatics*, **21**(15), 3301–3307.

Molinaro A, Lostritto K, Van Der Laan M (2010). "partDSA: Deletion/Substitution/Addition Algorithm for Partitioning the Covariate Space in Prediction." *Bioinformatics*, **26**(10), 1357–1363.

Montgomery D, Runger G (1993). "Gauge Capability and Designed Experiments. Part I: Basic Methods." *Quality Engineering*, **6**(1), 115–135.

Muenchen R (2009). *R for SAS and SPSS Users*. Springer.

Myers R (1994). *Classical and Modern Regression with Applications*. PWS-KENT Publishing Company, Boston, MA, second edition.

Myers R, Montgomery D (2009). *Response Surface Methodology: Process and Product Optimization Using Designed Experiments*. Wiley, New York, NY.

Neal R (1996). *Bayesian Learning for Neural Networks*. Springer-Verlag.

Nelder J, Mead R (1965). "A Simplex Method for Function Minimization." *The Computer Journal*, **7**(4), 308–313.

Netzeva T, Worth A, Aldenberg T, Benigni R, Cronin M, Gramatica P, Jaworska J, Kahn S, Klopman G, Marchant C (2005). "Current Status of Methods for Defining the Applicability Domain of (Quantitative) Structure–Activity Relationships." In "The Report and Recommendations of European Centre for the Validation of Alternative Methods Workshop 52," volume 33, pp. 1–19.

Niblett T (1987). "Constructing Decision Trees in Noisy Domains." In I Bratko, N Lavrač (eds.), "Progress in Machine Learning: Proceedings of EWSL–87," pp. 67–78. Sigma Press, Bled, Yugoslavia.

Olden J, Jackson D (2000). "Torturing Data for the Sake of Generality: How Valid Are Our Regression Models?" *Ecoscience*, **7**(4), 501–510.

Olsson D, Nelson L (1975). "The Nelder–Mead Simplex Procedure for Function Minimization." *Technometrics*, **17**(1), 45–51.

Osuna E, Freund R, Girosi F (1997). "Support Vector Machines: Training and Applications." *Technical report*, MIT Artificial Intelligence Laboratory.

Ozuysal M, Calonder M, Lepetit V, Fua P (2010). "Fast Keypoint Recognition Using Random Ferns." *IEEE Transactions on Pattern Analysis and Machine Intelligence*, **32**(3), 448–461.

Park M, Hastie T (2008). "Penalized Logistic Regression for Detecting Gene Interactions." *Biostatistics*, **9**(1), 30.

Pepe MS, Longton G, Janes H (2009). "Estimation and Comparison of Receiver Operating Characteristic Curves." *Stata Journal*, **9**(1), 1–16.

Perrone M, Cooper L (1993). "When Networks Disagree: Ensemble Methods for Hybrid Neural Networks." In RJ Mammone (ed.), "Artificial Neural Networks for Speech and Vision," pp. 126–142. Chapman & Hall, London.

Piersma A, Genschow E, Verhoef A, Spanjersberg M, Brown N, Brady M, Burns A, Clemann N, Seiler A, Spielmann H (2004). "Validation of the Postimplantation Rat Whole-embryo Culture Test in the International EC-VAM Validation Study on Three In Vitro Embryotoxicity Tests." *Alternatives to Laboratory Animals*, **32**, 275–307.

Platt J (2000). "Probabilistic Outputs for Support Vector Machines and Comparison to Regularized Likelihood Methods." In B Bartlett, B Schölkopf, D Schuurmans, A Smola (eds.), "Advances in Kernel Methods Support Vector Learning," pp. 61–74. Cambridge, MA: MIT Press.

Provost F, Domingos P (2003). "Tree Induction for Probability–Based Ranking." *Machine Learning*, **52**(3), 199–215.

Provost F, Fawcett T, Kohavi R (1998). "The Case Against Accuracy Estimation for Comparing Induction Algorithms." *Proceedings of the Fifteenth International Conference on Machine Learning*, pp. 445–453.

Quinlan R (1987). "Simplifying Decision Trees." *International Journal of Man–Machine Studies*, **27**(3), 221–234.

Quinlan R (1992). "Learning with Continuous Classes." *Proceedings of the 5th Australian Joint Conference On Artificial Intelligence*, pp. 343–348.

Quinlan R (1993a). "Combining Instance–Based and Model–Based Learning." *Proceedings of the Tenth International Conference on Machine Learning*, pp. 236–243.

Quinlan R (1993b). *C4.5: Programs for Machine Learning*. Morgan Kaufmann Publishers.

Quinlan R (1996a). "Bagging, Boosting, and C4.5." In "In Proceedings of the Thirteenth National Conference on Artificial Intelligence," .

Quinlan R (1996b). "Improved use of continuous attributes in C4.5." *Journal of Artificial Intelligence Research*, **4**, 77–90.

Quinlan R, Rivest R (1989). "Inferring Decision Trees Using the Minimum Description Length Principle." *Information and computation*, **80**(3), 227–248.

Radcliffe N, Surry P (2011). "Real–World Uplift Modelling With Significance–Based Uplift Trees." *Technical report*, Stochastic Solutions.

Rännar S, Lindgren F, Geladi P, Wold S (1994). "A PLS Kernel Algorithm for Data Sets with Many Variables and Fewer Objects. Part 1: Theory and Algorithm." *Journal of Chemometrics*, **8**, 111–125.

R Development Core Team (2008). *R: Regulatory Compliance and Validation Issues A Guidance Document for the Use of R in Regulated Clinical Trial Environments*. R Foundation for Statistical Computing, Vienna, Austria.

R Development Core Team (2010). *R: A Language and Environment for Statistical Computing*. R Foundation for Statistical Computing, Vienna, Austria.

Reshef D, Reshef Y, Finucane H, Grossman S, McVean G, Turnbaugh P, Lander E, Mitzenmacher M, Sabeti P (2011). "Detecting Novel Associations in Large Data Sets." *Science*, **334**(6062), 1518–1524.

Richardson M, Dominowska E, Ragno R (2007). "Predicting Clicks: Estimating the Click–Through Rate for New Ads." In "Proceedings of the 16th International Conference on the World Wide Web," pp. 521–530.

Ridgeway G (2007). "Generalized Boosted Models: A Guide to the gbm Package." URL http://cran.r-project.org/web/packages/gbm/vignettes/gbm.pdf.

Ripley B (1995). "Statistical Ideas for Selecting Network Architectures." *Neural Networks: Artificial Intelligence and Industrial Applications*, pp. 183–190.

Ripley B (1996). *Pattern Recognition and Neural Networks*. Cambridge University Press.

Robin X, Turck N, Hainard A, Tiberti N, Lisacek F, Sanchez JC, Muller M (2011). "pROC: an open-source package for R and S+ to analyze and compare ROC curves." *BMC Bioinformatics*, **12**(1), 77.

Robnik-Sikonja M, Kononenko I (1997). "An Adaptation of Relief for Attribute Estimation in Regression." *Proceedings of the Fourteenth International Conference on Machine Learning*, pp. 296–304.

Rodriguez M (2011). "The Failure of Predictive Modeling and Why We Follow the Herd." *Technical report*, Concepcion, Martinez & Bellido.

Ruczinski I, Kooperberg C, Leblanc M (2003). "Logic Regression." *Journal of Computational and Graphical Statistics*, **12**(3), 475–511.

Rumelhart D, Hinton G, Williams R (1986). "Learning Internal Representations by Error Propagation." In "Parallel Distributed Processing: Explorations in the Microstructure of Cognition," The MIT Press.

Rzepakowski P, Jaroszewicz S (2012). "Uplift Modeling in Direct Marketing." *Journal of Telecommunications and Information Technology*, **2**, 43–50.

Saar-Tsechansky M, Provost F (2007a). "Decision–Centric Active Learning of Binary–Outcome Models." *Information Systems Research*, **18**(1), 4–22.

Saar-Tsechansky M, Provost F (2007b). "Handling Missing Values When Applying Classification Models." *Journal of Machine Learning Research*, **8**, 1625–1657.

Saeys Y, Inza I, Larranaga P (2007). "A Review of Feature Selection Techniques in Bioinformatics." *Bioinformatics*, **23**(19), 2507–2517.

Schapire R (1990). "The Strength of Weak Learnability." *Machine Learning*, **45**, 197–227.

Schapire YFR (1999). "Adaptive Game Playing Using Multiplicative Weights." *Games and Economic Behavior*, **29**, 79–103.

Schmidberger M, Morgan M, Eddelbuettel D, Yu H, Tierney L, Mansmann U (2009). "State–of–the–Art in Parallel Computing with R." *Journal of Statistical Software*, **31**(1).

Serneels S, Nolf ED, Espen PV (2006). "Spatial Sign Pre-processing: A Simple Way to Impart Moderate Robustness to Multivariate Estimators." *Journal of Chemical Information and Modeling*, **46**(3), 1402–1409.

Shachtman N (2011). "Pentagon's Prediction Software Didn't Spot Egypt Unrest." *Wired*.

Shannon C (1948). "A Mathematical Theory of Communication." *The Bell System Technical Journal*, **27**(3), 379–423.

Siegel E (2011). "Uplift Modeling: Predictive Analytics Can't Optimize Marketing Decisions Without It." *Technical report*, Prediction Impact Inc.

Simon R, Radmacher M, Dobbin K, McShane L (2003). "Pitfalls in the Use of DNA Microarray Data for Diagnostic and Prognostic Classification." *Journal of the National Cancer Institute*, **95**(1), 14–18.

Smola A (1996). "Regression Estimation with Support Vector Learning Machines." *Master's thesis, Technische Universit at Munchen*.

Spector P (2008). *Data Manipulation with R*. Springer.

Steyerberg E (2010). *Clinical Prediction Models: A Practical Approach to Development, Validation, and Updating*. Springer, 1st ed. softcover of orig. ed. 2009 edition.

Stone M, Brooks R (1990). "Continuum Regression: Cross-validated Sequentially Constructed Prediction Embracing Ordinary Least Squares, Partial Least Squares, and Principal Component Regression." *Journal of the Royal Statistical Society, Series B*, **52**, 237–269.

Strobl C, Boulesteix A, Zeileis A, Hothorn T (2007). "Bias in Random Forest Variable Importance Measures: Illustrations, Sources and a Solution." *BMC Bioinformatics*, **8**(1), 25.

Suykens J, Vandewalle J (1999). "Least Squares Support Vector Machine Classifiers." *Neural processing letters*, **9**(3), 293–300.

Tetko I, Tanchuk V, Kasheva T, Villa A (2001). "Estimation of Aqueous Solubility of Chemical Compounds Using E–State Indices." *Journal of Chemical Information and Computer Sciences*, **41**(6), 1488–1493.

Tibshirani R (1996). "Regression Shrinkage and Selection via the lasso." *Journal of the Royal Statistical Society Series B (Methodological)*, **58**(1), 267–288.

Tibshirani R, Hastie T, Narasimhan B, Chu G (2002). "Diagnosis of Multiple Cancer Types by Shrunken Centroids of Gene Expression." *Proceedings of the National Academy of Sciences*, **99**(10), 6567–6572.

Tibshirani R, Hastie T, Narasimhan B, Chu G (2003). "Class Prediction by Nearest Shrunken Centroids, with Applications to DNA Microarrays." *Statistical Science*, **18**(1), 104–117.

Ting K (2002). "An Instance–Weighting Method to Induce Cost–Sensitive Trees." *IEEE Transactions on Knowledge and Data Engineering*, **14**(3), 659–665.

Tipping M (2001). "Sparse Bayesian Learning and the Relevance Vector Machine." *Journal of Machine Learning Research*, **1**, 211–244.

Titterington M (2010). "Neural Networks." *Wiley Interdisciplinary Reviews: Computational Statistics*, **2**(1), 1–8.

Troyanskaya O, Cantor M, Sherlock G, Brown P, Hastie T, Tibshirani R, Botstein D, Altman R (2001). "Missing Value Estimation Methods for DNA Microarrays." *Bioinformatics*, **17**(6), 520–525.

Tumer K, Ghosh J (1996). "Analysis of Decision Boundaries in Linearly Combined Neural Classifiers." *Pattern Recognition*, **29**(2), 341–348.

US Commodity Futures Trading Commission and US Securities & Exchange Commission (2010). *Findings Regarding the Market Events of May 6, 2010.*

Valiant L (1984). "A Theory of the Learnable." *Communications of the ACM*, **27**, 1134–1142.

Van Der Putten P, Van Someren M (2004). "A Bias–Variance Analysis of a Real World Learning Problem: The CoIL Challenge 2000." *Machine Learning*, **57**(1), 177–195.

Van Hulse J, Khoshgoftaar T, Napolitano A (2007). "Experimental Perspectives On Learning From Imbalanced Data." In "Proceedings of the 24th International Conference On Machine learning," pp. 935–942.

Vapnik V (2010). *The Nature of Statistical Learning Theory.* Springer.

Varma S, Simon R (2006). "Bias in Error Estimation When Using Cross–Validation for Model Selection." *BMC Bioinformatics*, **7**(1), 91.

Varmuza K, He P, Fang K (2003). "Boosting Applied to Classification of Mass Spectral Data." *Journal of Data Science*, **1**, 391–404.

Venables W, Ripley B (2002). *Modern Applied Statistics with S.* Springer.

Venables W, Smith D, the R Development Core Team (2003). *An Introduction to R.* R Foundation for Statistical Computing, Vienna, Austria, version 1.6.2 edition. ISBN 3-901167-55-2, URL http://www.R-project.org.

Venkatraman E (2000). "A Permutation Test to Compare Receiver Operating Characteristic Curves." *Biometrics*, **56**(4), 1134–1138.

Veropoulos K, Campbell C, Cristianini N (1999). "Controlling the Sensitivity of Support Vector Machines." *Proceedings of the International Joint Conference on Artificial Intelligence*, **1999**, 55–60.

Verzani J (2002). "simpleR – Using R for Introductory Statistics." URL http://www.math.csi.cuny.edu/Statistics/R/simpleR.

Wager TT, Hou X, Verhoest PR, Villalobos A (2010). "Moving Beyond Rules: The Development of a Central Nervous System Multiparameter Optimization (CNS MPO) Approach To Enable Alignment of Druglike Properties." *ACS Chemical Neuroscience*, **1**(6), 435–449.

Wallace C (2005). *Statistical and Inductive Inference by Minimum Message Length.* Springer–Verlag.

Wang C, Venkatesh S (1984). "Optimal Stopping and Effective Machine Complexity in Learning." *Advances in NIPS*, pp. 303–310.

Wang Y, Witten I (1997). "Inducing Model Trees for Continuous Classes." *Proceedings of the Ninth European Conference on Machine Learning*, pp. 128–137.

Weiss G, Provost F (2001a). "The Effect of Class Distribution on Classifier Learning: An Empirical Study." *Department of Computer Science, Rutgers University.*

Weiss G, Provost F (2001b). "The Effect of Class Distribution On Classifier Learning: An Empirical Study." *Technical Report ML-TR-44*, Department of Computer Science, Rutgers University.

Welch B (1939). "Note on Discriminant Functions." *Biometrika*, **31**, 218–220.

Westfall P, Young S (1993). *Resampling–Based Multiple Testing: Examples and Methods for P-Value Adjustment.* Wiley.

Westphal C (2008). *Data Mining for Intelligence, Fraud & Criminal Detection: Advanced Analytics & Information Sharing Technologies.* CRC Press.

Whittingham M, Stephens P, Bradbury R, Freckleton R (2006). "Why Do We Still Use Stepwise Modelling in Ecology and Behaviour?" *Journal of Animal Ecology*, **75**(5), 1182–1189.

Willett P (1999). "Dissimilarity–Based Algorithms for Selecting Structurally Diverse Sets of Compounds." *Journal of Computational Biology*, **6**(3), 447–457.

Williams G (2011). *Data Mining with Rattle and R : The Art of Excavating Data for Knowledge Discovery.* Springer.

Witten D, Tibshirani R (2009). "Covariance–Regularized Regression and Classification For High Dimensional Problems." *Journal of the Royal Statistical Society. Series B (Statistical Methodology)*, **71**(3), 615–636.

Witten D, Tibshirani R (2011). "Penalized Classification Using Fisher's Linear Discriminant." *Journal of the Royal Statistical Society. Series B (Statistical Methodology)*, **73**(5), 753–772.

Wold H (1966). "Estimation of Principal Components and Related Models by Iterative Least Squares." In P Krishnaiah (ed.), "Multivariate Analyses," pp. 391–420. Academic Press, New York.

Wold H (1982). "Soft Modeling: The Basic Design and Some Extensions." In K Joreskog, H Wold (eds.), "Systems Under Indirect Observation: Causality, Structure, Prediction," pt. 2, pp. 1–54. North–Holland, Amsterdam.

Wold S (1995). "PLS for Multivariate Linear Modeling." In H van de Waterbeemd (ed.), "Chemometric Methods in Molecular Design," pp. 195–218. VCH, Weinheim.

Wold S, Johansson M, Cocchi M (1993). "PLS–Partial Least-Squares Projections to Latent Structures." In H Kubinyi (ed.), "3D QSAR in Drug Design," volume 1, pp. 523–550. Kluwer Academic Publishers, The Netherlands.

Wold S, Martens H, Wold H (1983). "The Multivariate Calibration Problem in Chemistry Solved by the PLS Method." In "Proceedings from the Conference on Matrix Pencils," Springer–Verlag, Heidelberg.

Wolpert D (1996). "The Lack of a priori Distinctions Between Learning Algorithms." *Neural Computation*, **8**(7), 1341–1390.

Yeh I (1998). "Modeling of Strength of High-Performance Concrete Using Artificial Neural Networks." *Cement and Concrete research*, **28**(12), 1797–1808.

Yeh I (2006). "Analysis of Strength of Concrete Using Design of Experiments and Neural Networks." *Journal of Materials in Civil Engineering*, **18**, 597–604.

Youden W (1950). "Index for Rating Diagnostic Tests." *Cancer*, **3**(1), 32–35.

Zadrozny B, Elkan C (2001). "Obtaining Calibrated Probability Estimates from Decision Trees and Naive Bayesian Classifiers." In "Proceedings of the 18th International Conference on Machine Learning," pp. 609–616. Morgan Kaufmann.

Zeileis A, Hothorn T, Hornik K (2008). "Model–Based Recursive Partitioning." *Journal of Computational and Graphical Statistics*, **17**(2), 492–514.

Zhu J, Hastie T (2005). "Kernel Logistic Regression and the Import Vector Machine." *Journal of Computational and Graphical Statistics*, **14**(1), 185–205.

Zou H, Hastie T (2005). "Regularization and Variable Selection via the Elastic Net." *Journal of the Royal Statistical Society, Series B*, **67**(2), 301–320.

Zou H, Hastie T, Tibshirani R (2004). "Sparse Principal Component Analysis." *Journal of Computational and Graphical Statistics*, **15**, 2006.

Indicies

Computing

M. Kuhn and K. Johnson, *Applied Predictive Modeling*,
DOI 10.1007/978-1-4614-6849-3,
© Springer Science+Business Media New York 2013

General

M. Kuhn and K. Johnson, *Applied Predictive Modeling*,
DOI 10.1007/978-1-4614-6849-3,
© Springer Science+Business Media New York 2013